Obesity

Editor

ANGELA GOLDEN

NURSING CLINICS
OF NORTH AMERICA

www.nursing.theclinics.com

Consulting Editor
STEPHEN D. KRAU

December 2021 • Volume 56 • Number 4

ELSEVIER

1600 John F. Kennedy Boulevard • Suite 1800 • Philadelphia, Pennsylvania, 19103-2899

http://www.theclinics.com

NURSING CLINICS OF NORTH AMERICA Volume 56, Number 4
December 2021 ISSN 0029-6465, ISBN-13: 978-0-323-83522-0

Editor: Kerry Holland
Developmental Editor: Axell Ivan Jade M. Purificacion

Nursing Clinics of North America (ISSN 0029-6465) is published quarterly by Elsevier Inc., 360 Park Avenue South, New York, NY 10010-1710. Months of issue are March, June, September, and December. Periodicals postage paid at New York, NY and additional mailing offices. Subscription price per year is, $163.00 (US individuals), $669.00 (US institutions), $275.00 (international individuals), $692.00 (international institutions), $231.00 (Canadian individuals), $692.00 (Canadian institutions), $100.00 (US and Canadian students), and $135.00 (international students). To receive student/resident rate, orders must be accompanied by name of affiliated institution, date of term, and the signature of program/residency coordinator on institution letterhead. Orders will be billed at individual rate until proof of status is received. Foreign air speed delivery is included in all *Clinics* subscription prices. All prices are subject to change without notice. **POSTMASTER:** Send address changes to *Nursing Clinics*, Elsevier Health Sciences Division, Subscription Customer Service, 3251 Riverport Lane, Maryland Heights, MO 63043. **Customer Service: Telephone: 1-800-654-2452** (U.S. and Canada); **1-314-447-8871 (outside U.S. and Canada). Fax: 1-314-447-8029. E-mail: journalscustomerservice-usa@ elsevier.com** (for print support) and **journalsonlinesupport-usa@elsevier.com** (for online support).

Nursing Clinics of North America is covered in *EMBASE/Excerpta Medica, MEDLINE/PubMed (Index Medicus), Social Sciences Citation Index, Current Contents, ASCA, Cumulative Index to Nursing, RNdex Top 100,* and Allied Health Literature and International Nursing Index (INI).

Contributors

CONSULTING EDITOR

STEPHEN D. KRAU, PhD, RN, CNE
Associate Professor (Ret), Vanderbilt University School of Nursing, Nashville, Tennessee

EDITOR

ANGELA GOLDEN, DNP, FNP-C, FAANP
Owner and Clinician, NP from Home, LLC and NP Obesity Treatment Clinic, Flagstaff, Arizona

AUTHORS

MOHINI ARAS, MD
Division of Endocrinology, Weill Cornell Medicine, Obesity Medicine Fellow, Comprehensive Weight Control Center, New York, New York

NANCY T. BROWNE, MS, PPCNP-BC, FAANP, FAAN
Falmouth, Maine

MICHELLE I. CARDEL, PhD, MS, RD
Adjunct Professor, Department of Health Outcomes and Biomedical Informatics, University of Florida College of Medicine, Gainesville, Florida; WW International, Inc, Director of Global Clinical Research and Nutrition, New York, New York

AMANDA CHANEY, DNP, APRN, FAANP, AF-AASLD
Nurse Practitioner, Department of Transplant, Assistant Professor of Medicine, Mayo Clinic College of Medicine, Associate of Transplant Medicine, Chair, Advanced Practice Provider Subcommittee, Mayo Clinic, Jacksonville, Florida

LESLIE L. DAVIS, PhD, RN, ANP-BC, FAAN, FAANP, FACC, FAHA, FPCNA
Associate Professor of Nursing, The University of North Carolina at Chapel Hill, School of Nursing, Chapel Hill, North Carolina

NIKHIL V. DHURANDHAR, MS, LCEH, PhD, FTOS
Chairperson and Professor, Department of Nutritional Sciences, Texas Tech University, Lubbock, Texas

SATTARIA S. DILKS, DNP, PMHNP-BC, FAANP
Professor and Department Head, Graduate Nursing McNeese State University, Lake Charles, Louisiana

CANDICE FALLS, PhD, ACNP-BC
Assistant Professor, University of Kentucky, College of Nursing, Lexington, Kentucky

SHARON M. FRUH, PhD, RN, FNP-BC, FAANP
Professor, College of Nursing, University of South Alabama, Mobile, Alabama

ANGELA GOLDEN, DNP, FNP-C, FAANP
Owner and Clinician, NP from Home, LLC and NP Obesity Treatment Clinic, Flagstaff, Arizona

REBECCA J. GRAVES, PhD, NP-C
Associate Professor, Director of Special Projects and Evaluation, College of Nursing, University of South Alabama, Mobile, Alabama

CLARENCE C. GRAVLEE, PhD
Associate Professor, Department of Anthropology, University of Florida College of Liberal Arts and Sciences, Gainesville, Florida

TWILA STERLING GUILLORY, PhD, FNP-BC
Professor and MSN Coordinator, Graduate Nursing McNeese State University, Lake Charles, Louisiana

HEATHER R. HALL, PhD, RN, NNP-BC
Dean and Professor, College of Nursing, University of South Alabama, Mobile, Alabama

CAITLYN HAUFF, PhD
Assistant Professor of Health Promotion, Department of Health, Kinesiology, and Sport, University of South Alabama, Mobile, Alabama

RYAN HOLLEY-MALLO, PhD, DNP, NP-C, FAANP
Associate Professor, Graduate Nursing, School of Nursing, Averett University, Danville, Virginia

AMY BETH INGERSOLL, PA-C, MMS, FOMA
President, Arizona Obesity Organization, Phoenix, Arizona

CHRISTINE KESSLER, MN, CNS, ANP, BC-ADM, CDTC, FAANP
Metabolic Medicine Associates, King George, Virginia

THEODORE K. KYLE, RPh, MBA
ConscienHealth, Pittsburgh, Pennsylvania

DENISE G. LINK, PhD, WHNP-BC, FAAN, FAANP
Clinical Professor Emerita, Arizona State University Edson College of Nursing and Health Innovation, Phoenix, Arizona

SHEILA MELANDER, PhD, ACNP-BC, FCCM, FAANP, FAAN
Associate Dean of MSN & DNP Faculty & Practice Affairs, William S. & Elizabeth M. Morgan Professorship for Professional Nursing Practice, University of Kentucky, College of Nursing, Lexington, Kentucky

FAITH A. NEWSOME, BA
Doctoral Student, Department of Health Outcomes and Biomedical Informatics, University of Florida College of Medicine, Gainesville, Florida

MELISSA Z. NOLAN, MSN, RN
The University of North Carolina at Chapel Hill, School of Nursing, Chapel Hill, North Carolina

JOY PAPE, MSN, RN, FNP-C, CDCES, CFCN, FADCES
Division of Endocrinology, Weill Cornell Medicine, Clinical Nurse Practitioner, Certified Diabetes Care and Education Specialist, Comprehensive Weight Control Center, New York, New York

CHRISTY PERRY, DNP, PMHNP, ANP
Assistant Professor, Southeastern Louisiana University, School of Nursing, Baton Rouge, Louisiana

KRISTINA S. PETERSEN, PhD
Assistant Professor, Department of Nutritional Sciences, Texas Tech University, Lubbock, Texas

CRAIG PRIMACK, MD, FACP, FOMA, Dipl. ABOM
Physician/Co-Founder, Scottsdale Weight Loss Center, President, Obesity Medicine Association, Diplomate, American Board of Obesity Medicine, Scottsdale, Arizona

FATIMA CODY STANFORD, MD, MPH, MPA, MBA
Department of Medicine, Division of Endocrinology-Neuroendocrine, Massachusetts General Hospital, MGH Weight Center, Department of Pediatrics, Division of Endocrinology, Nutrition Obesity Research Center at Harvard (NORCH), Boston, Massachusetts

BEVERLY G. TCHANG, MD
Division of Endocrinology, Weill Cornell Medicine, Assistant Professor of Clinical Medicine, Comprehensive Weight Control Center, New York, New York

CHELSI WEBSTER, BS
Department of Nutritional Sciences, Texas Tech University, Lubbock, Texas

SUSAN G. WILLIAMS, PhD, RN
Assistant Professor, College of Nursing, University of South Alabama, Mobile, Alabama

Contents

Christy Perry, Twila Sterling Guillory, and Sattaria S. Dilks

Many psychiatric disorders are associated with obesity and include mood disorders, anxiety disorders, personality disorders, attention deficit hyperactivity disorder, binge eating disorders, trauma, bipolar disorder, and schizophrenia. According to National Obesity Observatory, there is evidence that both obesity and mental health disorders take up a significant portion of the global burden of disease. The bidirectional nature of obesity and mental illness indicates the importance of screening all persons being treated for either obesity or mental illnesses be screened for the other. Failure to do so may decrease the effectiveness of treatment for each one individually.

Craig Primack

Sleep is often misunderstood in its impact on many chronic diseases including obesity. Obesity and restorative sleep are intertwined processes. Poor sleep negatively affects the key hormones of weight and appetite regulation, thereby potentially increasing weight via mechanisms that increase hunger and lower metabolism, thereby making the successful treatment of obesity more difficult. Clinicians should consider a comprehensive sleep history and proper treatment or referral to a sleep specialist in conjunction with obesity treatment. Adequate restorative sleep is integral to a comprehensive obesity treatment program.

Candice Falls and Sheila Melander

The prevalence of obesity continues to rise and is caused by many factors. Obesity places patients at risk for high blood pressure, diabetes, heart disease, and cancer. Although obesity in the normal population is associated with increased morbidity and mortality, obesity in critically ill patients has lower mortality. This is referred to as the obesity paradox, and although not fully understood, involves several mechanisms that demonstrate a protective factor in critically ill obese patients. However, despite the benefit, the management of critically ill obese patients faces many challenges.

Nancy T. Browne

Pediatric obesity is a heterogeneous, chronic, relapsing disease associated with metabolic and psychosocial complications. Weight-based victimization, including unrelenting microaggressions, negatively impacts child mental and physical health. Evidence-based guidelines offer individualized, stepwise approaches to obesity treatment. Pediatric nurses positively impact children with obesity by providing affirmation, clinical management, and psychosocial support. Pediatric nurses are respected and positioned to present evidence-based obesity education, correct common obesity myths, sensitively address obesity-related bias and discrimination, and model person-first language and actions. This article shares how nurses in multiple practice areas can make a meaningful impact on the lives of children and adolescents with obesity.

The health outcomes of men are significantly worse, when compared with their female counterparts, for the top 15 leading causes of death nationwide. At this time, men are not actively engaged in the health care system, creating a challenge for those managing patients in the clinical setting. The premature morbidity and mortality of men financially burdens the health care system and places a financial strain in secondary and tertiary preventive care that is simply not sustainable. Obesity is a catalyst that fuels disease and is directly responsible for the pathogenesis for the disease claiming the lives of men nationwide.

Women who are obese are at risk for conditions that are different from those experienced by men. Some of these conditions are gender based; others are socially determined. In societies where appearance and being thin are valued and promoted in the media, advertising, literature, and other areas, women who are obese are subject to biases and stereotyping that impact them socially, financially, and academically. Obesity should be assessed and managed in the same way as other chronic disorders with patient-centered care, respect, and support from the health care team. Clinicians must approach the subject of weight with sensitivity.

Obesity is a multifactorial disease that disproportionally affects diverse racial and ethnic groups. Structural racism influences racial inequities in obesity prevalence through environmental factors, such as racism and discrimination, socioeconomic status, increased levels of stress, and bias in the health care delivery system. Researchers, clinicians, and policy makers must work to address the environmental and systematic barriers that contribute to health inequities in the United States. Specifically, clinicians should quantitatively and qualitatively assess environmental and social factors and proactively engage in patient-centered care to tailor available treatments based on identified needs and experiences.

Through four decades of rising obesity, health policy has been mostly ineffective. Prevention policies failed to reverse rising trends in prevalence, partly because they are often based on biased mental models about what should work to prevent obesity, rather than empiric evidence for what does work. Bias toward people living with obesity harms health, while contributing to poor access to effective care that might serve to improve it. Better public policy will come from an increased application of objective obesity science, research to fill knowledge gaps, and respect for the human dignity of people who live with obesity.

NURSING CLINICS OF NORTH AMERICA

SERIES OF RELATED INTEREST

Critical Care Nursing Clinics of North America
https://www.ccnursing.theclinics.com/
Advances in Family Practice Nursing
http://www.advancesinfamilypracticenursing.com/

THE CLINICS ARE AVAILABLE ONLINE!
Access your subscription at:
www.theclinics.com

Preface

Obesity's Impact

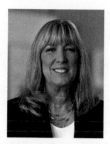

Angela Golden, DNP, FNP-C, FAANP
Editor

The rates of preobesity (overweight) and obesity are increasing worldwide.[1] The World Health Organization shows that obesity rates have tripled since 1975. The data showed 1.9 BILLION adults with preobesity and 650 million adults with obesity worldwide.[2] The cost to the global economy is staggering at 2 trillion dollars, as much as is spent on armed conflicts and smoking combined.[3] In the United States, 70% of adults have pre-obesity or obesity.[4] The World Health Organization has labeled this "globesity."[5]

For so long obesity has been seen as a simple calculation: "calories in and calories out," but current research now shows the pathophysiology is a process much more complex that the intake of excess calories. The Obesity Medicine Association (OMA) uses the definition that provides a concise overview of the complexity of obesity. Obesity is defined by OMA as a "chronic, relapsing, multi-factorial, neurobehavioral disease, wherein an increase in body fat promotes adipose tissue dysfunction and abnormal fat mass physical forces, resulting in adverse metabolic, biomechanical, and psychosocial health consequences."[6] With this in mind, the treatment of obesity must go beyond telling people to eat less and move more.

Obesity impacts almost every system of the body. Research has demonstrated more than 236 obesity-associated disorders, and 14 cancers are directly caused by obesity. Obesity poses a major health risk as the root of so many diseases and disorders. All health care providers need to be engaged in providing respectful and evidenced-based treatment to impact this global epidemic.

In this issue of *Nursing Clinics of North America*, there is a breadth of topics related to obesity, covering epidemiology, pathophysiology, and an overview of treatment. Authors then discuss how obesity impacts common diseases, such as cardiovascular, diabetes, NALFD and NASH, and psychiatric disorders. Obesity impacts populations differently as well and is addressed in the articles on minority disparities, men's health, women's health, and children. Finally, the issue brings to the forefront the role that health policy will play in the future of the treatment of obesity. With the pandemic

Nurs Clin N Am 56 (2021) xiii–xiv
https://doi.org/10.1016/j.cnur.2021.08.004
0029-6465/21/© 2021 Published by Elsevier Inc.

nature of obesity, the issue is designed to provide the reader with a full overview of what people living with obesity are facing and how nurses can impact the care of their patients living with obesity.

Angela Golden, DNP, FNP-C, FAANP
NP from Home
LLC and NP Obesity Treatment Clinic
Flagstaff, AZ, USA

PO Box 25959
Munds Park, AZ 86017, USA

E-mail address:
npfromhome@gmail.com

REFERENCES

1. World Health Organization Regional Office for Europe. Body mass index—BMI. Available at: https://www.euro.who.int/en/health-topics/disease-prevention/nutrition/a-healthy-lifestyle/body-mass-index-bmi. Accessed May 16, 2021.
2. World Health Organization. Obesity and overweight. Available at: https://www.who.int/news-room/fact-sheets/detail/obesity-and-overweight. Accessed May 16, 2021.
3. Swinburn BA, Kraak VI, Allender S, et al. The global syndemic of obesity, undernutrition, and climate change: the Lancet Commission report. Lancet 2019; 393(10173):791–846. https://doi.org/10.1016/S0140-6736(18)32822-8.
4. Centers for Disease Control and Prevention. Adult obesity facts. Available at: https://www.cdc.gov/obesity/data/adult.html. Accessed May 16, 2021.
5. World Health Organization. Controlling the global obesity epidemic. Available at: https://www.who.int/activities/controlling-the-global-obesity-epidemic. Accessed May 16, 2021.
6. Yeun M, Earle R, Kadambi N, et al. A systematic review and evaluation of current evidence reveals 236 obesity-associated disorders (ObAD). Presented at Obesity Week 2016. New Orleans, LA.

Key Causes and Contributors of Obesity: A Perspective

Nikhil V. Dhurandhar, MS, LCEH, PhD, FTOS*, Kristina S. Petersen, PhD,
Chelsi Webster, BS

KEYWORDS

- Etiology • Epidemiology • Risk factors • Prevention • Clinical management

KEY POINTS

- The body has multiple mechanisms to control energy intake and expenditure to maintain energy stores within a healthy range. Obesity is caused by an impairment in this regulation.
- Causative factors of obesity include monogenic defects, endocrine-related dysfunction, infections, and factors influencing hunger, satiety, or fat oxidation; such intrinsic impairment in energy balance is not based on behavior.
- Consumption of energy-dense food or large portion sizes, inadequate sleep duration or quality, physical inactivity and psychological health/well-being can contribute to weight gain.
- Multiple causative and contributory factors may be present in an individual, and the combination of such factors varies interindividually, leading to distinct expression of obesity in each individual. Understanding the multiple causes and contributors of obesity can help with individualized management of obesity.

OBESITY DEFINED

Obesity is a chronic disease with a multifactorial etiology that adversely affects multiple organs and physiologic functions. Clinically, obesity is diagnosed by body mass index (BMI), calculated as weight in kilograms divided by height in meters squared. BMI positively correlates with body fat content for most individuals. An individual with a BMI of 25 to 30 kg/m^2 is considered overweight, and a BMI of 30 kg/m^2 or greater is defined as obesity. For Asian individuals, BMI cutoffs for overweight and obesity are 23 kg/m^2 or greater and 25 kg/m^2 or greater, respectively. A BMI in the range of overweight or obesity indicates increasing health risk associated with excess body fat accumulation and resulting metabolic aberration. However, it does not explain what causes excess fat accumulation.

Traditionally, excess accumulation of body fat was assumed to result from greater energy intake and/or decreased energy expenditure.[1] However, to optimize obesity

Department of Nutritional Sciences, Texas Tech University, 1301 Akron Avenue, P.O. Box 41270, Lubbock, TX 79409, USA
* Corresponding author.
E-mail address: Nikhil.Dhurandhar@ttu.edu

Nurs Clin N Am 56 (2021) 449–464
https://doi.org/10.1016/j.cnur.2021.07.007
0029-6465/21/© 2021 Elsevier Inc. All rights reserved.

nursing.theclinics.com

prevention, treatment, and management, it is important to understand the upstream factors that lead to greater energy intake and/or decreased energy expenditure. Such an understanding of the causes of obesity (or excessive storage of energy) is crucial given the multifactorial nature of this disease and substantial interindividual variation. This article provides a focused overview of the known causes of obesity, factors that contribute to obesity, and the clinical importance of understanding obesity causes and contributors. The goal is to provide health care professionals, including nurses, with a concise summary of key causes and contributors to obesity to assist with clinical management.

CAUSES OF OBESITY

Most excess dietary energy is stored as fat in adipose tissue to provide an energy source in times of energy deficit. In addition, adipose tissue has multiple functions, including endocrine, paracrine, and some immune functions, as well as providing mechanical cushioning, protection, and thermal insulation.[2–4] However, too much or too little fat deposition is detrimental to health. For example, the reproductive ability of women can be impaired when stored body fat is excessive or too low.[5,6] Hence, several processes regulate fat storage within an optimal range, which varies among individuals.

Numerous factors regulate energy intake and expenditure and maintain body stores of excess energy within a range. Obesity results when one or more regulatory processes fail. Therefore, obesity is caused by impairment of mechanisms that regulate body fat stores, leading to excess fat accumulation. Thus, endogenous regulators of energy balance are primarily responsible for causing obesity; environmental factors such as food intake or activity are contributors not causes. In the sections that follow, key identified causes of obesity are described (**Table 1**).

Monogenic Causes

Although the regulation of energy stores is complex and incompletely understood, impairment in many known energy balance regulator genes is linked with obesity. For example, leptin is a hormone secreted by adipocytes to convey fat storage status to the brain. Greater leptin signaling indicates greater fat storage, prompting regulatory processes to decrease food intake or increase metabolic rate.[7,8] The opposite response is elicited if body fat declines. Decreased leptin signaling prompts the body to increase fat accumulation.[9] Genetic defects that impair leptin signaling because of an absence of leptin or leptin resistance can lead to excess fat accumulation, resulting in obesity.[10]

Another endogenous determinant of energy balance is the α-melanocyte-stimulating hormone, a neuropeptide involved in feeding behavior and energy homeostasis,[11] which requires the melanocortin 4 receptor (MC4R) for its action. A mutation in MC4R is linked with hyperphagia and obesity in 1% to 6% of individuals with early-onset severe obesity.[12] Although numerous other genes and single nucleotide polymorphisms have been implicated in excess body fat,[13] leptin and MC4R mutations are unequivocal examples of the strong effect a single gene can exert on body fat stores.

Endocrine-related Causes

Although endocrine system dysfunction may cause obesity in several ways, thyroid hormones, insulin, glucocorticoids, and growth hormone are some key hormones known to influence body fat storage.[14] Excess production of thyroid hormones can

Table 1
Specific prevention or treatment of causes and contributors of obesity

Causes	Treatment/Prevention Potential
Monogenic causes	
Absence of leptin/leptin resistance	Treatable
MC4R mutation	Treatable
Endocrine-related causes	
Thyroid conditions	Treatable
Growth hormone deficiency	Treatable
Excess glucocorticoids (Cushing's syndrome, long-term steroid therapy)	Treatable
Infectious causes (eg, human adenovirus 36)	Not modifiable by current technology
Causes influencing energy expenditure	
Brown adipose tissue deficiency/dysfunction	Not modifiable by current technology
Impaired fat oxidation in skeletal muscle	Not modifiable by current technology
Causes influencing food intake and processing	
Prader–Willi syndrome	Potentially treatable
Appetite hormone dysregulation	Not modifiable by current technology
Environmental chemicals	Not modifiable by current technology
Contributors	
Factors influencing energy intake	
Energy-dense foods	Preventable, modifiable
Large portion sizes	Preventable, modifiable
Ultraprocessed foods	Preventable, modifiable
Sleep duration and quality	Preventable, modifiable, treatable
Factors influencing energy expenditure	
Low physical activity levels	Preventable, modifiable
Sedentariness	Preventable, modifiable
Factors influencing energy intake and expenditure	
Psychological health and well-being	Potentially treatable
Tobacco cessation	Potentially preventable

lead to an increased metabolic rate and weight loss, whereas a deficiency can lead to weight gain, among other health issues. Growth hormone deficiency leads to fat mass gain, probably owing to decreased thermogenesis.[15] Excess glucocorticoids can result in weight gain and Cushing's syndrome.[16] In Cushing's syndrome, glucocorticoids interact with thyroid hormones and growth hormone, leading to a decreased metabolic rate and greater adipogenesis.[14]

Infectious Causes

Infections caused by microbes, including viruses,[17] bacteria, parasites, and scrapie agents, are linked to obesity.[18] Although most available experimental evidence is from animal models, strong observational evidence connects infection with certain adenoviruses and human obesity.[19] In particular, human adenovirus 36 causes obesity in animal models and is cross-sectionally associated with a greater risk of obesity and longitudinally linked with weight gain in adults and children.[20] The possibility that an infection can lead to obesity indicates the strong influence biology plays in obesity development.

Causes Influencing Energy Expenditure

Total daily energy requirement is determined by the aggregate of resting metabolic rate (RMR), diet-induced thermogenesis, and physical activity. Of these factors, RMR contributes 50% to 80% and has the greatest potential to influence the total daily energy requirement, followed by physical activity and diet-induced thermogenesis. In addition, the RMR varies considerably among individuals, and low RMR increases risk of weight gain.[21]

Although disease states such as hypothyroidism can decrease RMR, factors have been identified that may chronically influence energy expenditure in apparently healthy individuals and, as a result, increase energy stores. A potential key modulator is brown adipose tissue (BAT). Like white adipocytes, which store fat, brown adipocytes also contain lipid droplets but have a much higher number of mitochondria, which gives them a brown color. A key function of BAT is heat production and, in turn, energy expenditure. The presence of BAT in human adults was recognized after its identification in rodents and human infants. The amount of BAT in adult humans, measured by PET scan, is negatively associated with obesity.[22–24] This finding suggests that a lower BAT mass or its impaired functioning leads to a decreased resting energy expenditure and greater fat accumulation. Moreover, fat oxidation in skeletal muscle is impaired in obesity.[25] This decreased fat oxidation may result in greater fat stores over time.

Causes Influencing Food Intake and Processing

It is often thought that food causes obesity. However, food per se does not cause obesity in as much as water does not cause edema. It is impaired regulation of water balance that leads to water retention and edema. Similarly, impaired food intake regulation may lead to obesity. A good example of dysregulation of food intake is Prader–Willi syndrome, a genetic disorder marked by uncontrollable hunger and obesity in early childhood.[26] Besides genetic causes, food intake is physiologically regulated by hunger and satiety hormones. Onset of hunger is associated with high circulating levels of ghrelin, and as a meal progresses, satiety is induced with an increase in circulating levels of hormones such as peptide tyrosine tyrosine (PYY) and glucagon-like peptide-1, leading to meal termination. Dysregulation of this control, with greater stimulation of hunger by ghrelin or delayed onset of satiety because of a slower increase in PYY or glucagon-like peptide-1 in response to a meal, can influence energy intake, leading to obesity.[27–29] Indeed, this hunger and satiety hormone dysregulation is commonly observed in obesity.[30]

Potential Causes

Variations in anatomy or physiologic processes are associated with obesity. Specifically, accelerated gastric emptying (in approximately one-third of patients) and increased fasting gastric volume have been associated with obesity.[31] Faster gastric emptying has been associated with weight gain over a median of 4.4 years in young adults, with those exhibiting faster gastric emptying at baseline gaining 9.6 kg versus 2.8 kg for those with slower gastric emptying.[32] Stomach size is also positively associated with obesity.[31,33,34] The stomach has stretch receptors, which indicate fullness resulting from food intake,[35] so a larger sized stomach may accommodate more food before satiety is reached. Similarly, a slower intestinal transit time of food is associated with obesity,[36] likely because of increased digestion time, resulting in greater extraction of calories.

In rats with a genetic tendency for obesity, absorbed dietary fat is transported mainly to adipose tissue for storage,[37] whereas the absorbed fat is transported mainly to skeletal muscle for oxidation in genetically lean mice.[38,39] In humans with obesity, dietary fat undergoes relatively less oxidation and greater storage.[40]

Obesogens are synthetic chemicals that interfere with the endocrine system and are hypothesized to contribute to weight gain and obesity via several mechanisms, including disrupting energy metabolism.[41] Broadly, these include pesticides, food additives, plasticizers, and cosmetic or pharmaceutical additives. Specifically, some synthetic chemicals alter hormonal regulation of appetite and satiety, which may affect energy intake.[42] Furthermore, certain obesogens decrease resting energy expenditure or impair BAT thermogenesis, which may decrease total energy expenditure. Numerous obesogens have been identified, including potential mechanisms of action and effects on obesity (reviewed in[43]). However, most evidence regarding obesogens is epidemiologic or preclinical in design and, therefore, their exact contributions to human obesity remain unclear.

Causation cannot be inferred from these observational findings and future research in this area is required. Nonetheless, considering inborn defects that may predispose an individual to obesity can aid in identifying an effective obesity treatment strategy.

Weight Gain Regulation

The examples of causative factors of obesity discussed in this article highlight 2 key attributes of obesity. First, the nonvolitional nature of causative factors of obesity underscores the fallacy behind the perceived ease in preventing obesity. At this time, preventing many physiologic defects that lead to obesity is not feasible. Instead, efforts aimed at preventing weight gain may be more realistic. Second, the examples described demonstrate the multifactorial nature of obesity. Although excess fat accumulation may be common, depending on the cause, each type of obesity may have characteristically different expressions that affect risk of comorbidities. Additionally, within an individual, multiple causes of obesity may be present. This plurality of causes and variation in disease expression may be better described by the term obesities instead of obesity.

CONTRIBUTORS TO OBESITY

Energy balance is homeostatically regulated and defined as an equilibrium between energy intake from diet and energy expended to maintain bodily processes and during activities of daily living. However, factors that increase energy intake or promote positive energy balance do not necessarily lead to obesity. The development of obesity requires substantial, sustained, and cumulative positive energy balance leading to fat accumulation consistent with the definition of obesity (BMI >30 kg/m^2).

Individuals without a known predisposition to obesity seem to successfully maintain body weight under experimental conditions, likely through the regulation of energy intake and/or expenditure. Conversely, some individuals exposed to the same experimental conditions develop obesity. Therefore, this suggests an intrinsic defect(s) in energy balance regulation giving rise to long-term positive energy balance, resulting in excess adiposity and obesity.[44] This intrinsic inability combined with certain extrinsic factors can lead to excess weight gain and obesity.

The regulation of energy balance can be disrupted in all individuals, but there are some stark differences among individuals prone to obesity (ObP) versus those who seem resistant to obesity (ObR) under experimental conditions. Recently, George Bray described this very elegantly and comprehensively.[45] He presented substantial evidence from various clinical studies that forced overfeeding can increase fat accumulation, but the amount of weight or fat gain may be very different between ObR versus ObP individuals. Moreover, weight seems to quickly and relatively easily return to baseline in ObR individuals once experimental overfeeding is discontinued. Conversely, ObP individuals maintain the gained weight. These differences may be attributed to various factors, including lower nighttime fat oxidation or the ability to compensate for overfeeding in ObP individuals or a greater ability to sustain higher metabolic requirements in response to fasting in ObR individuals.[45] Although this evidence is informative to understanding obesity development, it is unclear how generalizable these findings are to development of obesity in free-living individuals exposed to the current food environment in the United States and other developed countries. Also, the age of obesity onset varies. Hence, it is difficult to predict if a person presently without obesity will develop it in the future. Following is a discussion of factors that may contribute to obesity (see **Table 1**). Factors that contribute to positive energy balance by affecting energy intake, expenditure, or both are described.

Key Contributors Influencing Energy Intake

Dietary factors
It is well documented that the US food supply does not align with dietary recommendations.[46] Numerous lines of evidence suggest chronic high intake of energy dense or ultraprocessed foods may result in the disruption of homeostatic mechanisms regulating energy intake. Similarly, large portion sizes might also alter regulatory mechanisms, giving rise to energy intake beyond physiologic needs. The abundance of ultraprocessed, energy-dense foods, as well as marketing practices that promote larger portion sizes, is increasing, and the potential contribution this makes to energy intake and body weight are described in these sections.

Energy density
Energy density refers to the number of calories per gram in a food or meal and, depending on the macronutrient and water composition, ranges from 0 to 9 kcal/g. A higher fat composition increases energy density (9 kcal/g), whereas carbohydrate and protein have a moderate effect on energy density (4 kcal/g). Water dilutes the energy density of most commonly consumed foods because of its noncaloric contribution to weight and volume (0 kcal/g). Concordant evidence shows energy intake increases with greater consumption of energy-dense foods.[47–49] Furthermore, a high energy density increases intake regardless of the macronutrient composition.[49] Increases in body weight are also observed in response to increases in energy density and the resulting increase in energy intake.[50] In clinical weight management, education focused on intake of foods with lower energy density decreases body weight.[51]

Portion size
In the United States, portion sizes of commonly consumed foods have been increasing since the 1970s.[52] Portion size is a known contributor to energy intake at eating occasions. In an 11-day randomized crossover trial, increasing portion sizes by 50% resulted in a mean daily increase in energy intake of approximately 400 kcal compared with standard portions.[53] Interestingly, this effect was not modified by baseline body weight or sex. Furthermore, no evidence of compensatory adjustments to energy intake occurred in response to increased caloric intake over the 11 days, suggesting regulatory mechanisms may be insufficient to maintain energy balance with this large portion size variation in these participants. This portion size effect has been observed consistently with a broad range of foods in adults and children in experimental and free-living conditions.[54] Restricting portion size is therefore a strategy used in weight management.

Ultraprocessing

At a population level, ultraprocessed foods account for approximately 55% of energy intake in US adults.[55] Ultraprocessed foods, defined by the NOVA classification system, are formulations made mostly or entirely from substances extracted from foods (eg, casein, lactose, whey, and gluten) or derived from processing of food constituents (eg, hydrogenated or interesterified oils, hydrolyzed proteins, soy protein isolate, maltodextrin, invert sugar, and high-fructose corn syrup), with little if any intact unprocessed or minimally processed foods.[56] From a consumer perspective, ultraprocessed foods are hyperpalatable and appealing and can be consumed with ease and convenience. They also have a long shelf-life.

Accumulating epidemiologic evidence shows that a higher intake of ultraprocessed foods is cross-sectionally and prospectively associated with greater risk of obesity.[57–60] These observational data are supported by findings of a randomized, crossover, inpatient feeding study that showed ad libitum calorie consumption was higher with exposure to an ultraprocessed diet compared with an isocaloric, macronutrient, and energy density matched unprocessed diet.[61] After 2 weeks of the ultraprocessed diet, body weight (0.9 kg) and fat mass (0.4 kg) increased compared with a decrease after the unprocessed diet (−0.9 and −0.3 kg, respectively). At present, the mechanistic underpinnings of the positive energy balance induced by the ultraprocessed diet are unclear. Interestingly, meal eating rate in grams (+7.4 g/min) and calories (+17 kcal/min) was higher with the ultraprocessed diet versus the unprocessed diet, which may result in greater energy intake before the onset of satiety signaling and passive overconsumption.[61] Evidence suggests that limiting the intake of ultraprocessed food may be a strategy to avoid positive energy balance, but it is important to acknowledge the time, skill, expense, and other resources needed to prepare meals from minimally processed foods.

Although we have discussed energy density, portion size, and ultraprocessing as separate concepts, in reality, the US population is exposed to a food supply abundant in energy dense ultraprocessed foods in large portion sizes. Therefore, with regard to ingestive behavior, these factors co-occur, and the impact may be additive. Patient education focused on concepts of energy density and portion size may assist in obesity management.[51]

Sleep duration and quality

The American Academy of Sleep Medicine and the Sleep Research Society recommend adults regularly sleep for 7 or more hours per night.[62] Short sleep duration (<7 hours/night) is prospectively associated with higher relative risk of obesity in both adults and children.[63,64] At present, the relationship between short sleep duration and obesity has been characterized incompletely. Still, a number of aberrations caused by inadequate sleep that impact energy intake and expenditure plausibly contribute to obesity.[65] Under experimental conditions, total sleep deprivation (not sleeping for a 24-hour period) decreased activity in the appetitive evaluation regions within the frontal cortex and insula cortex of the brain and amplified activity within the amygdala during a food desire task compared with adequate sleep duration (8 hours).[66] Furthermore, relative to the adequate sleep condition, sleep deprivation increased the proportion of "wanted" food items with a high caloric content. This study suggests that sleep deprivation affects neurocognitive function in ways that may alter food selection and choice.

It is also plausible that diet impacts sleep quality and duration, which might contribute to obesity. Diet quality could influence sleep via dietary components such as tryptophan, a precursor to melatonin and serotonin that affects sleep quality and duration.[67] Currently, the totality of available evidence does not support a shift in energy metabolism (ie, resting energy expenditure) as a result of short sleep duration, and overall energy expenditure is generally higher with sleep restriction because of energy needed to maintain wakefulness.[65] Observational evidence is mixed regarding the relationship between sleep duration and physical activity.[65] It is likely that a bidirectional relationship exists between sleep duration and quality and physical activity. Higher activity levels are associated with better sleep quality,[68] and worse sleep quality and duration is associated with tiredness and fatigue, which may limit activity.

Key Contributors Influencing Energy Expenditure

Positive energy balance may result from the influence of factors that affect energy expended. Total energy expenditure is determined by the RMR, diet-induced thermogenesis, and physical activity-related energy expenditure. Physical activity-related energy expenditure is composed of exercise-related activity energy expenditure (eg, walking, running, sports) and non–exercise-related activity energy expenditure (non-exercise activities of daily living). It should be noted that total energy balance results from an interplay of many individual factors, and it is difficult to draw conclusions about energy balance without information about all its components. For instance, unless energy intake is known, it is not possible to accurately infer whether a person is in positive or negative energy balance at a given level of physical activity. In these sections, factors that can contribute to positive energy balance by affecting energy expenditure are described.

Exercise-related activity energy expenditure

The 2018 Physical Activity Guidelines for Americans recommend all adults, including those with chronic conditions or disabilities who are able, accumulate at least 150 to 300 min/wk of moderate-intensity physical activity.[69] For weight management, more than 300 min/wk of moderate-intensity activity is recommended, as well as muscle-strengthening activities to assist in maintaining lean body mass. Currently, approximately one-fourth of US adults meet physical activity guidelines.[70] Prospective epidemiologic evidence shows that lower physical activity levels are associated with a higher risk of obesity.[71]

Individual-, interpersonal-, environmental-, and policy-level factors contribute to time spent physically active. At the individual level, age, health status, self-efficacy, and motivation are associated with physical activity.[72] However, environmental factors such as the built environment (eg, community walkability, parks, pedestrian safety), natural environment (eg, weather, day-light time), and social environment (eg, organizational practices, neighborhood crime) may also influence physical activity levels. At present, some evidence shows a higher physical activity level is associated with greater neighborhood walkability and access to recreation facilities, trails, or parks.[73] However, less evidence supports this translating into a lower risk of obesity.

Non–exercise-related activity energy expenditure

Non–exercise-related activity accounts for a large proportion of total energy expenditure, substantially greater than exercise-related activity expenditure, but is the most varied component of energy expenditure. Generally, energy expenditure owing to non–exercise-related activity is 300 to 2000 kcal/d.[74] An inverse relationship exists between sedentary time and non–exercise-related activity energy expenditure. Thus, higher levels of sedentary time result in diminished non–exercise-related activity energy expenditure.

Sedentary time is defined as any waking behavior characterized by low levels of energy expenditure that occurs while sitting, reclining, or lying. For the first time, the 2018 iteration of the Physical Activity Guidelines for Americans acknowledged the health risks associated with sedentary behavior and benefits associated with decreasing time spent being sedentary.[69] Greater sedentary time is consistently and prospectively associated with a higher risk of obesity.[75] Higher sedentary behavior during childhood and adolescence is a strong predictor of obesity in adulthood.

Key Contributors Influencing Energy Intake and Expenditure

Psychological health and well-being

Psychological health and well-being may contribute to weight gain. Psychological conditions such as depression and anxiety are likely reciprocally related to obesity risk. For example, depression is related to an increased risk of obesity, and obesity is associated with a higher risk of depression.[76,77] Chronic stress exposure is also associated with obesity. Chronic stress is defined as cumulative, repeated, or prolonged stress exposure. Chronic stress is associated with poorer diet quality and a sedentary lifestyle, which may contribute to obesity development. However, stress may also cause physiologic alterations that contribute to obesity.

Stress causes increased cortisol levels that stimulate fat storage and affect dietary behaviors.[78] Specifically, cortisol influences brain regions implicated in reward and appetite. Cortisol upregulates neuropeptide Y, an appetite and reward inducer, and dysregulates insulin and leptin, which results in increased appetite and reward.[78] Gastrointestinal hormones known to affect hunger and satiety are also affected by stress. A recent systematic review and meta-analysis of 10 clinical trials showed that experimentally induced stress acutely increased plasma ghrelin levels, and individuals with obesity had a stronger, more prolonged response.[79] Multiple biological pathways contribute to complex interrelations between stress, diet, and obesity, and the relevance of a patient's psychological state, including health and well-being should be considered in weight management. Kubzansky and colleagues[80] published some brief questions clinicians can ask patients to assess well-being and statements that can be used to promote positive psychological well-being in clinic visits.

Use of tobacco products

The US Food and Drug Administration defines tobacco products as cigarettes, cigarette tobacco, roll-your-own tobacco, smokeless tobacco products, electronic cigarettes (e-cigarettes) or electronic nicotine delivery systems, cigars, hookah (also called waterpipe tobacco), pipe tobacco, nicotine gels, and dissolvables.[81] In 2018, 19.7% of US adults over 18 years of age used any tobacco product and nearly 4% reported use of 2 or more tobacco products.[82] Although the use of tobacco products has numerous detrimental health effects and cessation is indicated for all individuals,[83] cessation is associated with weight gain. Nicotine increases energy expenditure by increasing sympathetic drive and thermogenesis.[84] Additionally, nicotine suppresses appetite through the modulation of appetite-regulating hormones (PYY, orexin, neuropeptide Y). Nicotine replacement during tobacco product cessation can assist in preventing weight gain.[84]

CLINICAL RELEVANCE OF UNDERSTANDING CAUSES OF OBESITY

As for any chronic illness, the multiple causes of obesity must be investigated with the intention of developing possible prevention or treatment approaches. The plurality of causes and contributors underscores that the BMI of an individual is the net result of multiple factors that may influence energy stores. Hence, a more complete understanding of these factors increases the efficacy of obesity prevention or treatment strategies.

Most importantly, it is necessary to differentiate between modifiable and nonmodifiable risk factors for obesity, keeping in mind that the many factors considered nonmodifiable today may eventually become modifiable. For example, the absence of leptin or MC4R deficiency was considered nonmodifiable in the past. However, both can now be treated effectively with leptin or setmelanotide, respectively.[85,86] Additionally, identifying pathologic conditions that lead to weight gain and obesity, such as hypothyroidism or Cushing's syndrome, is important so underlying conditions can be treated and further contribution to weight gain prevented. Thus, identifying these conditions in people with obesity becomes clinically very relevant.

Excess energy intake may result from the dysregulation of feeding behavior owing to accelerated gastric emptying or suboptimal functioning of satiety or hunger hormones,[30] leading to food cravings, excessive and/or frequent hunger, or delayed satiety. This point is relevant because weight loss treatment relies on creating substantial and sustained negative energy balance and decreasing energy intake is a key approach to achieving negative energy balance. Fortunately, medications approved by the US Food and Drug Administration for weight loss may selectively address these conditions.[87] One could select a medication that mainly decreases hunger,[88] food cravings,[89] or fat digestion in a meal or one that increases satiety.[90] This process can be greatly facilitated by understanding patient feeding behavior. A targeted inquiry specifically to determine if a person feels hungrier, craves certain foods, or feels less full can guide in selecting an appropriate weight loss medication.[91]

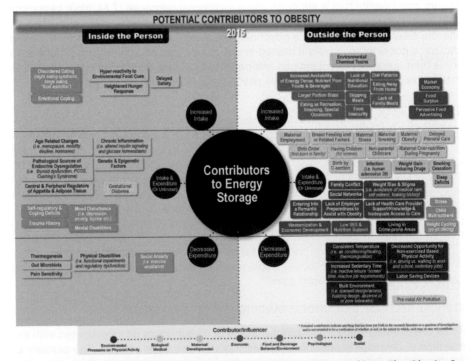

Fig. 1. Potential* contributors to obesity. SES, socioeconomic status. (*From* The Obesity Society. January 22, 2016. Available at: https://www.facebook.com/TheObesitySociety/photos/have-you-seen-our-infographic-on-potential-contributors-to-obesity-see-it-at-htt/10153370347378543/ Accessed April 12, 2021.)

Similarly, treatment can be targeted for patients with accelerated gastric emptying because they have significantly better weight loss responses to treatments that delay gastric emptying, such as glucagon-like peptide-1 receptor analogs or intragastric balloons.[31,92,93]

CLINICAL RELEVANCE OF UNDERSTANDING CONTRIBUTORS OF OBESITY

Weight loss treatment for obesity involves a decrease in energy intake and/or increases in energy expenditure to create a chronic, substantial negative energy balance. As described, energy intake and expenditure are influenced by a number of factors, some of which are potentially modifiable (**Fig. 1**). As a part of patient assessment, potentially modifiable, actionable factors should be points of inquiry to inform obesity management. For example, open-ended questions may be used to gain understanding of a patient's context and typical daily schedule, including time spent physically active or doing nonexercise activity as part of work, social, or household tasks; sedentary time; sleep habits; and usual food choices and meal timing. Psychological health assessment is relatively routine, and most electronic health record systems have depression screening instruments embedded for point-of-care use. A patient's experience of stress may also be assessed by a question such as, "On a scale of 1 to 10, how would you rate your feelings of stress today (or over the past few months)? Can you tell me why you chose ___?"[80] Information gained from assessing potential contributors to obesity may help identify individualized behavior change targets that may measurably impact body weight. In consultation with the patient as part of shared decision-making, SMART (specific, measurable, achievable, realistic, and timed) goal(s) should be agreed upon and appropriate counseling and plans for follow-up made to facilitate behavior change.

SUMMARY

Obesity is a chronic disease with a multifactorial etiology that leads to structural abnormalities, physiologic derangements, and functional impairments that impact health and well-being. We posit that obesity is caused by impairment of mechanisms that regulate body fat stores leading to excess fat accumulation. A number of primary factors cause obesity directly by impairing the regulation of hunger, satiety, digestive processes, adipose tissue fat storage, and RMR, which can result in a positive energy balance and accumulation of excess body fat. For the most part, these primary factors are under nonvolitional control. In addition, several other factors contribute to obesity by influencing energy intake, expenditure, or both. Impairment in the function of primary factors seems necessary for contributors to promote obesity. Most factors classified as contributors have an unclear role in "causing" obesity. Nonetheless, in clinical settings, a better understanding of obesity's causes and contributors may assist in effective weight management.

CLINICS CARE POINTS

- When treating obesity, recognize that it is not due to a lack of willpower. Obesity results from impaired regulation of fat storage.
- To effectively treat obesity, identify and address the contributors to weight gain that are modifiable.
- Approaches for preventing or treating obesity should focus on monitoring body fat content.

DISCLOSURE

The authors report no relevant commercial or financial conflicts of interest.

REFERENCES

1. Meldrum DR, Morris MA, Gambone JC. Obesity pandemic: causes, consequences, and solutions—but do we have the will? Fertil Sterility 2017;107(4): 833–9.
2. Nedergaard J, Cannon B. Brown adipose tissue as a heat-producing thermoeffector. Handb Clin Neurol 2018;156:137–52.
3. Alexander CM, Kasza I, Yen CLE, et al. Dermal white adipose tissue: a new component of the thermogenic response. J lipid Res 2015;56(11):2061–9.
4. Scheja L, Heeren J. The endocrine function of adipose tissues in health and cardiometabolic disease. Nat Rev Endocrinol 2019;15(9):507–24.
5. Mintziori G, Nigdelis MP, Mathew H, et al. The effect of excess body fat on female and male reproduction. Metabolism 2020;107:154193.
6. Bohler H Jr, Mokshagundam S, Winters SJ. Adipose tissue and reproduction in women. Fertil sterility 2010;94(3):795–825.
7. Triantafyllou GA, Paschou SA, Mantzoros CS. Leptin and hormones: energy homeostasis. Endocrinol Metab Clin North Am 2016;45(3):633–45.
8. Considine RV, Sinha MK, Heiman ML, et al. Serum immunoreactive-leptin concentrations in normal-weight and obese humans. N Engl J Med 1996;334(5):292–5.
9. Müller MJ, Enderle J, Pourhassan M, et al. Metabolic adaptation to caloric restriction and subsequent refeeding: the Minnesota Starvation Experiment revisited. Am J Clin Nutr 2015;102(4):807–19.
10. Montague CT, Farooqi IS, Whitehead JP, et al. Congenital leptin deficiency is associated with severe early-onset obesity in humans. Nature 1997;387(6636): 903–8.
11. Shipp SL, Cline MA, Gilbert ER. Recent advances in the understanding of how neuropeptide Y and α-melanocyte stimulating hormone function in adipose physiology. Adipocyte 2016;5(4):333–50.
12. Doulla M, McIntyre AD, Hegele RA, et al. A novel MC4R mutation associated with childhood-onset obesity: a case report. Paediatr Child Health 2014;19(10):515–8.
13. Moustafa JSE-S, Froguel P. From obesity genetics to the future of personalized obesity therapy. Nat Rev Endocrinol 2013;9(7):402.
14. Weaver JU. Classical endocrine diseases causing obesity. Obes Metab 2008;36: 212–28.
15. Kreitschmann-Andermahr I, Suarez P, Jennings R, et al. GH/IGF-I regulation in obesity – mechanisms and practical consequences in children and adults. Horm Res Paediatrics 2010;73(3):153–60.
16. Geer EB, Lalazar Y, Couto LM, et al. A prospective study of appetite and food craving in 30 patients with Cushing's disease. Pituitary 2016;19(2):117–26.
17. Voss JD, Dhurandhar NV. Viral infections and obesity. Curr Obes Rep 2017;6(1): 28–37.
18. Dhurandhar NV, Bailey D, Thomas D. Interaction of obesity and infections. Obes Rev 2015;16(12):1017–29.
19. Akheruzzaman M, Hegde V, Dhurandhar NV. Twenty-five years of research about adipogenic adenoviruses: a systematic review. Obes Rev 2018;20(4):499–509.
20. Xu MY, Cao B, Wang DF, et al. Human adenovirus 36 infection increased the risk of obesity: a meta-analysis update. Medicine (Baltimore) 2015;94(51):e2357.

21. Ravussin E. Low resting metabolic rate as a risk factor for weight gain: role of the sympathetic nervous system. Int J Obes Relat Metab Disord 1995;19:S8–9.
22. Cypess AM, Lehman S, Williams G, et al. Identification and importance of brown adipose tissue in adult humans. N Engl J Med 2009;360(15):1509–17.
23. van Marken Lichtenbelt WD, Vanhommerig JW, Smulders NM, et al. Cold-activated brown adipose tissue in healthy men. N Engl J Med 2009;360(15):1500–8.
24. Saito M, Okamatsu-Ogura Y, Matsushita M, et al. High incidence of metabolically active brown adipose tissue in healthy adult humans: effects of cold exposure and adiposity. Diabetes 2009;58(7):1526–31.
25. Berggren JR, Boyle KE, Chapman WH, et al. Skeletal muscle lipid oxidation and obesity: influence of weight loss and exercise. Am J Physiol Endocrinol Metab 2008;294(4):E726–32.
26. Khan MJ, Gerasimidis K, Edwards CA, et al. Mechanisms of obesity in Prader-Willi syndrome. Pediatr Obes 2018;13(1):3–13.
27. le Roux CW, Batterham RL, Aylwin SJ, et al. Attenuated peptide YY release in obese subjects is associated with reduced satiety. Endocrinology 2006; 147(1):3–8.
28. Verdich C, Toubro S, Buemann B, et al. The role of postprandial releases of insulin and incretin hormones in meal-induced satiety–effect of obesity and weight reduction. Int J Obes Relat Metab Disord 2001;25(8):1206–14.
29. Castorina S, Barresi V, Luca T, et al. Gastric ghrelin cells in obese patients are hyperactive. Int J Obes (Lond) 2021;45(1):184–94.
30. Lean MEJ, Malkova D. Altered gut and adipose tissue hormones in overweight and obese individuals: cause or consequence? Int J Obes (2005) 2016;40(4): 622–32.
31. Acosta A, Camilleri M, Shin A, et al. Quantitative gastrointestinal and psychological traits associated with obesity and response to weight-loss therapy. Gastroenterology 2015;148(3):537–46.e4.
32. Pajot G, Camilleri M, Calderon G, et al. Association between gastrointestinal phenotypes and weight gain in younger adults: a prospective 4-year cohort study. Int J Obes 2020;44(12):2472–8.
33. Granström L, Backman L. Stomach distension in extremely obese and in normal subjects. Acta Chir Scand 1985;151(4):367–70.
34. Geliebter A. Gastric distension and gastric capacity in relation to food intake in humans. Physiol Behav 1988;44(4–5):665–8.
35. Carmagnola S, Cantù P, Penagini R. Mechanoreceptors of the proximal stomach and perception of gastric distension. Am J Gastroenterol 2005;100(8):1704–10.
36. Nguyen NQ, Debreceni TL, Burgess JE, et al. Impact of gastric emptying and small intestinal transit on blood glucose, intestinal hormones, glucose absorption in the morbidly obese. Int J Obes (Lond) 2018;42(9):1556–64.
37. Jackman MR, Kramer RE, MacLean PS, et al. Trafficking of dietary fat in obesity-prone and obesity-resistant rats. Am J Physiol Endocrinol Metab 2006;291(5): E1083–91.
38. Jensen MD. Fate of fatty acids at rest and during exercise: regulatory mechanisms. Acta Physiol Scand 2003;178(4):385–90.
39. Bessesen DH, Rupp CL, Eckel RH. Trafficking of dietary fat in lean rats. Obes Res 1995;3(2):191–203.
40. Westerterp KR. Dietary fat oxidation as a function of body fat. Curr Opin Lipidol 2009;20(1):45–9.
41. Grün F, Blumberg B. Environmental obesogens: organotins and endocrine disruption via nuclear receptor signaling. Endocrinology 2006;147(6):s50–5.

42. Heindel JJ, Blumberg B. Environmental obesogens: mechanisms and controversies. Annu Rev Pharmacol Toxicol 2019;59:89–106.

43. Amato AA, Wheeler HB, Blumberg B. Obesity and endocrine-disrupting chemicals. Endocr Connect 2021;10(2):R87–105.

44. Jastreboff AM, Kotz CM, Kahan S, et al. Obesity as a disease: the Obesity Society 2018 Position Statement. Obesity 2019;27(1):7–9.

45. Bray GA. The pain of weight gain: self-experimentation with overfeeding. Am J Clin Nutr 2020;111(1):17–20.

46. Miller PE, Reedy J, Kirkpatrick SI, et al. The United States food supply is not consistent with dietary guidance: evidence from an evaluation using the Healthy Eating Index-2010. J Acad Nutr Diet 2015;115(1):95–100.

47. Bell EA, Castellanos VH, Pelkman CL, et al. Energy density of foods affects energy intake in normal-weight women. Am J Clin Nutr 1998;67(3):412–20.

48. Rolls BJ, Bell EA, Castellanos VH, et al. Energy density but not fat content of foods affected energy intake in lean and obese women. Am J Clin Nutr 1999;69(5):863–71.

49. Bell EA, Rolls BJ. Energy density of foods affects energy intake across multiple levels of fat content in lean and obese women. Am J Clin Nutr 2001;73(6):1010–8.

50. Stubbs R, Johnstone A, O'Reilly L, et al. The effect of covertly manipulating the energy density of mixed diets on ad libitum food intake in 'pseudo free-living' humans. Int J Obes 1998;22(10):980–7.

51. Rolls B. Dietary energy density: applying behavioural science to weight management. Nutr Bull 2017;42(3):246–53.

52. Young LR, Nestle M, Flegal K, et al. Reducing portion sizes to prevent obesity. Am J Prev Med 2012;43(5):565.

53. Rolls BJ, Roe LS, Meengs JS. The effect of large portion sizes on energy intake is sustained for 11 days. Obesity 2007;15(6):1535–43.

54. English L, Lasschuijt M, Keller KL. Mechanisms of the portion size effect. What is known and where do we go from here? Appetite 2015;88:39–49.

55. Zhang Z, Jackson SL, Martinez E, et al. Association between ultraprocessed food intake and cardiovascular health in US adults: a cross-sectional analysis of the NHANES 2011-2016. Am J Clin Nutr 2021;113(2):428–36.

56. Monteiro CA, Cannon G, Moubarac JC, et al. The UN Decade of Nutrition, the NOVA food classification and the trouble with ultra-processing. Public Health Nutr 2018;21(1):5–17.

57. Machado PP, Steele EM, Levy RB, et al. Ultra-processed food consumption and obesity in the Australian adult population. Nutr Diabetes 2020;10(1):39.

58. Pestoni G, Habib L, Reber E, et al. Ultraprocessed Food consumption is strongly and dose-dependently associated with excess body weight in Swiss women. Obesity (Silver Spring) 2021;29(3):601–9.

59. Konieczna J, Morey M, Abete I, et al. Contribution of ultra-processed foods in visceral fat deposition and other adiposity indicators: prospective analysis nested in the PREDIMED-Plus trial. Clin Nutr 2021;40(6):4290–300.

60. Rauber F, Chang K, Vamos EP, et al. Ultra-processed food consumption and risk of obesity: a prospective cohort study of UK Biobank. Eur J Nutr 2020;60(4):2169–80.

61. Hall KD, Ayuketah A, Brychta R, et al. Ultra-processed diets cause excess calorie intake and weight gain: an inpatient randomized controlled trial of ad libitum food intake. Cell Metab 2019;30(1):67–77.e63.

62. Panel CC, Watson NF, Badr MS, et al. Recommended amount of sleep for a healthy adult: a joint consensus statement of the American Academy of Sleep Medicine and Sleep Research Society. J Clin Sleep Med 2015;11(6):591–2.

63. Li L, Zhang S, Huang Y, et al. Sleep duration and obesity in children: a systematic review and meta-analysis of prospective cohort studies. J Paediatr Child Health 2017;53(4):378–85.

64. Zhou Q, Zhang M, Hu D. Dose-response association between sleep duration and obesity risk: a systematic review and meta-analysis of prospective cohort studies. Sleep Breath 2019;23(4):1035–45.

65. St-Onge M-P, Grandner MA, Brown D, et al. American Heart Association Obesity, Behavior Change, Diabetes, and Nutrition Committees of the Council on Lifestyle and Cardiometabolic Health; Council on Cardiovascular Disease in the Young; Council on Clinical Cardiology; and Stroke Council. Sleep duration and quality: impact on lifestyle behaviors and cardiometabolic health: a scientific statement from the American Heart Association. Circulation 2016;134(18):e367–86.

66. Greer SM, Goldstein AN, Walker MP. The impact of sleep deprivation on food desire in the human brain. Nat Commun 2013;4(1):1–7.

67. St-Onge M-P, Zuraikat FM. Reciprocal roles of sleep and diet in cardiovascular health: a review of recent evidence and a potential mechanism. Curr Atheroscler Rep 2019;21(3):11.

68. Buman MP, Hekler EB, Bliwise DL, et al. Exercise effects on night-to-night fluctuations in self-rated sleep among older adults with sleep complaints. J Sleep Res 2011;20(1pt1):28–37.

69. Piercy KL, Troiano RP, Ballard RM, et al. The physical activity guidelines for Americans. JAMA 2018;320(19):2020–8.

70. Virani SS, Alonso A, Aparicio HJ, et al. Heart disease and stroke statistics—2021 update: a report from the American Heart Association. Circulation 2021;143(8): e254–743.

71. Cleven L, Krell-Roesch J, Nigg CR, et al. The association between physical activity with incident obesity, coronary heart disease, diabetes and hypertension in adults: a systematic review of longitudinal studies published after 2012. BMC public health 2020;20:1–15.

72. Bauman AE, Reis RS, Sallis JF, et al. Correlates of physical activity: why are some people physically active and others not? Lancet 2012;380(9838):258–71.

73. Dixon BN, Ugwoaba UA, Brockmann AN, et al. Associations between the built environment and dietary intake, physical activity, and obesity: a scoping review of reviews. Obes Rev 2020;22(4):e13171.

74. Hamilton MT, Hamilton DG, Zderic TW. Role of low energy expenditure and sitting in obesity, metabolic syndrome, type 2 diabetes, and cardiovascular disease. Diabetes 2007;56(11):2655–67.

75. Thorp AA, Owen N, Neuhaus M, et al. Sedentary behaviors and subsequent health outcomes in adults: a systematic review of longitudinal studies, 1996–2011. Am J Prev Med 2011;41(2):207–15.

76. Luppino FS, de Wit LM, Bouvy PF, et al. Overweight, obesity, and depression: a systematic review and meta-analysis of longitudinal studies. Arch Gen Psychiatry 2010;67(3):220–9.

77. Mannan M, Mamun A, Doi S, et al. Prospective associations between depression and obesity for adolescent males and females-a systematic review and meta-analysis of longitudinal studies. PLoS One 2016;11(6):e0157240.

78. Michels N. Biological underpinnings from psychosocial stress towards appetite and obesity during youth: research implications towards metagenomics, epigenomics and metabolomics. Nutr Res Rev 2019;32(2):282–93.

79. Bouillon-Minois J-B, Trousselard M, Thivel D, et al. Ghrelin as a biomarker of stress: a systematic review and meta-analysis. Nutrients 2021;13(3):784.

80. Kubzansky LD, Huffman JC, Boehm JK, et al. Positive psychological well-being and cardiovascular disease: JACC health promotion series. J Am Coll Cardiol 2018;72(12):1382–96.

81. The facts on the FDA's new tobacco rule. U.S. Food & Drug Administration. 2016. Available at: https://www.fda.gov/consumers/consumer-updates/facts-fdas-new-tobacco-rule. Accessed March 29, 2021.

82. Creamer MR, Wang TW, Babb S, et al. Tobacco product use and cessation indicators among adults—United States, 2018. Morbidity mortality weekly Rep 2019; 68(45):1013.

83. Barua RS, Rigotti NA, Benowitz NL, et al. 2018 ACC expert consensus decision pathway on tobacco cessation treatment: a report of the American College of Cardiology Task Force on Clinical Expert Consensus Documents. J Am Coll Cardiol 2018;72(25):3332–65.

84. Kos K. Cardiometabolic morbidity and mortality with smoking cessation, review of recommendations for people with diabetes and obesity. Curr Diabetes Rep 2020; 20(12):1–9.

85. Paz-Filho G, Wong M-L, Licinio J. Ten years of leptin replacement therapy. Obes Rev 2011;12(5):e315–23.

86. Clément K, van den Akker E, Argente J, et al. Efficacy and safety of setmelanotide, an MC4R agonist, in individuals with severe obesity due to LEPR or POMC deficiency: single-arm, open-label, multicentre, phase 3 trials. Lancet Diabetes Endocrinol 2020;8(12):960–70.

87. Pilitsi E, Farr OM, Polyzos SA, et al. Pharmacotherapy of obesity: available medications and drugs under investigation. Metabolism 2019;92:170–92.

88. Highlights of prescribing information: qsymia (phentermine-topiramate extended-release), U.S. Food and Drug Administration. Mountain View (CA): VIVUS, Inc; 2012. Available at: https://www.accessdata.fda.gov/drugsatfda_docs/label/2012/022580s000lbl.pdf. Accessed April, 2021.

89. Highlights of prescribing information: Contrave, U.S. Food and Drug Administration. La Jolla (CA): Orexigen Therapeutics, Inc.; 2020. Available at: https://www.accessdata.fda.gov/drugsatfda_docs/label/2020/200063s015lbl.pdf. Accessed April, 2021.

90. Highlights of prescribing information: Saxenda, U.S. Food and Drug Administration. Novo Nordisk; 2018. Available at: https://www.accessdata.fda.gov/drugsatfda_docs/label/2018/206321s007lbl.pdf. Accessed April, 2021.

91. Acosta A, Camilleri M, Abu Dayyeh B, et al. Selection of antiobesity medications based on phenotypes enhances weight loss: a pragmatic trial in an obesity clinic. Obesity (Silver Spring). 2021;29(4):662–71.

92. Halawi H, Khemani D, Eckert D, et al. Effects of liraglutide on weight, satiation, and gastric functions in obesity: a randomised, placebo-controlled pilot trial. Lancet Gastroenterol Hepatol 2017;2(12):890–9.

93. Gómez V, Woodman G, Abu Dayyeh BK. Delayed gastric emptying as a proposed mechanism of action during intragastric balloon therapy: results of a prospective study. Obesity 2016;24(9):1849–53.

Pathophysiology of Obesity

Christine Kessler, MN, CNS, ANP, BC-ADM, CDTC

KEYWORDS

- Obesity • Epigenetics • Adipose tissue • Adipokines • Appetite regulation
- Energy balance • Metabolic adaptation • Chronotype

KEY POINTS

- The pathogenesis of obesity is complex but primarily involves a sustained, positive energy balance with enlargement (and defense) of the body's fat mass.
- Adipose tissue comprises a highly active, secretory organ involved in lipid storage/metabolism, insulin sensitivity, and hormone release, which, when subjected to hypertrophy-induced apoptosis, leads to systemic inflammation impaired metabolism and multiple complications.
- Genetic, epigenetic, and developmental factors are greatly influenced by numerous environmental factors to promote obesity risk that can be a focus for obesity prevention and treatment.
- It is time to abandon the outdated paradigm of obesity pathogenesis as simply the behavioral problem of "eating too much and moving too little."

INTRODUCTION

Obesity has long been assumed the consequence of unhealthy lifestyle choices and negative behavior traits, such as gluttony, self-indulgence, laziness, and lack of willpower that leads to excessive energy consumption, in the presence of reduced energy expenditure, resulting in undue weight gain. In other words, a person simply eats too much and moves to little.[1] These erroneous assumptions fail to recognize growing, scientific evidence confirming obesity as a complex, chronic, progressive disease that results from impairment of several physiologic processes. Chief among these impaired biological interactions is failure of normal weight and energy homeostasis, leading to an increase in body fat mass. Misunderstanding the heterogeneity of the underlying causes of obesity can lead to medical and public bias, intervention inertia, and less effective treatment strategies.[2]

Although there is no medical consensus regarding the definition of obesity, the Obesity Medicine Association (OMA) offers the most precise description of obesity as "a chronic, relapsing, multifactorial, neurobehavioral disease, wherein an increase in body fat promotes adipose tissue dysfunction and abnormal fat mass physical

Metabolic Medicine Associates, 6315 Vista Court, King George, VA 22485, USA
E-mail address: ckessler@maranatha.net

Nurs Clin N Am 56 (2021) 465–478
https://doi.org/10.1016/j.cnur.2021.08.001
0029-6465/21/© 2021 Elsevier Inc. All rights reserved.

forces, resulting in adverse metabolic, biomechanical, and psychosocial health consequences."[3] To promote clarity, the American Association of Clinical Endocrinologists recently proposed a new diagnostic term for obesity, "Adiposity-Based Chronic Disease."[2,4] Obesity is also defined and categorized by a variety of assessment methods. Body mass index (BMI) (weight in kg/height in m^2), is currently the most widely used formula to define overweight (BMI 25–29.9 kg/m^2) and obesity (BMI $\geq$30 kg/m^2), with lower weight threshold targets for Asian individuals. Although not a true measure of body fat mass in comparison with lean muscle mass, BMI is considered simple to use in health screenings.[1] Regardless of how obesity is defined, the prevalence of this disease continues to rise unabated since its sudden emergence as a health care problem in 1980.

MECHANISMS OF OBESITY PATHOGENESIS

It is becoming clear that obesity is primarily a dysfunction of energy homeostasis, rather than an insidious, passive accumulation of excess body fat (abnormal energy storage). What is less clear is how chronic energy imbalances cause a chain of altered biochemical signaling to occur, leading to an increase in body weight and subsequent biological defense of the resulting expansion of body fat mass. To fully comprehend the complex pathogenesis of obesity requires an integrated review of obesity-related genetic, developmental, behavioral, and environmental (epigenetic) influences, as well as an exploration of fat mass regulation, central and peripheral influences on energy homeostasis, the neuroscience of feeding behavior, and the hedonic food reward system. Although genes play an important role in determining individual susceptibility to obesity, a high genetic obesity risk does not always translate into actual obesity development; thus, signifying the complex interplay between genetic susceptibility and the influence of an obesogenic environment (such as, high-risk eating behaviors, socioeconomic factors, intrauterine trauma, childhood stress, an evening chronotype, and endocrine-disrupting chemicals).[5–11] An in-depth look at the impact of gene-environment interactions on obesity development is beyond the scope of this article.

Adult body weight is usually quite stable and refractory to transient changes in energy balance (positive or negative) and obesogenic environmental conditions, indicating that body weight and fat mass are actively regulated and defended like other body tissues (eg, blood cells). This understanding supports the notion that obesity is a disease, which shifts the blame for obesity development from the person to the broken physiology. Essentially, the underlying pathology of obesity involves 2 linked, but distinct, processes: a sustained positive energy balance (energy intake > energy expenditure) and an upward resetting of the body weight "set point" that promotes abnormal adipose tissue (body fat) production and function.

ADIPOSE TISSUE PHYSIOLOGY AND REGULATION

Contrary to long-held misconceptions, adipose tissue is a complex, highly active metabolic and endocrine organ that plays a critical role in regulating numerous biological operations that influence most of the body's function.[12,13] Histologically, it is a loose connective tissue (collagen and reticular fibers) comprised mostly of adipocytes. Within this connective tissue matrix are found nerve fibers, stromovascular cells (vascular endothelial cells), immune cells (eg, macrophages), lymph nodes, fibroblasts, and preadipocytes (undifferentiated adipose cells). Adipocytes also express receptors for several hormones, cytokines, and growth factors, as well as produce a number of peptides/hormones (referred to as "adipokines" or "adipocytokines"), which allow adipose tissue to communicate with other tissues and organs (eg, endothelium, skeletal muscle, and central nervous system) (**Fig. 1**).[14] Dysregulation of the body's fat mass is involved in the pathogenesis of a variety of metabolic and immunologic disorders.

The presence of adiposity (abnormal fat mass) and obesity depend on the size and number of adipocytes, the last being regulated through *adipogenesis.* The size of adipocytes and adipose tissue mass is controlled and rigorously defended by the body.[13] Approximately 10% of fat cells are reproduced annually, and their collective mass is determined by a genetic set point. Adipocytes are classified as white adipose tissue (WAT) or brown adipose tissue (BAT), each with molecular, anatomic, and functional differences.[15] WAT is the most abundant fat type and may contribute up to 50% of total body mass in those with obesity.[16]

White Adipose Tissue

For many years, the singular role of energy (lipid) storage was attributed to WAT. Studies have now expanded the role of WAT to include control of energy metabolism and secretion of hormones and inflammatory/immune-modulating adipokines that play a role in appetite regulation, adipogenesis, immunity, neuroendocrine function, glucose metabolism, reproduction, blood pressure control, and other metabolic processes.[15,17] Beta-adrenergic receptors on cell membranes of WAT respond to catecholamine stimulation by releasing fatty acids to help meet the body's energy needs.[18] Adipose tissue not only plays a role in lipid metabolism but also a pivotal role in insulin sensitivity through its secretions of hormones and cytokines that either promote insulin sensitivity (eg, leptin and adiponectin) or impair insulin sensitivity (eg, resistin and retinol-binding protein 4).[14]

WAT is further categorized as either subcutaneous (SAT) or visceral adipose (VAT). VAT accounts for 10% to 20% of WAT and is mostly found among vital organs within the abdominal and thoracic cavities, depositing primarily in and around the omentum, liver, mesentery, heart, and mediastinum. This deleterious fat depot contributes to *visceral adiposity.* VAT is also the most hormonally active and inflammatory fat type, which, if overly abundant, is associated with significant metabolic impairments.[19]

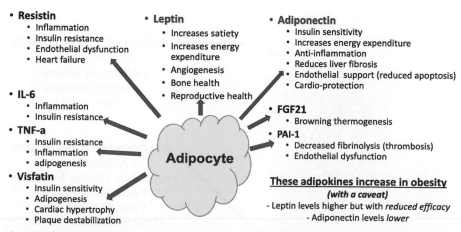

Fig. 1. Selected adipokine metabolic activities. Among them, leptin and adiponectin are metabolically protective (IL-6, TNF-α, PAI-1 [plasminogen activating inhibitor)], FGF21 [fibroblast growth factor 21]).

SAT is a superficial fat layer deposited in the upper body (arm, breast, abdomen) and lower body (gluteofemoral region). Comprising approximately 80% of WAT mass, SAT operates primarily as a lipid storage depot, but is heavily involved with energy metabolism and appears to be significantly less inflammatory than VAT.[16]

There are other differences between VAT and SAT besides their respective depot location within the body. For example, VAT and SAT differ in appearance; SAT appears heterogeneous, composed mainly of small, multilocular adipocytes, whereas WAT appears more uniform and is composed mostly of large unilocular adipocytes. In addition, VAT increases in mass primarily through *hypertrophy* (cell expansion) of existing adipocytes, whereas SAT mostly grows via hyperplasia (increasing the number) of adipocytes (**Fig. 2**). Hypertrophic VAT adipocytes are more pathogenic to cardiometabolic health. This is because an overexpansion of adipocytes leads to cell apoptosis causing the mobilization of macrophages and the release of free fatty acids, reactive oxygen species, and inflammatory cytokines (eg, tumor necrosis factor [TNF] α, interleukin (IL)-6, resistin, and monocyte chemoattractant protein-1), leading to chronic, low-grade systemic inflammation and a host of metabolic derangements.[16,19] In addition, hypertrophied VAT exhibits a limited ability to synthesize and release a key anti-inflammatory adipokine, *adiponectin*, an important, endogenous, insulin sensitizer. Hypertrophied and dysfunctional VAT is sometimes referred to as "sick fat" or *adiposopathy*.[16] In contrast to this, SAT exhibits less lipolysis and free fatty acids release, while promoting greater adiponectin release and insulin sensitivity.

Brown Adipose Tissue

Brown adipocytes are metabolically active tissue located in cervical and subclavicular regions, making up approximately 2% of the body's fat mass.[14] BAT is rich in energy-producing mitochondria (hence the brown color) that are involved in heat production via *nonshivering thermogenesis* (increased energy expenditure). More precisely, brown adipocytes convert chemically stored energy, in the form of fatty acids and glucose, into heat through nonshivering thermogenesis. This plays an important role in newborns who have decreased ability to maintain body temperature because of their body's high surface area–to-volume ratio and lower muscle mass that deprives them the ability to generate sufficient heat via *shivering* thermogenesis.[20]

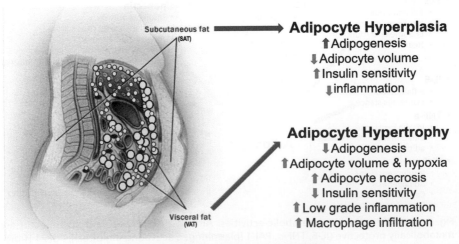

Adipocyte Hyperplasia
⬆Adipogenesis
⬇Adipocyte volume
⬆Insulin sensitivity
⬇inflammation

Adipocyte Hypertrophy
⬇Adipogenesis
⬆Adipocyte volume & hypoxia
⬆Adipocyte necrosis
⬇Insulin sensitivity
⬆Low grade inflammation
⬆Macrophage infiltration

Subcutaneous fat (SAT)

Visceral fat (VAT)

Fig. 2. WAT. Adipocyte hyperplasia versus adipocyte hypertrophy.

In adults, eating and exposure to mild cold can activate BAT. Genetic variants of the FTO gene have been linked to lower amounts of BAT in humans.[15,21]

Beige ("brite") adipose tissues are brownlike adipocytes that have mitochondria and thermogenic capacity but are found interspersed within SAT. These adipocytes are increased and activated by chronic cold, long-term therapy with peroxisome proliferator-activated receptor gamma agonists (such as pioglitazone), or by exercise-induced skeletal muscle release of the hormones *irisin* and *lactate*.[14,21] There appears to be a beneficial relationship between greater *angiogenesis* (blood vessel proliferation) and beige adipocyte development. Pro-angiogenic conditions help in propagating beige adipose tissue, which in turn improves systemic glucose homeostasis, even in the presence of obesity.[22] Recent studies have shed further light on the activation of BAT and beige adipocytes. *Leptin,* a WAT-derived, satiety hormone that regulates body weight and energy expenditure, has been shown to activate brown and beige fat. This is believed to occur through stimulation of the beta2-adrenergic receptors responsible for the release of stored lipids from WAT.[20]

Precipitators of Dysfunctional White Adipose Tissue Adipogenesis

Over the past decade, more has been learned about what/how various internal and external mechanisms impact adipogenesis and adipocyte deposition that may lead to adiposopathy, obesity, and adiposity-related metabolic disturbances. Three prominent mechanisms are presented here.

Sirtuins

Sirtuins (SIRT 1–7) are a family of 7 nicotinamide adenine dinucleotide (NAD)-dependent proteins involved in cell survival, senescence, metabolism, and genome stability. Sirtuins are also known for their role in longevity.[23,24] Of these, SIRT1 and SIRT6 have the more prominent metabolic regulatory roles, involving metabolism (eg, glucose and lipid metabolism), insulin sensitivity, inflammation, development, and reproduction, which ultimately affect the processes of aging and disease. Both sirtuins play a significant role in regulating adipogenesis and the maturation and remodeling of WAT and BAT, as well as energy metabolism through the activation of BAT (nonshivering thermogenesis). SIRT3 also plays a part in BAT metabolism. If there is cold exposure, SIRT3 expression is upregulated in BAT leading to thermogenesis. Diet can also affect sirtuin activation. In response to a positive energy balance (caloric excess) or high fat intake, SIRT1 may downregulate, increasing the risk of obesity (via adipocyte hypertrophy), insulin resistance, type 2 diabetes mellitus, fatty liver, and cardiovascular diseases.[23,24] On a curious note, resveratrol, a polyphenol found in red wine, directly or indirectly, activates SIRT1 in fat and other cells and that appears to trigger fat loss and confer some protection against high-fat–induced obesity and metabolic derangements.[24]

Cortisol excess

Chief among adipogenic disruptors is the impact of elevated circulating levels of *cortisol* (a glucocorticoid secreted by the adrenal gland) that is observed in chronic, high-stress situations, impaired sleep, and hyperstimulation of the adrenal gland or hypothalamic-pituitary-adrenal axis. Hypercortisolism at either the systemic or local level (fat cell cortisone) appears to have a significant impact on expansion and deposition of VAT, although the mechanisms for this has not been fully elucidated. At the same time, beneficial SAT mass can become depleted. Mounting evidence has revealed that disordered (or flattened) circadian variation in cortisol levels is positively associated with an upper body fat distribution. In addition, abnormal diurnal cortisol rhythms, in the presence of a highly variable eating schedule, can increase the risk of visceral adipocyte hypertrophy. In some individuals, increased VAT could be considered a maladaptive response to stress.[25]

Disordered sleep

Sleep is another area of risk for impaired adipogenesis. Shortened or disrupted sleep (whether self-induced due to night-shift work or late-night activities, untreated sleep apnea, or other sleep disorders), has been found to increase cortisol levels and cause fat mass dysregulation, contributing to insulin resistance, glucose intolerance, systemic inflammation, immunologic impairment, and metabolic upheaval.[26–28] Along with an increase in cortisol levels and altered central and peripheral hunger hormone-signaling, impaired sleep also increases adipocyte-derived inflammatory cytokines while decreasing satiety hormones (such as leptin), thyroid-stimulating hormone, and adiponectin, a potent fat-derived anti-inflammatory hormone.[29] Chronic sleep deficiency (fewer than 6 hours a night) increases propensity for weight gain and adiposopathy with greater VAT. It has been estimated that BMI may increase by 1.22 kg/m for each hour of sleep lost.[30]

Two sleep-related eating disorders may also contribute abnormal adipogenesis: *night eating syndrome*, defined as consuming at least 25% of caloric intake after the evening meal at least twice a week for more than 3 months, and *sleep-related eating disorder*, a dysfunctional eating pattern that is thought to be a form of sleepwalking, whereby an individual, after an arousal from primary sleep, begins to unconsciously consume food and even inedible or toxic substances.[31]

ENERGY HOMEOSTASIS

The body's energy metabolism, adiposity, and weight are carefully held in balance by central neural networks using dynamic feedback loops involving multiple, coordinated central and peripheral bio-hormonal circuits, each linked to the gut, pancreas, and adipose tissue.[15] Factors impacting weight include energy intake-expenditure balance, lipid storage, and glucose usage, which are under the control of different neuroendocrine systems, such as the gut-brain axis and metabolic hormones.[32,33]

Appetite Regulation

The brain is involved in overseeing energy metabolism and monitoring information from the body and the environment to determine the sufficiency of the body's nutrient supply and make a decision whether to eat or not. The melanocortin system, within the hypothalamus, houses the most pivotal neuronal pathways involved in the regulation of food intake. This system is composed of a number of melanocortin receptors (MCR) and circuits with the capability of sensing signals from an astounding array of nutrients, hormones, and afferent neural inputs. It is here that the brain perceives and responds to orexigenic (hunger) and anorexigenic (satiety) signals and evokes adaptive eating behaviors and metabolic changes to control short-term food (energy) intake and long-term energy balance to help maintain and defend the body's fat mass.[34,35]

Interconnected areas in the brain and hypothalamus work as a core processor for the control of ingestive behaviors, gastrointestinal responses to food, and activities of other peripheral organs involved in energy storage and utilization. Typically, the body's "need to feed" is driven by 2 things: the metabolic energy and tissue reparative requirements with corresponding peripheral signals sent to the hypothalamus via the circulation or vagus nerve/brain stem, as well as feedback from the "food reward" system sent by neural signals from outside the hypothalamic appetite-regulatory area.[36]

Gut-brain axis

The 2 sets of neurons most involved in feeding behaviors lie within the appetite-regulatory area of the brain, specifically within the arcuate nucleus of the hypothalamus: the *agouti-related peptide/neuropeptide Y [AgRP/NPY]*) and *proopiomelanocortin/ cocaine and amphetamine regulated transcript [POMC/CART]*). These neurons are stimulated, or inhibited, by peripheral signals from the gut (incretins), WAT (leptin), and circulating hormones and metabolites (primarily insulin) (**Fig. 3**). Dozens of peripheral hormones are known to regulate appetite and food intake.[37] Ghrelin, a pro-hunger incretin released from the stomach, stimulates the AgRP neurons, prompting food-seeking behaviors. The POMC/CART neurons are stimulated by various satiety hormones, of which several also tandemly *suppress* AgRP/NPY hunger neurons. Gut incretins provide a hormonal "report" to the hypothalamus about ingested food (gut-brain-axis) so that energy homeostasis centers can make adjustments to better balance energy metabolism (food intake and energy expenditure).[36,37]

The most potent satiety hormones are leptin and insulin, which, along with satiety gut incretins, are stimulated by eating. Carbohydrates appear to induce a stronger hormonal response than does dietary fat. Although circulating levels of strong hunger-reducing hormones are often elevated in those with obesity, their actions are believed to be inhibited due to obesity-related, hypothalamic inflammation ("the obese brain"). In obesity, leptin levels can be quite elevated, as leptin levels increase proportionately to increased adipose mass and leptin resistance.

A "deregulation" of the gut-brain axis may likely be a starting point for obesity pathogenesis. Once the balance of the gut-brain axis is broken, an expansion of white adipocytes (both in cell size and number) ensues, and adiposity spreads into ectopic locations as both VAT and SAT.[37] As obesity develops, the mechanisms that control energy metabolism and central neural feedback networks (especially with gut incretins) are blunted and unable to protect against, or reverse, diet-induced obesity.[37] Following this, the brain establishes a higher weight set point, and biological

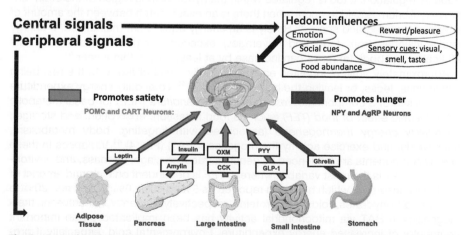

Fig. 3. Central and peripheral control mechanisms of appetite regulation: These signals will promote hunger and food seeking or increase satiety and a sensation of fullness. In the arcuate nucleus of the hypothalamus: NPY (neuropeptide Y), AgRP (Agouti-related protein), POMC (pro-opiomelanocortin/) CART neurons (cocaine- and amphetamine-related transcript neurons). Peripheral hormones: CCK, cholecystokinin; GLP-1, glucagonlike peptide-1; OXM, oxyntomodulin; PYY, peptide YY. (*Data from* Saladin, K. Anatomy & Physiology: The Unity of Form and Function. 8th Ed. McGraw Hill; 2018.)

processes act to maintain the new weight set point and greater body fat mass. This makes losing weight, or maintaining body weight after weight loss, more difficult.[36]

Hedonic reward pathway

Central input from the frontal cortex, ventral, dorsal striatum, and amygdala also influences eating behaviors and is associated with increased food-craving. The anticipation, sight, and taste of food can overcome self-control. A way to distinguish between sustenance-driven feeding and hedonistic reward-driven feeding is that sustenance feeding will halt once sufficient energy and nutrients have been consumed, whereas hedonic feeding might continue. Reward-driven feeding is more pronounced when consuming highly palatable and high-energy food, such as fat.[38] If a high amount of fat is eaten with sucrose, or with something that has a sweet taste, the satiety response may be blunted. It has also been found that endocannabinoids, lipid-based neurotransmitters that are expressed throughout the central, vertebral, and peripheral nervous systems and involved in a cognition, immune responses, reproduction, and sleep, are also implicated in weight control by its effects on appetite and energy metabolism. Consumption of palatable foods, such as food containing fat and sucrose, will stimulate endocannabinoid release, which will promote increased hunger and adipogenesis.[39]

This hedonistic, neural input has been found to be more active in those with obesity versus lean individuals, in those unable to resist tempting food or beverages, and in those with less post-bariatric surgery weight loss. Furthermore, dopamine release in the mid-brain mesolimbic dopaminergic pathway, has been associated with carbohydrate addiction and the hedonic reward system. Carbohydrate addiction drives poor nutrient choices, leading to excessive caloric intake and increased obesity risk.[38]

Energy Balance

Energy balance is the difference between energy intake and energy expenditure. Like appetite regulation, it too is regulated within the hypothalamic region of the brain. Energy equilibrium is said to occur when there is an exact match between the amount of energy consumed and spent.[40] Rarely is an energy equilibrium maintained. If energy intake (calories from food and beverages) exceeds energy expenditure by just 20 kcal a day, body fat mass can increase by at least 1 kg within a year.[41]

Approximately 90% of ingested energy is readily metabolized, with the rest being lost in urine, feces, or leaving the body via the skin.[40] Total daily energy expenditure is composed of 3 components: *resting energy expenditure (REE)* (or basal metabolic rate), *thermic effect of food (TEF)* (such as food ingestion, absorption, and storage), *nonactivity energy thermogenesis* (associated with fidgeting, body metabolism, housework), and exercise activity thermogenesis (EAT) **(Fig. 4)**.[41] Variances in these energy components are influenced by genetics, race, sex, age, fat mass, and environment.[40,41] EAT is the most variable, whereas TEF is dependent on type and amount of nutrients consumed, which has been reported as 5% to 10%, 0% to 3%, and 20% to 30% for carbohydrates, lipids, and proteins, respectively. Recently, nonshivering thermogenesis in BAT via mitochondrial activity has been implicated as an important contributor of increased energy expenditure. Environmental cold, especially if prolonged, can induce increased energy expenditure, ranging from 2% to 17% elevations in both REE and TEF.[21,40,42] Those with an obesity phenotype have reduced BAT levels and activity.[43] As with energy intake, regulation of energy expenditure is insured by interactive cortical cognitive, reward, and autonomic circuits in the brain. Obesity results from neuroendocrine derangements and an imbalance between energy intake and expenditure in genetically and environmentally disfavored individuals.[43]

ENERGY METABOLISM

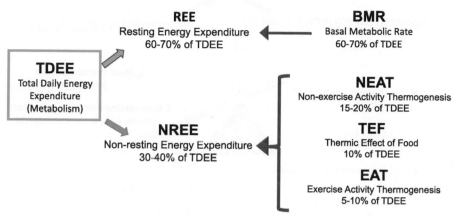

Fig. 4. Components of energy expenditure and metabolism. Energy components vary with age, gender, body size, and composition.

METABOLIC ADAPTATION AND DEFENSE OF BODY FAT MASS

Most people who have intentionally engaged in successful weight loss strategies to combat overweight or obesity have experienced the frustration of regaining much of that lost weight. *Weight regain* is believed to occur in more than 80% of those who have succeeded in losing weight. This frustrating phenomenon is called "metabolic adaptation" or "adaptive thermogenesis," and appears to occur after periods of negative energy balance.[44,45] Following a period of weight loss that stalls after several months, a progressive increase in weight ensues in most people.[44] Studies have shown that more than half of the lost weight is regained within 2 years.[44,46] There is no consensus on what triggers this adaptation, although many researchers believe that some sort of *genetic fat mass set point* may drive weight regain.[47] Neurohormonal changes have been found during weight regain that correspond with increased hunger and a positive energy balance; this includes *decreased* levels of satiety hormones (leptin, insulin, cholecystokinin), a *rise* in hunger hormones (ghrelin), and a *plunge* in the basal metabolic rate (REE) by 15%. The significant fall in REE during weight loss is due to the loss of metabolically active tissue (VAT) and some degree of muscle mass (**Fig. 5**).[38,48]

Many biological mechanisms are initiated to defend the body's fat mass once the set point has been surpassed. The onset of reactive metabolic slowing is an adaptive response to compensate for the decreased food energy intake and/or the increased energy expenditure experienced during early weight loss. There is also modification in the reward system that creates an addiction, like state via reward circuits in the brain areas of the melanocortin, opioid and endocannabinoid networks, and the dopamine mesolimbic system. The ensuing metabolic adaptation is essentially caused by an inefficiency of the neuroendocrine system that is supposed to control energy metabolism.[47,48]

ANATOMIC AND METABOLIC EFFECTS OF OBESITY

The excess adiposity seen in obesity can cause more than 100 complications through *anatomic* and *metabolic* effects. Increased adipose tissue mass can put anatomic

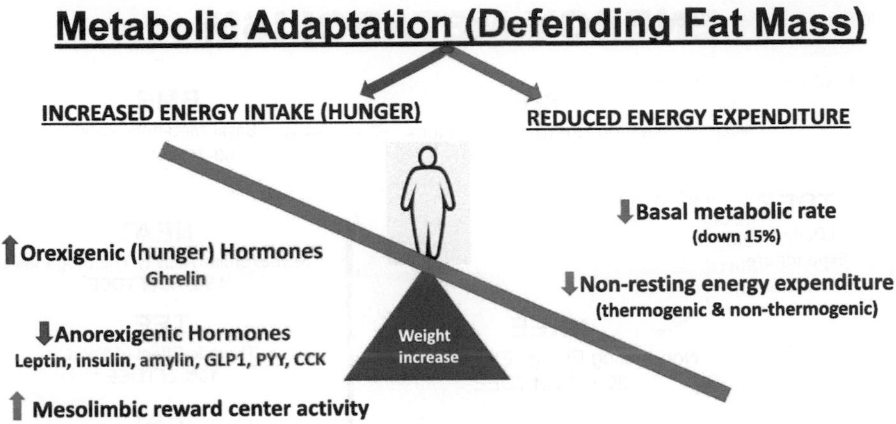

Metabolic Adaptation (Defending Fat Mass)

INCREASED ENERGY INTAKE (HUNGER)

REDUCED ENERGY EXPENDITURE

⬇Basal metabolic rate
(down 15%)

⬆Orexigenic (hunger) Hormones
Ghrelin

⬇Non-resting energy expenditure
(thermogenic & non-thermogenic)

⬇Anorexigenic Hormones
Leptin, insulin, amylin, GLP1, PYY, CCK

Weight increase

⬆ Mesolimbic reward center activity

Fig. 5. Metabolic adaptation of adipose tissue mass via metabolically induced positive energy balance. CCK, cholecystokinin; GLP-1, glucagonlike peptide 1; PYY, peptide YY. (*Data from* Sumithran P, Proietto J. Clin Sci (Lond). 2013;124:231-241.)

strain on various sites and organs leading to obstructive sleep apnea, hypoventilation syndromes, and musculoskeletal osteoarthritis pain in the back and weight-bearing joints.[49] In addition, increased intra-abdominal pressure related to a large fat mass can cause gastroesophageal reflux disease and Barrett's esophagus.[49,50]

As mentioned previously, an overexpansion of visceral adipose tissue mass is linked to increased secretion of proinflammatory adipokines that promote systemic, low-grade inflammation, known as "meta-inflammation," and immune system dysregulation. These potent adipose-related cytokines (TNF-α, IL-1, and IL-6) have been implicated in endothelial dysfunction, cardiometabolic disease, pulmonary disorders (eg, asthma), pain syndrome, malignancy, and severe infectious disease in individuals with obesity.[7,49]

Apoptosis of lipid-containing visceral adipocytes release high levels of free fatty acids as well as ceramides (lipid intermediates), which in turn promote insulin resistance, nonalcoholic fatty liver disease, dyslipidemia, and cardiovascular disease, further contributing to type 2 diabetes, polycystic ovaries, and metabolic syndrome (**Fig. 6**).[50] In addition, obesity is strongly associated with chronic kidney disease due to progressive glomerulosclerosis from adiposity-induced inflammation and fat compression of the renal system.[49]

Several large studies have ascertained that both the degree of fat mass excess and its location in the body can profoundly impact mortality. In the Framingham heart study, a prospective cohort study, men and women (aged 40 years and nonsmokers) lived 5.8 and 7.1 years less than their nonobese counterparts.[51] The INTERHEART study, as well as others, demonstrated that high waist fat distribution (visceral adiposity) is associated with higher risk of acute myocardial infarction, especially in perimenopausal women.[52] An increased risk of ischemic and hemorrhagic stroke has also been associated with obesity, although hemorrhagic stroke is more often seen in men than in women. In addition, studies have linked central adiposity to greater prediction of stroke mortality.[52]

Obesity has long been associated with psychopathy, particularly depression and anxiety. Several things are thought to cause this association, such as dealing with public stigma and bias regarding the excess weight, low self-esteem, adiposity-related chronic illnesses, pain syndromes, comorbid psychiatric disorders, chronic drug use, and poor sleep quality. Recent studies show that women with obesity were more likely to suffer

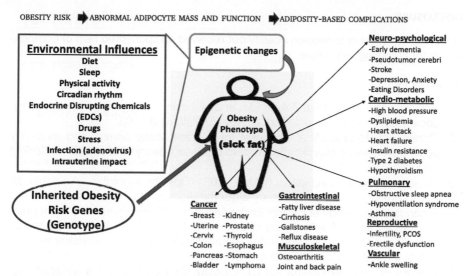

Fig. 6. Obesity risk and complications.

depression and anxiety than men with obesity or nonobese men and women. There also appears to be a bidirectional relationship with regard to mood disorders due to impact on and by eating behaviors.[53] New evidence has found that the links between energy homeostasis, adipocyte metabolism, stress, inflammation, and neuroendocrine responses are shared biological mechanisms between obesity and depression. Neurodegenerative diseases, like dementia, have also been associated with obesity, although the underlying mechanism for this is not fully known.[54]

SUMMARY

Obesity continues a relentless march across the globe with little pause. Researchers are beginning to unlock the complicated interplay among obesity, its ensuing inflammation, and downstream complications. From emerging evidence, it is clear that obesity is a chronic, inflammatory, multifactorial disease of maladaptive adipose tissue mass involving complex links among genetics, hormones, and the environment. Understanding the intricate pathogenesis of obesity and its sequela will go a long way to discovering better treatment options and lessen anti-obesity bias.

CLINICS CARE POINTS

1. Understanding that obesity is a chronic, progressive, relapsing, multifactorial disease and not the character flaw of simply overeating should allay medical bias and a delay in treatment.

2. The chronicity of obesity and weight loss–induced metabolic adaptation will necessitate lifelong anti-obesity interventions.

3. A nonobese, overweight person who presents with visceral adiposity should be considered at metabolic risk and anti-obesity lifestyle interventions begun.

4. Because persistently high cortisol levels and altered body rhythms may contribute to abnormal adipogenesis, it is important to ascertain the patient's length and quality of sleep, shiftwork, and chronic stress levels.

DISCLOSURE

NovoNordisk speaker bureau on obesity but received no sponsored help or compensation for authoring this article.

REFERENCES

1. Schwartz MW, Seeley RJ, Zeltser LM, et al. Obesity pathogenesis: an endocrine society scientific statement. Endocr Rev 2017;38(4):267–96.
2. Garvey WT, Mechanick JI. Proposal for a scientifically correct and medically actionable disease classification system (ICD) for obesity. Obesity (Silver Spring) 2020;28(3):484–92.
3. Obesity Medical Association (OMA). 2021 Obesity Algorithm. Available at: https://obesitymedicine.org/obesity-algorithm/Accessed on March 22, 2021.
4. American Association of Clinical Endocrinologists. Comprehensive clinical practice guidelines for medical care of patients with obesity ©. 2016. Available at. https://pro.aace.com/disease-state-resources/nutrition-and-obesity/clinical-practice-guidelines/comprehensive-clinical. Accessed on February 28, 2021.
5. Centers of Disease Control (CDC). Obesity data and statistics. Available at: https://www.cdc.gov/obesity/data/index.html. Accessed on March 10, 2021.
6. Ng M, Fleming T, Robinson M, et al. Global, regional, and national prevalence of overweight and obesity in children and adults during 1980-2013: a systematic analysis for the Global Burden of Disease Study 2013. Lancet 2014; 384(9945):746.
7. Heymsfield SB, Wadden TA. Mechanisms, pathophysiology, and management of obesity. N Engl J Med 2017;376(15):1492.
8. Brandkvist M, Bjørngaard JH, Ødegård RA, et al. Quantifying the impact of genes on body mass index during the obesity epidemic: longitudinal findings from the HUNT Study. BMJ 2019;366:l4067.
9. Thaker VV. Genetic and epigenetic causes of obesity. Adolesc Med State Art Rev 2017;28(2):379–405.
10. Chin J. The biology and genetic of obesity—a century of inquiries. N Engl J Med 2014;370(20):1874–7.
11. Khera AV, Chaffin M, Wade KH, et al. Polygenic prediction of weight and obesity trajectories from birth to adulthood. Cell 2019;177(3):587–96, e9.
12. Stephens JM. The fat controller: adipocyte development. Plos Biol 2012;10(11): e1001436.
13. Frayn K, Karpe F, Fielding B, et al. Integrative physiology of human adipose tissue. Int J Obes 2003;27:875–88.
14. Kahn CR, Wang G, Lee KY. Altered adipose tissue and adipocyte function in the pathogenesis of metabolic syndrome. J Clin Invest 2019;129(10):3990–4000.
15. Rogge MM, Gautam B. Biology of obesity and weight regain: implications for clinical practice. J Am Assoc Nurse Pract 2017;29(S1):S15–29.
16. Kwok K, Lam K, Xu A. Heterogeneity of white adipose tissue: molecular basis and clinical implications. Exp Mol Med 2016;48:e215.
17. Uranga R, Keller J. The complex interactions between obesity, metabolism and the brain. Front Neurosci 2019;13:513.
18. Bartness T, Liu Y. Neural innervations of white adipose tissue and control of lipolysis. Front Neuroendocrinol 2014;35(4):473–93.
19. Blondin DP, Nielsen S, Kuipers EN, et al. Human brown adipocyte thermogenesis is driven by β2-AR stimulation. Cell Metab 2020;32(2):287–300.e7.

20. Gregor M, Hotamisligil G. Inflammatory mechanisms in obesity. Annu Rev Immunol 2011;29:415–45.
21. Sidossis L, Kajimura S. Brown and beige fat in humans: thermogenic adipocytes that control energy and glucose homeostasis. J Clin Invest 2015;125(2):478–86.
22. Min SY, Kady J, Nam M, et al. Human "brite/beige" adipocytes develop from capillary networks, and their implantation improves metabolic homeostasis in mice. Nat Med 2016;22:312–8.
23. Kurylowicz A. In search of new therapeutic targets in obesity treatment: sirtuins. Int J Mol Sci 2016;17(4):572.
24. Li X. SIRT1 and energy metabolism. Acta Biochim Biophys Sin (Shanghai) 2013; 45(1):51–60.
25. Lee MJ, Pramyothin P, Karastergiou K, et al. Deconstructing the roles of glucocorticoids in adipose tissue biology and the development of central obesity. Biochim Biophys Acta 2014;1842(3):473–81.
26. Duraccio KM, Krietsch KN, Chardon ML, et al. Poor sleep and adolescent obesity risk: a narrative review of potential mechanisms. Adolesc Health Med Ther 2019; 10:117–30.
27. Geiker NRW, Astrup A, Hjorth MF, et al. Does stress influence sleep patterns, food intake, weight gain, abdominal obesity and weight loss interventions and vice versa? Obes Rev 2018;19(1):81–97.
28. Bayon V, Leger D, Gomez-Merino D, et al. Sleep debt and obesity. Ann Med 2014;46(5):264–72.
29. Lucassen EA, Rother KI, Cizza G. Interacting epidemics? sleep curtailment, insulin resistance, and obesity. Ann N Y Acad Sci 2012;1264(1):110–34.
30. Covassin N, Singh P, Somers VK. Keeping up with the clock: circadian disruption and obesity risk. Hypertension 2016;68(5):1081–90.
31. Depner CM, Stothard ER, Wright KP Jr. Metabolic consequences of sleep and circadian disorders. Curr Diab Rep 2014;14(7):507.
32. Ghanemi A, Yoshioka M, St-Amand J. Broken energy homeostasis and obesity pathogenesis: the surrounding concepts. J Clin Med 2018;7(11):453.
33. Buhmann H, le Roux CW, Bueter M. The gut-brain axis in obesity. Best Pract Res Clin Gastroenterol 2014;28(4):559–71.
34. Gadde KM, Martin CK, Berthoud HR, et al. Obesity: pathophysiology and management. J Am Coll Cardiol 2018;71(1):69–84.
35. Lean M, Malkova D. Altered gut and adipose tissue hormones in overweight and obese individuals: cause or consequence? Int J Obes 2016;40:622–32.
36. Suzuki K, Simpson K, Minnion J, et al. The role of gut hormones and the hypothalamus in appetite regulation. Endocr J 2010;57:359–72.
37. Ghanemi A, Yoshioka M, St-Amand J. Broken energy homeostasis and obesity pathogenesis: the surrounding concepts. J Clin Med 2018;7(11):453.
38. Pucci A, Batterham RL. Endocrinology of the gut and the regulation of body weight and metabolism. In: Feingold KR, Anawalt B, Boyce A, et al, editors. Endotext [Internet]. South Dartmouth (MA): MDText.com, Inc.; 2000. Available from: https://www.ncbi.nlm.nih.gov/books/NBK556470/.
39. Horn H, Böhme B, Dietrich L, et al. Endocannabinoids in body weight control. Pharmaceuticals (Basel) 2018;11(2):55.
40. Lam YY, Ravussin E. Analysis of energy metabolism in humans: a review of methodologies. Mol Metab 2016;5(11):1057–71.
41. Oussaada SM, van Galen KA, Cooiman MI, et al. The pathogenesis of obesity. Metabolism 2019;92:26–36.

42. Trexler ET, Smith-Ryan AE, Norton LE. Metabolic adaptation to weight loss: implications for the athlete. J Int Soc Sports Nutr 2014;11(1):7.
43. Hall KD. Metabolic adaptations to weight. Obesity (Silver Spring) 2018;26(5):790–1.
44. Richard D. Cognitive and autonomic determinants of energy homeostasis in obesity. Nat Rev 2015;11:489–501.
45. Fothergill E, Guo J, Howard L, et al. Persistent metabolic adaptation 6 years after "The Biggest Loser" competition. Obesity (Silver Spring) 2016;24(8):1612–9.
46. Halpern B. Response to "Metabolic adaptation is not observed after 8 weeks of overfeeding but energy expenditure variability is associated with weight recovery". Am J Clin Nutr 2019;110(6):1513.
47. Müller MJ, Bosy-Westphal A, Heymsfield SB. Is there evidence for a set point that regulates human body weight? F1000. Med Rep 2010;2:59.
48. Sumithran P, Prendergast LA, Delbridge E, et al. Long-term persistence of hormonal adaptations to weight loss. N Engl J Med 2011;365(17):1597–604.
49. Ansari S, Haboubi H, Haboubi N. Adult obesity complications: challenges and clinical impact. Ther Adv Endocrinol Metab 2020;11. 2042018820934955.
50. Segula D. Complications of obesity in adults: a short review of the literature. Malawi Med J 2014;26(1):20–4.
51. Peeters A, Barendregt JJ, Willekens F, et al. Obesity in adulthood and its consequences for life expectancy: a life-table analysis. Ann Intern Med 2003;138:24–32.
52. Xue R, Li Q, Geng Y, et al. Abdominal obesity and risk of CVD: a dose–response meta-analysis of thirty-one prospective studies. Br J Nutr. 2021:1-11.
53. Değirmenci T, Kalkan-Oğuzhanoğlu N, Sözeri-Varma G, et al. Psychological symptoms in obesity and related factors. Noro Psikiyatr Ars 2015;52(1):42–6.
54. Ouakinin SRS, Barreira DP, Gois CJ. Depression and obesity: integrating the role of stress, neuroendocrine dysfunction and inflammatory pathways. Front Endocrinol (Lausanne) 2018;9:431.

Weight Bias and Stigma
Impact on Health

Sharon M. Fruh, PhD, RN, FNP-BC, FAANP[a],*,
Rebecca J. Graves, PhD, NP-C[b], Caitlyn Hauff, PhD[c],
Susan G. Williams, PhD, RN[d], Heather R. Hall, PhD, RN, NNP-BC[e]

KEYWORDS

- Obesity bias and stigma • Weight discrimination • People-first language
- Explicit bias • Implicit bias

KEY POINTS

- Weight bias and stigma is present in media, education, employment, and health care
- Weight bias and stigma are evident across all professionals in the health care industry, including physicians, nurses, dietitians, and mental health care providers.
- People-first language is critical to reducing bias and discrimination.
- It is important to use specific strategies to reduce obesity bias and stigma: clinic setting in the waiting room and the examination room.

Weight bias and stigma exist in a variety of realms in our society, and it is sad that it is often viewed as a socially acceptable form of discrimination.[1–3] For decades, those in the Western culture have had trouble understanding and accepting preobesity and obesity as a disease state, considering it a condition brought on by lack of willpower or self-control, and thus, we find both implicit and explicit forms of bias being perpetuated in an assortment of landscapes when it comes to discussing weight.[1,4,5] As researchers and health care providers, it is important to delineate the differences between weight bias and weight stigma, and the differences between implicit and explicit forms of bias. Awareness and sensitivity of these personal issues surrounding weight should be approached in a culturally competent and inclusive manner.

Brownell and colleagues[6] suggest that although both bias and stigma are connected to prejudice, the experience of prejudice differs based on whether one is

[a] College of Nursing, University of South Alabama, 5721 USA Drive North, Mobile, AL 36688, USA; [b] College of Nursing, University of South Alabama, 5721 USA Drive North, HAHN 2037 F, Mobile, AL 36688, USA; [c] Department of Health, Kinesiology, and Sport, College of Education and Professional Studies, University of South Alabama, HKS 1020, 171 Student Services Drive, Mobile, AL 36688, USA; [d] College of Nursing, University of South Alabama, 161 North Section Street Suite C, Fairhope, AL 36532, USA; [e] College of Nursing, University of South Alabama, 5721 USA Drive North, Room 3068, Mobile, AL 36688, USA
* Corresponding author.
E-mail address: sfruh@southalabama.edu

Nurs Clin N Am 56 (2021) 479–493
https://doi.org/10.1016/j.cnur.2021.07.001
0029-6465/21/© 2021 Elsevier Inc. All rights reserved.

stigmatized or the target of bias. Weight bias refers to instances wherein individuals receive negative or unreasonable judgments about their person based on their body size or weight, with prejudice being a potential outcome.[6] Typically, weight bias manifests as a negative attitude, assumption of a stereotype, or a verbal or physical attack toward someone of differing body size.[7] In addition, weight bias may be embedded in our physical[8] and social environments,[1] specifically when considering elements such as medical equipment and furniture, physical examination space, and language.

Comparatively, weight stigma refers to situations in which an individual is labeled with certain personality or behavioral characteristics because of their perceived body size or weight. Therefore, an individual becomes a target of prejudice.[6] Those that are stigmatized for having a larger body size are devalued, ostracized, and often criticized in society because they do not fit the societal standard for beauty or the socially constructed norm of an ideal body.[2,6,9] The resulting prejudice further leads to weight-based discrimination, which may present as microaggressions or explicit inequitable treatment.[10] Occurrences of weight stigma are not uncommon and have been documented in numerous settings, including, but not limited to health care, education, employment, and media portrayals.[1,2,6] The problem with the pervasiveness of weight stigma is that it ultimately results in the unfair treatment of those with larger body sizes, negatively impacting physical health, mental health, self-esteem, and well-being. In recent years, weight bias and weight stigma have evolved into social justice issues. We must view misconceptions regarding body size through this lens to best address the issues plaguing our society and develop best practices that are inclusive and supportive of body diversity.

Both weight bias and stigma can occur implicitly or explicitly. Implicit bias refers to instances wherein the bias operates at the subconscious level. Individuals form negative preconceptions about individuals of larger body sizes.[11] Frequently, implicit bias is an automatic, unconscious response and might occur as an initial thought or reaction toward viewing someone in the audience of question. For example, several researchers[12–14] have used the Implicit Association Test (IAT) to measure implicit weight bias in a variety of contexts. The IAT measures how quickly individuals can pair concepts with specific attributes—in this case, pairing the attributes of "good" and "bad" with the target variables of "fat" and "thin."[15,16] When measuring implicit weight bias, researchers assess the speed and accuracy in which each participant can correctly categorize the attributes and words together (eg, categorize fat/good and thin/bad). Implicit weight bias becomes evident when participants are able to categorize "fat" with "bad" attributes more efficiently than being able to accurately and quickly categorize "fat" with "good" attributes.[16] Owing to our own bias and societal perceptions, what many researchers have found is that we make automatic associations more easily when categorizing "thin" with "good" words and "fat" with "bad" words,[11,16,17] thus perpetuating implicit bias toward those with preobesity or obesity. While implicit bias often occurs only at the subconscious level (meaning this is not bias on which we outwardly act), those negative thoughts, feelings, and attitudes are still present and influence our perceptions toward individuals of larger body sizes.

Explicit bias, on the other hand, refers to actions (physical, verbal, or nonverbal) or thoughts that are outward, intentional, and operate at a conscious level.[11] Those engaging in explicit bias hold negative attitudes and prejudices toward groups of individuals and are well aware of the opinions, beliefs, and perceptions they hold.[18] Explicit bias often occurs in the form of discrimination as a result of a deliberate thought. Much of the explicit bias experienced by individuals of larger body sizes comes in the form of stereotyping, specifically, believing that individuals with preobesity or obesity are lazy, lack willpower and self-control, and are unmotivated.[5,6,12,19]

Many of these stereotypes stem from decades of socially constructed norms about ideal body sizes and our society's continual celebration of those meeting the "thin" or "muscular" ideal.[20] The result of explicit bias for those with larger body sizes varies, but researchers have documented that bias impacts employment, communication, and treatment in a variety of settings, including health care.[1,2,6,16]

Despite society's unrealistic ideal standards for bodies, the rates of preobesity and obesity have been on the rise for the past decade, so much so that our country has deemed obesity to be an epidemic.[1,21,22] As the rates of preobesity and obesity have increased, so too have the rates of bias and stigmatization toward individuals of larger body sizes.[1,10] Unlike racial bias or bias against those with physical or mental disabilities, there has been no Civil Rights Act or Americans with Disabilities Act to protect individuals of larger body sizes against discrimination in the workplace, education, or health care (to name a few). In fact, weight bias remains a common form of discrimination in our nation.[10] Individuals rationalize that weight is an acceptable form of discrimination because of the perception surrounding the controllability of one's weight.[5,10] Weight is believed to be an attribute of our bodies over which we have control, and it is, therefore, our personal choices, self-control (or lack thereof), and lifestyles that influence our body weight and size.[2,5] The belief that weight is in one's control is true to an extent, yet, it is important to understand the multifaceted and complex nature of obesity to gain a full understanding of this condition. Weight is influenced by a multitude of factors, including, but not limited to, personal behaviors, the environment, social factors, genetics/biology, and cultural elements.[6] It is trivial to believe that weight is the sole result of someone's personal choices and lack of self-control when they find themselves in an environment that is laden with energy-dense food that is affordable, accessible, and convenient. Despite recognizing that obesity is a complex issue, society still discriminates against those with preobesity and obesity because of the group norms that are embedded in our infrastructure. Weight discrimination has resulted in negative physical and mental health outcomes, avoidance of health treatment, unfair treatment by doctors and nurses, loss of employment opportunities, and decreased academic performance.[1,2,6,10,16] As long as society continues to encourage unrealistic body standards, the prevalence of weight discrimination will persist, because those in larger body sizes will not fit the norm of a body that is socially acceptable.

WEIGHT BIAS AND STIGMA IN SPECIFIC ENVIRONMENTS
Media

One arena in which we witness substantial explicit weight bias is within the media. Television shows and movies are notorious for depicting those with larger body sizes as disheveled, unorganized, lacking in personality, undesirable, and deserving of poor treatment.[12,23,24] Those with preobesity and obesity are often the target of many jokes in the media, further perpetuating the stereotype that larger bodies are unacceptable and not welcome in our society.

In both traditional and social media, the normalization of weight bias, stigma, and discrimination are evident and falsely infer social acceptability of bias and stigma. Pearl and colleagues[25] noted the stigmatization of individuals with obesity in media and entertainment sources, including talk shows, cartoons, movies, and comedies. In addition, weight stigma is often portrayed in movies and television shows that are popular among children and teens.[26] Much entertainment created for children upholds stereotypes of body size, planting the seeds of both implicit and explicit bias early in life. In print media, acceptability and practice of weight bias toward obesity and people with obesity increased when participants were given fictional scientific news articles that promoted negative perceptions of obesity as a whole when compared with participants provided with news articles that did not promote negative scientific information.[27]

Jeon and colleagues[28] determined that the cloak of anonymity on social media emboldened some commenters on YouTube videos of individuals with obesity in online dating. Two-thirds of the comments were negative and attacking, frequently using words that were insulting, derogatory, mocking, and profane.

Education

Children with preobesity or obesity often experience weight stigma presented as bullying. Teachers and parents have noted that bullying based on body size is more prevalent than bullying based on other characteristics, including sexual orientation and disability.[29,30] In postsecondary education, the higher a female students' body mass index (BMI), the less likely she was to be in a romantic relationship.[31]

Children experience weight bias from educators in addition to their peers. Educators in middle schools and high schools assigned lower grades on the same papers to students they believed to have preobesity compared with those without obesity or preobesity.[32] The teachers also perceived that students with preobesity needed more tutoring assistance, had to put forth more effort, and had lower grades than students without obesity or preobesity. Individuals enrolled in health and physical education programs at a university had both implicit and explicit bias against children with obesity, rating the children as being more self-conscious and less healthy and having lower self-satisfaction and confidence.[33]

Employment

Despite equal or higher qualifications for a position, applicants with obesity seeking employment are frequently overlooked compared with other applicants without obesity.[34] Employees with obesity have higher rates of discrimination than individuals with a typical weight and often report lower wages, fewer promotion opportunities, and increased termination.[34] Remarkably, there is no federal protection for those who experience weight bias in employment because weight is not an included characteristic under US Civil Rights protections unless obesity contributes to disability. However, there is one state (Michigan) that has enacted protections against weight discrimination in the workplace. Lack of protection by federal law is consistent in most nations of the world.[34]

Health Care

Health care providers, including those who work specifically in obesity care, are not immune to demonstrations of weight bias and stigma.[35–38] Indeed, bias and stigma are evident across all professionals in the health care industry, including physicians, nurses, dietitians, and mental health care providers.[13,14,39,40] Individuals with obesity ranked physicians as the second, after family members, most frequent source of weight bias.[41]

Unfortunately, weight bias and stigma may be learned behaviors from educational programs of health care professions. Medical students reported witnessing weight bias by faculty when observing interactions with patients with obesity.[11] Even more disturbing, some faculty used negative, stigmatic language referring to patients with obesity during the medical students' education. In the same study, third-year medical students with higher levels of weight bias were less likely to provide appropriate, patient-centered care to patients with obesity.[11] Nurse practitioner (NP) students witnessed similar patterns with family NP preceptors.[42] In addition, these NP students identified areas of stigma by other members of the health care teams, such as calling out weights of patients without discretion and using judgmental, stigmatic adjectives and language when referring to the patients.[42]

As discussed previously, weight bias exists both explicitly and implicitly. Although both forms of bias interfere with a compassionate, patient-centered relationship between an individual with obesity and his/her health care provider,[14,40] it is possible that implicit bias can be a more insidious obstacle. Individuals with obesity who perceive bias are less likely to seek care, including preventive care and screening.[40,43] Women with obesity report higher levels of avoidance in seeking health care,[40] potentially delaying early detection of breast or cervical cancer, hypertension, and/or diabetes. Additionally, perceived weight stigma often prevents seeking care for obesity and other obesity-related conditions, including musculoskeletal pain and mobility concerns.[40] Health care providers often report a perception that patients who have obesity are less likely to adhere to wellness plans,[44] often attributing the characteristics of laziness, lack of motivation, and noncompliance.[11]

Through implicit bias, well-meaning providers who want to encourage patients with obesity to improve their health cannot conceptualize that their bias may prevent therapeutic, patient-centered care.[45] Individuals with obesity who experience and internalize weight stigma are more likely to exhibit unhealthy eating and weight control behaviors, such as increased binge eating, frequency of eating, and portion sizes and are less likely to engage in physical activity.[46–49] Thus, the relationship between the patient and the health care provider can become counterproductive in the goal of improving the health of the patient. There is also evidence that people who experience weight bias have a higher incidence of development of obesity and increased weight and body size.[50,51]

Individuals who experience weight bias have higher levels of stress compared with those who do not,[52] accompanied by increased levels of cortisol and inflammation. Physiologic actuation of bias, thus, places recipients at a higher risk for cardiovascular disease.[52]

The physical environment of health care also presents a bias. Health care offices that are not appropriately suited for the care of an individual with obesity introduce bias for individuals with obesity, occurring with the sizes of gowns, the sizes of blood pressure cuffs, and the setting, atmosphere, and procedure by which an individual is weighed.[42]

PEDIATRIC OBESITY BIAS

According to the United States Centers for Disease Control and Prevention, prevalence of obesity in children and adolescents is 18.9% for those in the lowest income group.[53] The middle-income group is at 19.9%, and the highest income group is at 10% prevalence for having obesity.[53] Non-Hispanic Caucasians and Asians, as well as Hispanic pediatric patients, were also in the lowest category of having obesity. The National Health and Nutrition Survey confirms that children/adolescents with obesity are measured by a BMI at or more than the 95th percentile for their ages.[54] In 2017 to 2018, the cumulative average of children/adolescents with obesity was 19.3%, with boys at 20.5% and girls at 18%. Adolescents aged 12 to 19 years had the highest cumulative numbers, with 21% having obesity. Males again had a higher prevalence at 21.2% and females at 19.2%.[54,55]

In 2013, the American Medical Association recognized obesity as a disease and not just a result of personal choices.[56] This way of understanding obesity, unfortunately, has not been adopted by all medical professionals.[57] Severe obesity is the most rapidly growing disease, affecting as many as 5 million children. If this trend continues, as many as 57% of children today may have obesity as adults by the age of 35 years, creating significant health risks.[58]

When a pediatric patient has obesity, there is often a stigmatized experience that follows. Puhl and colleagues[59] found that when children/adolescents experience weight bias or stigma, they begin to internalize their feelings related to their weight status, weight loss attempts, and eating habits. Adverse outcomes may result leading to psychological, behavioral, and physical manifestations. Many children/adolescents may experience weight stigma from well-meaning family members who do not know how to properly help their children/adolescents manage their weight.[60,61] Furthermore, stigma or bias can come from peers, teachers, school nurses, health care professionals, social media, and traditional media.[11,43] Pediatric health care providers and office support staff may consider that the child/adolescent's weight gain is controllable. To further complicate the issue, many professional health care workers do not use "people-first" language (eg, using "the child who has obesity" instead of using "the overweight, obese, morbidly obese, or fat child").[62]

Palad and colleagues[26] encourage health care professionals who are providing medical care when working with pediatric patients to provide support, acceptance, and appreciation for their individual and unique personalities. Some children and adolescents may prefer their weight status to be described as "plus-size" instead of being called "fat, large, or obese."[63] Working with anyone who has a weight issue required adaptation of the intervention to individual characteristics and preferences. When implementing weight management with a child or adolescent, there must be multiple factions addressed in the treatment process including psychological, physical, mental, and emotional health. Otherwise, issues such as stigma, negativism, and unwillingness to participate in a program may greatly affect the treatment process.[64]

Weight-Related Teasing

Often when children or adolescents have obesity, they may be teased or bullied in the school, neighborhood, or even church. This type of detrimental treatment can cause psychological harm, which can be more damaging than the physiologic harm of obesity.[65] Some adults may think gently teasing children about their weight may nudge the child to eat less, exercise more, and motivate the child to be mindful of his or her weight. Instead, this talk from a loved one can propagate the opposite behavior, causing some children/adolescents to eat more, hide food, or binge eat to soothe the negative feelings that are created from the ongoing, sometimes relentless teasing.[66,67]

In a systematic review, Day and colleagues[68] found that when adolescents are teased or victimized because of their weight, they have a greater likelihood of having body image disturbances and other psychological issues such as binge eating, purging, dietary restriction, and unhealthy weight control. Being bullied and not getting regular exercise were significantly associated with poor physical and psychosocial quality of life.[69] Furthermore, having difficulty finding size-/age-appropriate clothing was also significantly correlated with lower quality of life in children.[69]

CLINICAL IMPLICATIONS

It is important for health care providers to support individuals diagnosed with preobesity or obesity and their families. Providers need to be mindful to use people-first language (**Table 1**). Specific strategies can be used by providers in their practice setting

Table 1	
People-First Language is critical to reducing bias and discrimination	
Example of People-First Language	**Example of Non-People-First Language**
A 43-y-old female patient with obesity	A 43-y-old obese female patient
A study related to children with obesity	A study of obese children

The term "obese" should never be used in conversations or written form. A helpful handout is available at People-First Language for Obesity: https://www.obesityaction.org/wp-content/uploads/People-First.pdf.

to reduce obesity bias and stigma (**Box 1**). Therapeutic conversations with patients can be started by providers by carefully choosing their words (**Box 2; Table 2**).

Patients with these diagnoses are at risk for stigma and bias, specifically toward individuals of larger body sizes. The risks for these individuals are not a new occurrence or phenomenon. Society continues to blame the individual's lack of control or willpower that reinforces weight as an acceptable form of discrimination, despite the many attempts to explain preobesity and obesity as a disease resulting from a myriad of complex social, environmental, and biological influences. Thus, health care providers continue to care for individuals with larger bodies who have been devalued and shamed, resulting in negative physical and mental health outcomes. Health care providers should ensure spaces or equipment support for individuals of larger body sizes (**Box 3**). As nurses, we can connect health care providers working in our environments with the education and resources available related to reducing weight bias This step may help improve the understanding of weight bias and change the way we look at individuals who have preobesity or obesity.

Box 1
A general list of strategies to reduce obesity bias and stigma

1. *Identifying your own bias:* The Obesity Society has helpful questions to identify bias; the Rudd Center has an 8-module tool kit self-assessment course to help prevent obesity bias in providers.

2. *Promoting positive perceptions of individuals with obesity:* When individuals are provided with information regarding obesity as a complex disease with multiple causes (genetic, biological, and no controllable aspects), their negative attitudes decreased.

3. *Advancing your knowledge:* Providers who have greater knowledge in obesity management offer more comprehensive care and treat patients confidently.

4. *Understanding the patient's point of view:* Patients may have a long history of negative experiences with health care providers in nonsupportive office environments; they may have also tried to lose weight repeatedly and feel frustrated trying once again.

5. *Taking online educational programs:* When health care providers and students complete online educational materials, it can help reduce obesity bias.

6. *Motivational interviewing:* This effective strategy viewed by patients as less threatening is associated with greater patient adherence and outcomes.

7. *Demonstrating respect and compassion:* Providers need to communicate with patients respectfully and compassionately.

Data from Puhl RM, Schwartz MB, Brownell KD. Impact of perceived consensus on stereotypes about obese people: a new approach for reducing bias. Health Psychol 2005;24(5):517–25 and Fruh SM, Nadglowski J, Hall HR, et al. Obesity stigma and bias. J Nurse Pract 2016;12(7);425–32.

> **Box 2**
> **Language to be considered before discussing weight with patients; improved health should be made the reason for the discussion**
>
> What words would you like me to use when we talk about weight?
>
> How do you feel about your weight?
>
> Can we talk about your weight today?
>
> Do I have permission to discuss your weight?
>
> Would you be willing to have a discussion about your weight?
>
> *Data from* Fruh SM, Nadglowski J, Hall HR, et al. Obesity stigma and bias. J Nurse Pract 2016;12(7):425–32.

When health care providers care for children or adolescents diagnosed with obesity, it is important to understand the home environment of the patient through communication with parents/caregivers. It is critical that parents and other adults close to the child do not use weight-based teasing or shaming with children. Weight-based teasing plays a role in negative mental health and may lead to increased eating and long-term emotional problems. Parents often think that they are helping the child through teasing and shaming. This form of teasing is detrimental and should never be used on any individual.

Health care providers should offer parents education and resources necessary to create a healthy home environment (see Fruh and colleagues[70]). It is vital to address the importance of a healthy home environment. Having healthy activity patterns, healthy home food offerings, and specific bedtime routines may make a significant difference in obesity management.[71] If counseling, psychological therapy, and behavioral changes are not included in the plan of treatment, efforts to change habits that have started at a very early age may be futile. A review by Alman and colleagues[72] found that treating pediatric patients with a lifestyle intervention that included diet, exercise, and behavioral modification therapy was the most successful. Other researchers also recommend examining weight status, weight bias, bullying, and other barriers to successful treatment such as economic status. If a family cannot

Table 2
Strategies to reduce obesity bias and stigma: compassionate and respectful communication

Encouraged terms	Discouraged Terms
Weight	Morbidly obese
Unhealthy weight	Obese
Overweight	Fat
Preobesity	Heaviness
Body mass index	Large size
Excessive energy stores	Chubby
Affected by obesity	Plump
Eating habits/nutrition	Big size
Physical activity	Diet
Healthy habits	Exercise

Adapted from Bays HE, et al. 2020. Available at: https://obesitymedicine.org/obesity-algorithm/. Accessed March 26, 2021.

Box 3
Strategies to reduce obesity bias and stigma: clinic setting

Waiting room:
- Seating without armrests
- Wider chairs to accommodate all sizes
- Adequate space between each chair
- Avoid publications that contain offensive or discriminating images
- Respectful and compassionate communication with office staff

Equipment:
- Proper size gowns
- Sturdy, wide examination tables with sturdy stool or step with handles
- Measuring tape
- Appropriate vaginal speculum sizes
- Blood pressure cuffs in all sizes
- High-capacity weight scales (225–315 kg) in a private location (never call out weights)
- Hand-held Doppler assessment of the fetal heart rate may not be feasible in some cases before 16 to 20 weeks; sometimes, transabdominal ultrasonography is necessary.
- Bathrooms equipped with hand rails that can comfortably accommodate individuals of all sizes
- Laboratory draw chair that will comfortably accommodate all individuals

Data from Fruh SM, Nadglowski J, Hall HR, et al. Obesity stigma and bias. J Nurse Pract 2016;12(7):425–32.

---

afford healthy foods or lives in a neighborhood where there are few stores to purchase healthy food, it may be difficult to change the weight status of a child without significant efforts by a caring and actively involved health care professional.[73] Srivastava and colleagues[73] further recommend using the socioecological framework so that all areas of potential barriers to treatment can be examined before starting a treatment program. When assessing children or adolescents, completing a screening measure related to any form of bullying, teasing, or victimization is an important first step to understand what the child may be experiencing.[74]

It is vital for programs training health care providers and continuing education opportunities to include content related to obesity bias, obesity prevention, and obesity management. It is important for nursing programs to implement the most current evidence related to obesity bias prevention, obesity prevention, and obesity management in course objectives and student learning outcomes for undergraduate and graduate programs. In addition, nursing faculty may also consider including this content in the clinical course components. Students will have an opportunity to care for patients of all body sizes across the lifespan and from primary care/wellness and acute care settings, including the intensive care unit.[75] Including the latest evidence-based obesity management care is essential for nursing education.

Within the health care setting, continuing education for nurses and health care providers is a good place to begin to strategically focus on reducing obesity bias and providing high-quality obesity management and care. Continuing education objectives that are relevant to health care providers caring for patients with obesity is paramount. Encouraging the directors of workplace environments to become educated on obesity bias may be an initial place to start with helping to change bias at an organizational level. Educating health care providers with the latest evidence and guidelines on obesity management is a core strategy to be implemented throughout the clinical setting.[75]

CLINICS CARE POINTS

- Weight stigma results in the unfair treatment of those with larger body sizes, negatively impacting physical health, mental health, self-esteem, and well-being.
- Weight discrimination has resulted in negative physical and mental health outcomes, avoidance of health treatment, unfair treatment by doctors and nurses, loss of employment opportunities, and decreased academic performance.
- Individuals with obesity ranked physicians as the second, after family members, most frequent source of weight bias.
- Providers with higher levels of weight bias are less likely to provide appropriate, patient-centered care to patients with obesity.
- Individuals with obesity who perceive bias are less likely to seek care, including preventive care and screening (ie, routine care and cancer screening).
- Women with obesity report higher levels of avoidance in seeking health care.
- Individuals with obesity who experience and internalize weight stigma are more likely to exhibit unhealthy eating and weight control behaviors, such as increased binge eating, frequency of eating, and portion sizes and are less likely to engage in physical activity.
- Adolescents are teased or victimized because of their weight; they have a greater likelihood of having body image disturbances and other psychological issues such as binge eating, purging, dietary restriction, and unhealthy weight control.

FUNDING SOURCE

NIH/NCATS CTSA Grant UL1TR003096.

DISCLOSURE

The authors have no disclosures.

HELPFUL RESOURCES

Obesity Action Coalition: https://www.obesityaction.org/
Stop Obesity Alliance: https://stop.publichealth.gwu.edu/
Obesity Care Advocacy Network: https://obesitycareadvocacynetwork.com/
National Obesity Care Week: https://www.obesitycareweek.org/
Obesity Medicine Association: https://obesitymedicine.org/
The Obesity Society: https://www.obesity.org/
Rudd Center for Food Policy and Obesity: https://uconnruddcenter.org/
Health at Every Size Approach: https://asdah.org/health-at-every-size-haes-approach/
National Eating Disorder Association: https://www.nationaleatingdisorders.org/

WEB SITES

Centers for Disease Control and Prevention: Pediatric obesity tips for parents: https://www.cdc.gov/healthyweight/children/index.html.
Centers for Disease Control and Prevention: Healthy eating tips
https://www.cdc.gov/healthyweight/healthy_eating/index.html.
Centers for Disease Control and Prevention: Preventing weight gain
https://www.cdc.gov/healthyweight/prevention/index.html.
Centers for Disease Control and Prevention: Physical activity for a healthy weight

https://www.cdc.gov/healthyweight/physical_activity/index.html.

Mayo Clinic: Childhood obesity: https://www.mayoclinic.org/diseases-conditions/childhood-obesity/diagnosis-treatment/drc-20354833.

Parents: Help kids lose weight: https://www.parents.com/kids/teens/weight-loss/help-kids-lose-weight/

National Institute of Health: Helping your child who is overweight: https://www.niddk.nih.gov/health-information/weight-management/helping-your-child-who-is-overweight.

Very Well Health: Weight loss help for kids who are not losing weight: https://www.verywellhealth.com/help-with-weight-loss-for-kids-who-cant-lose-weight-2633987.

Very Well Family: Weight management guide for children with preobesity: https://www.verywellfamily.com/weight-management-guide-2632244.

REFERENCES

1. Pearl RL. Weight bias and stigma: public health implications and structural solutions. Soc Issues Policy Rev 2018;12(1):146–82.
2. Puhl RM, Brownell KD. Psychosocial origins of obesity stigma: toward changing a powerful and pervasive bias. Obes Rev 2003;4(4):213–27.
3. Ramos Salas X, Alberga AS, Cameron E, et al. Addressing weight bias and discrimination: moving beyond raising awareness to creating change. Obes Rev 2017;18(11):1323–35.
4. Alberga AS, Russell-Mayhew S, von Ranson KM, et al. Weight bias: a call to action. J Eat Disord 2016;4(1):34.
5. Crandall CS. Prejudice against fat people: ideology and self-interest. J Personal Soc Psychol 1994;66(5):882–94.
6. Brownell KD, Puhl RM, Schwartz MB, et al. Weight bias: nature, consequences, and remedies. New York: Guilford Publications; 2005.
7. Nutter S, Russell-Mayhew S, Ellard JH, et al. Reducing unintended harm: addressing weight bias as a social justice issue in counseling through justice motive theory. Prof Psychol Res Pract 2020;51(2):106–14.
8. Carels RA, Latner J. Weight stigma and eating behaviors. An introduction to the special issue. Appetite 2016;102:1–2.
9. Tomiyama AJ, Carr D, Granberg EM, et al. How and why weight stigma drives the obesity 'epidemic' and harms health. BMC Med 2018;16(1):123.
10. Diedrichs PC, Puhl R. Weight bias: prejudice and discrimination toward overweight and obese people. In: Sibley CG, Barlow FK, editors. *The cambridge handbook of the psychology of prejudice.* Cambridge handbooks in psychology. Cambridge (United Kingdom): Cambridge University Press; 2016. p. 392–412.
11. Phelan SM, Dovidio JF, Puhl RM, et al. Implicit and explicit weight bias in a national sample of 4,732 medical students: the medical student CHANGES study. Obesity 2014;22(4):1201–8.
12. Karsay K, Schmuck D. "Weak, Sad, and Lazy Fatties": Adolescents' explicit and implicit weight bias following exposure to weight loss reality TV shows. Media Psychol 2019;22(1):60–81.
13. Panza GA, Armstrong LE, Taylor BA, et al. Weight bias among exercise and nutrition professionals: a systematic review. Obes Rev 2018;19(11):1492–503.
14. Phelan SM, Puhl RM, Burgess DJ, et al. The role of weight bias and role-modeling in medical students' patient-centered communication with higher weight standardized patients. Patient Educ Couns 2021. https://doi.org/10.1016/j.pec.2021.01.003.

15. Greenwald AG, McGhee DE, Schwartz JLK. Measuring individual differences in implicit cognition: the implicit association test. J Personal Soc Psychol 1998; 74(6):1464–80.
16. Hinman NG, Burmeister JM, Kiefner AE, et al. Stereotypical portrayals of obesity and the expression of implicit weight bias. Body Image 2015;12:32–5.
17. Schwartz MB, Chambliss HO, Brownell KD, et al. Weight bias among health professionals specializing in obesity. Obes Res 2012;11(9):1033–9.
18. Puhl RM, Schwartz MB, Brownell KD. Impact of perceived consensus on stereotypes about obese people: a new approach for reducing bias. Health Psychol 2005;24(5):517–25.
19. Tomiyama AJ, Finch LE, Belsky ACI, et al. Weight bias in 2001 versus 2013: contradictory attitudes among obesity researchers and health professionals. Obesity 2015;23(1):46–53.
20. Thompson JK, Stice E. Thin-ideal internalization: mounting evidence for a new risk factor for body-image disturbance and eating pathology. Curr Dir Psychol Sci 2001;10(5):181–3.
21. Flegal KM, Kruszon-Moran D, Carroll MD, et al. Trends in obesity among adults in the United States, 2005 to 2014. JAMA 2016;315(21):2284.
22. Hales CM, Carroll MD, Fryar CD, et al. Prevalence of obesity and Severe obesity among adults: United States, 2017–2018. National Center for Health Statistics; 2020. p. 8. Available at: https://www.cdc.gov/nchs/products/databriefs/db360.htm.
23. Greenleaf C, Klos L, Hauff C, et al. "Unless you puke, faint, or die, keep going!" exploring weight stigma in the gym on the biggest loser. Fat Stud 2019;8(2):110–26.
24. Wanniarachchi VU, Mathrani A, Susnjak T, et al. A systematic literature review: what is the current stance towards weight stigmatization in social media platforms? Int J Human-Computer Stud 2020;135:102371.
25. Pearl RL, Puhl RM, Brownell KD. Positive media portrayals of obese persons: impact on attitudes and image preferences. Health Psychol 2012;31(6):821–9.
26. Palad CJ, Yarlagadda S, Stanford FC. Weight stigma and its impact on paediatric care. Curr Opin Endocrinol Diabetes Obes 2019;26(1):19–24.
27. Frederick DA, Saguy AC, Sandhu G, et al. Effects of competing news media frames of weight on antifat stigma, beliefs about weight and support for obesity-related public policies. Int J Obes 2016;40(3):543–9.
28. Jeon YA, Hale B, Knackmuhs E, et al. Weight stigma goes viral on the internet: systematic assessment of YouTube comments attacking overweight men and women. Interact J Med Res 2018;7(1):e6.
29. Bradshaw CP, Waasdorp TE, O'Brennan LM, et al. Teachers' and education support professionals' perspectives on bullying and prevention: findings from a National Education Association Study. Sch Psych Rev 2013;42(3):280–97.
30. Puhl RM, Latner JD, O'Brien K, et al. Cross-national perspectives about weight-based bullying in youth: nature, extent and remedies. Pediatr Obes 2016;11(4):241–50.
31. van Woerden I, Brewis A, Hruschka D, et al. Young adults' BMI and changes in romantic relationship status during the first semester of college. PLoS One 2020;15(3):e0230806.
32. Finn KE, Seymour CM, Phillips AE. Weight bias and grading among middle and high school teachers. Br J Educ Psychol 2020;90(3):635–47.

33. Lynagh M, Cliff K, Morgan PJ. Attitudes and beliefs of nonspecialist and specialist trainee health and physical education teachers toward obese children: evidence for "anti-fat" bias. J Sch Health 2015;85(9):595–603.

34. Puhl RM, Latner JD, O'Brien KS, et al. Potential policies and laws to prohibit weight discrimination: public views from 4 countries. Milbank Q 2015;93(4): 691–731.

35. Moulder R, Schvartz D, Goodlett DR, et al. Proteomics of diabetes, obesity, and related disorders. Proteomics Clin Appl 2018;12(1):1600134.

36. Mackey C, Plegue MA, Deames M, et al. Family physicians' knowledge, attitudes, and behaviors regarding the weight effects of added sugar. SAGE Open Med 2018;6. 2050312118801245.

37. Glauser TA, Roepke N, Stevenin B, et al. Physician knowledge about and perceptions of obesity management. Obes Res Clin Pract 2015;9(6):573–83.

38. Sabin JA, Marini M, Nosek BA. Implicit and explicit anti-fat bias among a large sample of medical doctors by bmi, race/ethnicity and gender. PLoS One 2012; 7(11):e48448.

39. Pearl RL, Schulte EM. Weight bias during the COVID-19 pandemic. Curr Obes Rep 2021. https://doi.org/10.1007/s13679-021-00432-2.

40. Alberga AS, Edache IY, Forhan M, et al. Weight bias and health care utilization: a scoping review. Prim Health Care Res Dev 2019;20:e116.

41. Hebl MR, Xu J. Weighing the care: physicians' reactions to the size of a patient. Int J Obes 2001;25(8):1246–52.

42. Hauff C, Fruh SM, Graves RJ, et al. NP student encounters with obesity bias in clinical practice. Nurse Pract 2019;44(6):41–6.

43. Phelan SM, Burgess DJ, Yeazel MW, et al. Impact of weight bias and stigma on quality of care and outcomes for patients with obesity. Obes Rev 2015;16(4): 319–26.

44. Puhl RM, Phelan SM, Nadglowski J, et al. Overcoming weight bias in the management of patients with diabetes and obesity. Clin Diabetes 2016;34(1):44–50.

45. Rubino F, Puhl RM, Cummings DE, et al. Joint international consensus statement for ending stigma of obesity. Nat Med 2020;26(4):485–97.

46. Vartanian LR, Porter AM. Weight stigma and eating behavior: a review of the literature. Appetite 2016;102:3–14.

47. Major B, Hunger JM, Bunyan DP, et al. The ironic effects of weight stigma. J Exp Soc Psychol 2014;51:74–80.

48. Pearl RL, Puhl RM, Dovidio JF. Differential effects of weight bias experiences and internalization on exercise among women with overweight and obesity. J Health Psychol 2015;20(12):1626–32.

49. Pearl RL, Puhl RM, Himmelstein MS, et al. Weight stigma and weight-related health: associations of self-report measures among adults in weight management. Ann Behav Med 2020;54(11):904–14.

50. Jackson SE, Beeken RJ, Wardle J. Perceived weight discrimination and changes in weight, waist circumference, and weight status. Obesity 2014;22(12):2485–8.

51. Sutin AR, Terracciano A. Perceived weight discrimination and obesity. PLoS One 2013;8(7):e70048.

52. Tomiyama AJ. Weight stigma is stressful. A review of evidence for the cyclic obesity/weight-based stigma model. Appetite 2014;82:8–15.

53. Centers for Disease Control and Prevention. Childhood obesity facts: prevalence of childhood obesity in the United States. Overweight Obesity. 2021. Available at: https://www.cdc.gov/obesity/data/childhood.html. Accessed April 2, 2021.

54. Fryar CD, Carroll MD, Afful J. Prevalence of overweight, obesity, and Severe obesity among children and adolescents aged 2–19 years: United States, 1963–1965 through 2017–2018. 2020. Available at: https://www.cdc.gov/nchs/data/hestat/obesity-child-17-18/obesity-child.htm. Accessed March 24, 2021.

55. Fryar CD, Carroll MD, Ogden CL. Prevalence of overweight, obesity, and extreme obesity among adults aged 20 and over: United States, 1960–1962 through 2013–2014. National Center for Health Statistics; 2019. Available at: https://www.cdc.gov/nchs/data/hestat/obesity_adult_13_14/obesity_adult_13_14.htm. Accessed January 22, 2019.

56. Stoner L, Cornwall J. Did the American Medical Association make the correct decision classifying obesity as a disease? Australas Med J 2014;7(11):462–4.

57. Tsai AG, Histon T, Kyle TK, et al. Evidence of a gap in understanding obesity among physicians. Obes Sci Pract 2018;4(1):46–51.

58. Ward ZJ, Long MW, Resch SC, et al. Simulation of growth trajectories of childhood obesity into adulthood. N Engl J Med 2017;377(22):2145–53.

59. Puhl RM, Himmelstein MS, Quinn DM. Internalizing weight stigma: prevalence and sociodemographic considerations in US adults. Obesity (Silver Spring) 2018;26(1):167–75.

60. Lydecker JA, Riley KE, Grilo CM. Associations of parents' self, child, and other "fat talk" with child eating behaviors and weight. Int J Eat Disord 2018;51(6):527–34.

61. Spiel EC, Rodgers RF, Paxton SJ, et al. 'He's got his father's bias': Parental influence on weight bias in young children. Br J Dev Psychol 2016;34(2):198–211.

62. Bajaj SS, Stanford FC. Dignity and respect: people-first language with regard to obesity. Obes Surg 2021. https://doi.org/10.1007/s11695-021-05304-1.

63. Puhl RM, Himmelstein MS, Armstrong SC, et al. Adolescent preferences and reactions to language about body weight. Int J Obes 2017;41(7):1062–5.

64. Kyle TK, Puhl RM. Putting people first in obesity. Obesity (Silver Spring) 2014;22(5):1211.

65. Stanford FC, Kyle TK. Respectful language and care in childhood obesity. JAMA Pediatr 2018;172(11):1001.

66. Pont SJ, Puhl R, Cook SR, et al, Section on Obesity, The Obesity Society. Stigma experienced by children and adolescents with obesity. Pediatrics 2017;140(6):e20173034.

67. Fields LC, Brown C, Skelton JA, et al. Internalized weight bias, teasing, and self-esteem in children with overweight or obesity. Child Obes 2020;17(1):43–50.

68. Day S, Bussey K, Trompeter N, et al. The impact of teasing and bullying victimization on disordered eating and body image disturbance among adolescents: a systematic review. Trauma Violence Abuse 2021. https://doi.org/10.1177/1524838020985534.

69. Gunawardana S, Gunasinghe CB, Harshani MS, et al. Physical and psychosocial quality of life in children with overweight and obesity from Sri Lanka. BMC Public Health 2021;21(1):86.

70. Fruh S, Williams S, Hayes K, et al. A practical approach to obesity prevention: healthy home habits. J Am Assoc Nurse Pract 2021. https://doi.org/10.1097/JXX.0000000000000556.

71. Williams BD, Whipps J, Sisson SB, et al. Associations between health-related family environment and objective child sleep quality. J Paediatr Child Health 2021. https://doi.org/10.1111/jpc.15372.

72. Alman KL, Lister NB, Garnett SP, et al. Dietetic management of obesity and se-vere obesity in children and adolescents: a scoping review of guidelines. Obes Rev 2021;22(1):e13132.
73. Srivastava G, Browne N, Kyle TK, et al. Caring for US children: barriers to effec-tive treatment in children with the disease of obesity. Obesity 2021;29(1):46–55.
74. Le LK-D, Barendregt JJ, Hay P, et al. Prevention of eating disorders: a systematic review and meta-analysis. Clin Psychol Rev 2017;53:46–58.
75. Shea JM, Gagnon M. Working with patients living with obesity in the intensive care unit: a study of nurses' experiences. Adv Nurs Sci 2015;38(3):E17–37.

Current Evidence-Based Treatment of Obesity

Amy Beth Ingersoll, PA-C, MMS, FOMA

KEYWORDS

- Obesity • Evidence-based • Obesity treatment • Obesity management

KEY POINTS

- Obesity is a chronic, progressive, relapsing disease state that requires chronic management.
- Obesity management is comprehensive in nature, containing 4 key elements of nutrition, physical activity, behavioral intervention, and clinical management.
- Obesity management is ever-evolving, and understanding of this complex disease continues to progress, leading health care providers to always be updating themselves on current best practices for management of obesity.
- Health care providers play a key role in an individual's long-term management of this complex disease state.

INTRODUCTION

Obesity is a chronic, progressive, and relapsing disease state in which comprehensive, long-term management is clinically appropriate. It is imperative that all health care providers (HCPs) have an understanding and foundation of current evidence-based treatment to support individuals affected by preobesity and obesity.

DISCUSSION

As the understanding of the complexity behind the disease of obesity continues to expand, it is imperative that HCPs understand current evidence-based treatment of individuals affected by preobesity or obesity. Current evidence-based treatment includes a comprehensive approach that focuses on long-term management. This comprehensive approach focuses on management, including nutrition, physical activity, behavioral intervention, and for many patients, medications. Devices and surgical interventions are considered for appropriate patients as well.

Arizona Obesity Organization, Phoenix, AZ, USA
E-mail address: amy.beth.ingersoll@gmail.com

Nurs Clin N Am 56 (2021) 495–509
https://doi.org/10.1016/j.cnur.2021.07.011
0029-6465/21/© 2021 Elsevier Inc. All rights reserved.

GUIDELINES

Current guidelines recommend having an individualization of a comprehensive approach, including use of behavioral intervention to support nutritional guidance and counseling of increasing physical activity as a foundation of care. Recommendations include the use of Food and Drug Administration (FDA)-approved pharmacotherapy when clinically appropriate, and referral to obesity management specialist and/or bariatric surgery (**Fig. 1**). A comprehensive approach utilization of 4 areas of management, including clinical management, nutrition, behavioral change, and physical activity, is the foundation of evidence-based management for obesity. Nutritional guidance should be individualized with a goal of long-term sustainability. The HCP's role is to help guide an individual toward the best nutrition plan the individual can follow and maintain long term. There is a need for movement and physical activity that the individual can implement and maintain over the years as well. HCPs use behavioral interventions to guide the individual on lifestyle and clinical management of preobesity and obesity. These components will be implemented over a period of time to allow for the comprehensive nature of clinical management. Pharmacotherapy, devices, and/or bariatric surgery support the nutritional, behavioral, and physical activity components and help to treat the complexity of this chronic disease.

NUTRITION

Nutrition is one of the aspects of comprehensive care and clinical management when creating a long-term care plan for individuals with preobesity or obesity. There are a variety of eating plans that could be used, and helping to guide and support individuals with an understanding of how to use food as a nutritional tool to treat this chronic disease is an important part of care (**Table 1**). When talking with individuals, education should always be focused on finding an eating plan they can sustain long term and work into their daily routine, while helping to support their health goals.

Low-carbohydrate nutrition has had a great deal of attention and research over the years. Low carbohydrate has been known over the years as Keto, Atkins, and Paleo. A reduced-carbohydrate nutrition guide will have 50 to 150 g of carbohydrates as part of the total caloric intake for the day, with the focus on reduction in carbohydrates, and focus on an increase in protein and fat macronutrients. A very-low-carbohydrate eating plan is defined as less than 50 g of carbohydrates. Examples of low- and very-low-carbohydrate nutrition guides include the ketogenic diet, Atkins, and paleo. Evidence has shown that reduction in carbohydrates helps to improve metabolic

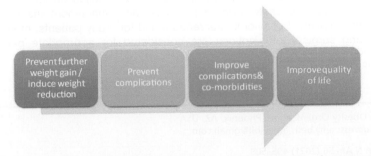

Fig. 1. How the severity of disease state progresses, and the intensity of treatment modalities should be adjusted accordingly.[5]

Table 1
Types of nutrition plan and clinical benefits

Eating Plan	Definition	Metabolic Benefits
Reduced-carbohydrate nutrition plan	Defined as 50–150 g of carbohydrates/d Very-low carbohydrate nutrition guide is defined as <50 g of carbohydrate/d	Improvement in fasting glucose, fasting insulin, and reduction in triglycerides Reduction in blood pressure Increase in HDL
Reduced-fat nutrition plan	Defined as 10%–30% of total caloric intake comes from fat	With reduction in weight, a reduction in fasting glucose, insulin, and a modest improvement in blood pressure may be seen
Mediterranean nutrition plan	Encourages intake of whole foods, including vegetables, fruit, legumes, whole grains, nuts and seeds, healthy fats, small intake of red wine, and moderate consumption of seafood, fermented dairy products (cheese and yogurt), poultry, red meat, and eggs Removal of sugar-sweetened beverages, processed meats, refined grains, refined oils, added sugars, and ultraprocessed foods	Evidence has shown support in reduction in CVD disease risk, reduction in inflammatory markers, protection against Parkinson, dementia, and Alzheimer, along reduction in premature all-cause mortality
Reduced calorie nutrition plan	Low-calorie nutrition guide will provide a 500-kcal reduction in total caloric intake, between 1000 and 1600 kcal/d Very-low-calorie diets (VLCD) are defined as <800 kcal/d	Improvement in metabolic markers, including fasting glucose, fasting insulin, and triglycerides There is a potential for benefit of improvement in HDL and reduction in LDL Reduction in blood pressure is commonly seen in VLCD eating plans
Whole food/plant-based nutrition plan	Consumption of plant-based, whole foods. No animal products	Improvement in metabolic markers, reduction in blood pressure, reduction in visceral adiposity, some evidence supporting potential for reduction in premature all-cause mortality

(*continued on next page*)

Table 1 (continued)		
Time-restricted feeding/ intermittent fasting	Variety of ways to implement Alternate day fasting with reduction in calories on alternating days 16/8 (16 h of fasting, 8 h restricted eating) 12/12 (12 h of fasting, 12 h restricted eating) 18/6 (18 h of fasting, 6 h restricted eating)	Longer fasting periods have shown evidence of reduction in inflammatory markers, reduction in visceral adiposity, improvement in metabolic markers, reduction in blood pressure. Intermittent fasting has shown evidence of improvement in blood pressure, decrease of inflammatory markers, improvement in insulin resistance, and improvement in gut microbiome

markers and reduce insulin levels. Benefits from a reduced carbohydrate nutrition guide have shown improvement in HgA_{1c}, reduction in cholesterol levels with improvement in high-density lipoprotein (HDL), and reduction in triglycerides, as well as up to a 10% reduction in weight. A reduced carbohydrate nutrition plan, specifically, a very-low-carbohydrate plan, provides an improved sense of satiety.

A low-fat nutrition plan, such as the DASH diet, has been a nutritional style that has been around for years. A low-fat nutrition plan recommends fat intake to be between 15% and 20% of total caloric intake for the day. The evidence of health benefits from a reduced fat nutrition plan has been shown to decrease total and low-density lipoprotein (LDL) cholesterol by 10% to 20%, and improvement in blood pressure, and a 5% to 10% reduction in weight.[1,2]

Mediterranean style of nutrition focuses on whole foods with a focus on healthy fats and reduction in added sugars and processed foods. Mediterranean style nutrition focuses on daily consumption of vegetables, fruit, whole grains, and healthy fats, weekly intake of fish, poultry, beans, and eggs, with moderate portions of dairy products, and a limitation of consumption of red meat. Consumption of sugar-sweetened beverages, processed meats, refined grains, refined oils, added sugars, and ultraprocessed foods is discouraged from the dietary intake. The current studies focus mainly on the cardiovascular benefits, and evidence shows the clinical benefits from the Mediterranean style of nutrition includes improvement in cardiac disease, reduction in inflammatory markers, protection against Parkinson, dementia, and Alzheimer, and an overall reduction in all causes of death, including malignancy.[3,4]

Whole food/plant based is focused on clean eating and on helping to focus on consumption of whole food, no animal products, with no processed or ultraprocessed foods in this type of nutritional plan. This type of eating plan focuses on consumption of plant-based, whole foods. The evidence that is currently available shows improvement in metabolic markers, reduction in blood pressure, and reduction in visceral adiposity, and there is some evidence that shows there may be a reduction in premature all-cause mortality.[5,6]

Time-restricted eating and intermittent fasting have a variety of potential meal patterns and variation in days and timing of fasting. There are some studies that looked at alternate-day fasting that varies from fasting to reduction in caloric intake on alternating days.[2,7] Intermittent fasting is a popular time-restricted pattern, and studies have looked at a variation of timing, including 16/8 (16 hours of fasting, 8 hours restricted feeding), 12/12 (12 hours of fasting, 12 hours of restricted feeding), and 18/6 (18 hours fasting, 6 hours eating with restricted eating). One of the most popular fasting plans is 16 hours of fasting with an 8 hour of eating timeframe. The evidence shows potential for reduction in inflammatory markers, reduction in visceral adiposity, improvement in metabolic markers, and reduction in blood pressure. Studies have shown that utilization of intermittent fasting can lead to clinical benefits, including improvement in blood pressure, decrease in inflammatory markers, reduction in insulin resistance, improvement in gut microbiome, and reduction in weight.[8–11]

Reduced calorie food plans include a low-calorie nutrition plan that is focused on reduction in total calories versus focus on a macronutrient. Low-calorie nutrition is between 800 and 1600 kcal/d and is what we have in the past seen as the typical "diet" mindset around a nutrition plan. In clinical practice, a low-calorie nutrition plan can be supplemented with use of meal replacement for structure and stimulus control. Studies have shown evidence of remission of type 2 diabetes, and short-term success in reduction in weight, but as we understand, obesity is a long-term, chronic progressive disease state with metabolic adaptation that occurs. This may be a difficult eating plan for an individual to maintain, as reduction in calories over time in individuals has a reduction in their resting metabolic rate. This reduction in calories may no longer be realistic.[5,12–15]

A very-low-calorie nutrition plan is a very structured eating plan, commonly seen in obesity-management centers, that commonly will use meal replacement shakes for this nutrition guide. This limits total caloric intake to less than 800 kcal/d while keeping total protein intake around 70 to 100 g per day. Studies have shown evidence of short-term reduction in weight and improvement in metabolic markers.[5,16] A very-low-calorie nutrition plan may be helpful for short-term management with the idea to adapt to a nutrition guide that is sustainable for long-term management.

The A-to-Z study was a comprehensive study that showed a variety of eating plans. Individuals followed 1 of 4 types of eating plans.[1] What this study shows is that there were some participants who gained weight, and some who had a reduction in weight in every category of eating plans. This study helps us to show that there is a great need to individualize nutritional recommendations, and that there is potential to adapt their nutritional plan pending their outcomes.

The literature is clear that there is no one eating plan that works for everyone. The best nutrition guide is the nutrition plan the individual can maintain long term. As an HCP, your goal is to help to guide them through options for an eating plan.

PHYSICAL ACTIVITY

Physical activity is an important tool to know how to implement and optimize while working with individuals. Studies have shown that exercise minimally impacts active reduction in weight, with an ability to account for around 10% of the weight reduced.[17–20]

There is vast amount of evidence supporting the incredible amount of health benefits from activity that goes beyond the scale.[17] The understanding of the role of physical activity with management of obesity is the clear delineation to help an individual understand the role of physical activity with a long-term care plan. Activity is a critical component to long-term management of obesity because of the complexities of metabolic adaptation that lead to a reduction in metabolic rate.

Current guidelines recommend 150 minutes of moderate aerobic activity per week. A key clarification is there is minimal evidence showing that the 150 min/wk contributed to significant reduction in weight, but the studies have shown that physical activity for long-term management and maintenance is an additional 250 to 300 minutes above baseline guidelines.[21,22] With these numbers in mind, it is important to start this conversation of physical activity early so that there can be a gradual increase in physical activity throughout the management that will support the potential of ~400 minutes of physical activity weekly for support of long-term management.

Resistance training is another component of a physical activity plan. Resistance training helps to preserve lean muscle mass during active reduction in weight. There are studies as well that show resistance training may help to improve metabolic markers by reduction of visceral adiposity.[17] There is a need to make sure individuals understand how to implement resistance training without injury. Depending on the complexity of an individual's health, there may be benefit of a referral to a specialist to help with support of a physical activity plan, that is, exercise physiologist, physical therapist.

In a clinical setting, utilization of a physical activity prescription can be helpful to have a written prescription for activity goals. This is also a place the authors bring in their utilization of behavioral change to help support physical activity education. A common acronym for a physical activity prescription is FITTE, which stands for: Frequency, Intensity, Time, Type, and Enjoyment (**Fig. 2**). The frequency will detail how often for a given timeframe that activity will be done. The intensity is the level of physical demand of the activity, which will vary from person to person. The time is the specific amount of time the patient will engage in that activity. The type of activity helps to specify what exact activity will be completed during that timeframe. Enjoyment is likely one of the most important aspects of this prescription. When we were kids, we use to have this type of activity that we simply called "play." It was fun, enjoyable, something we looked forward to without being a chore. Finding a type of physical activity that is enjoyable is key for an individual to be successful with long-term implementation of physical activity needs.

BEHAVIORAL INTERVENTION

Behavioral intervention will help to guide and direct lifestyle changes around nutritional planning and physical activity. Self-monitoring is a tool that can be used to help support individuals with behavioral intervention. Self-monitoring helps to identify barriers, helps identify patterns, and helps the individual to better self-reflect on understanding barriers that are impacting their ability to achieve long-term goals. There are studies that provide evidence that many individuals have greater success in reduction in weight when monitored more frequently.[18,23,24]

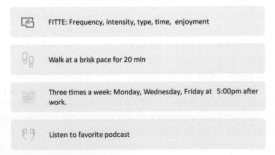

FITTE: Frequency, intensity, type, time, enjoyment

Walk at a brisk pace for 20 min

Three times a week: Monday, Wednesday, Friday at 5:00pm after work.

Listen to favorite podcast

Fig. 2. FITTE physical activity prescription.

Motivational interviewing is a process that can allow the clinician to guide patients. It is a form of patient-centered communication that explores and resolves issues with a focus on goals to support long-term management and change. Motivational interviewing is a form of shared decision making, allowing the individual to actively participate in their treatment plan.

Tools that can be beneficial are prescriptions and using SMART goals. Eating plan and physical activity prescriptions have been shown through studies to guide individuals through successful long-term management.[18,23,25] Using the acronym SMART: Specific, Measurable, Achievable, Realistic, Timely can also help with setting specific and measurable goals to support long-term management (**Table 2**).

Other techniques to help with behavioral interventions include the 5 A's. The 5 A's provide a structure that can be used for intensive behavioral therapy and counseling around obesity. There are 2 variations of 5 A's that include: Ask, Assess, Advise, Agree, and Assist (**Table 3**). Medicare has a slightly different version of the 5 A's that are used with their intensive behavioral therapy, which stands for Assess, Advice, Agree, Assist, and Arrange.

PHARMACOTHERAPY

When reviewing pharmacotherapy, it is important to be aware of goals of treatment. The focus on the management of obesity is beyond simply the number on the scale. Although a reduction in weight of 5% to 10% is a goal of management, it is important that we understand the goal of management is improvement in the disease of obesity and its complications and comorbidities (**Fig. 3**). Beyond the scale, an improvement in obesity-related complications within 6 months may include reducing cardiovascular risk factors, preventing and/or delaying the onset of type 2 diabetes mellitus (T2DM) , optimizing of body mass index (BMI) to help reduce pressure on joints, and improvement of patient's overall health and quality of life.

Most of the current pharmacologic interventions are to be used in conjunction with or as adjunct therapy to lifestyle interventions for patients 18 years and older with BMI greater than or equal to 30 kg/m^2 or BMI 27 kg/m^2 with comorbidities. Liraglutide is now approved for patients 12 to 17 years old who have a body weight of 60 kg with an initial BMI corresponding to 30 kg/m^2 or greater for adults. All antiobesity medications are contraindicated during pregnancy and lactation, and a pregnancy test at baseline for all women of reproductive age is recommended.

Similar to the individualization of nutrition and physical activity plan, patients may respond differently to medications. If a patient does not have success or has side effects with 1 medication, consider another.

Current FDA-approved medication includes those that are approved for short-term use and those that have been approved for chronic use. It is important to clarify that

Table 2	
Behavioral change using SMART acronym	
Meaning	**Example**
Specific	"I am going to walk Monday, Wednesday, and Friday."
Measurable	"I am going to start with 10 minutes of walking."
Achievable	"Currently I am walking once a week, so this seems like a realistic goal."
Relevant	"I have found since COVID my activity has greatly decreased. I really want a way to create a long-term sustainable plan for staying active."
Timely	"I will start this week."

Table 3 The 5 As of obesity management	
Ask	Ask permission to discuss weight
Assess	Assess for stage of obesity Assess barriers to care Assess for obesity-related complications Assess for motivation for change
Advise	Advise on benefit of clinically meaningful management of obesity and reduction in weight Advise on chronic nature of disease state Advise on evidence-based treatment available
Agree	Agree on care plan Agree on SMART goal Agree on short-term management goal of obesity Agree on long-term management goal of obesity
Assist	Assist with providing resources for management Assist with schedule a follow-up office visit Assist with referral to specialist to support comprehensive care

the short-term therapies came to the market when obesity was not seen as a chronic disease state.

Short-term antiobesity medications are in the class of sympathomimetics, including Phentermine, Diethylpropion, Phendimetrazine, and Benzphetamine (**Table 4**). The common side effects seen in this class of medications include insomnia, palpitations, tachycardia, dizziness, tremor, changes in taste, gastrointestinal side effects, headache, restlessness, and increase in blood pressure. Contraindications for this class of medication include cardiovascular disease (CVD), uncontrolled hypertension, glaucoma, hyperthyroidism, seizures, pregnancy/breastfeeding, history of drug abuse, monoamine oxidase (MAO) inhibitors, anxiety disorders. These medications are schedule IV medications, and it is important as a clinician you understand your local state laws as well as prescribing laws.

Endocrine Society Statement on Long-Term Use of Phentermine

Phentermine has been a long-studied medication, and the Endocrine Society has an important statement for HCP to understand discussion of and prescribing for long-term use in which they state that if an individual has no history of CVD, no psychiatric/substance abuse history, has been informed about therapies that are approved for long-term use, has no clinically significant increase in pulse and blood pressure,

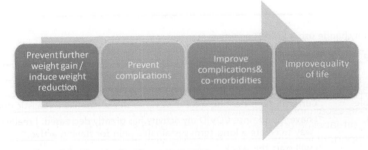

Fig. 3. Goals of antiobesity medication treatment.

Table 4
Short-term medications for obesity management

Medication	Class/Mechanism of Action	Side Effects	Contraindications/ Cautions
Phentermine	Sympathomimetic amines, increases satiety	Insomnia, palpitations, tachycardia, dizziness, tremor, changes in taste, gastrointestinal side effects, headache, restlessness, and increase in blood pressure	History of CVD, administration during or within 14 d following the administration of MAO inhibitors, hyperthyroidism, glaucoma, history of drug abuse, hypersensitivity, & pregnancy/nursing
Diethylpropion	Sympathomimetic amines, increases satiety	Insomnia, palpitations, tachycardia, dizziness, tremor, changes in taste, gastrointestinal side effects, headache, restlessness, and increase in blood pressure	History of CVD, administration during or within 14 d following the administration of MAO inhibitors, hyperthyroidism, glaucoma, history of drug abuse, hypersensitivity, & pregnancy/nursing
Phendimetrazine	Sympathomimetic amines, increases satiety	Insomnia, palpitations, tachycardia, dizziness, tremor, changes in taste, gastrointestinal side effects, headache, restlessness, and increase in blood pressure	History of CVD, administration during or within 14 d following the administration of MAO inhibitors, hyperthyroidism, glaucoma, history of drug abuse, hypersensitivity, & pregnancy/nursing
Benzphetamine	Sympathomimetic amines, increases satiety	Insomnia, palpitations, tachycardia, dizziness, tremor, changes in taste, gastrointestinal side effects, headache, restlessness, and increase in blood pressure	History of CVD, administration during or within 14 d following the administration of MAO inhibitors, hyperthyroidism, glaucoma, history of drug abuse, hypersensitivity, & pregnancy/nursing

and sees reduction in weight while being prescribed phentermine, this medication can safely be prescribed. It is recommended that the clinician monitors the patient monthly during dose escalation and then quarterly once on a stable dose, and clearly documents the off-label nature of prescribing phentermine long-term in the medical record. It is also important to notate the HCP is familiar with their state prescribing laws around phentermine.[26]

FDA-approved antiobesity medications for long-term management of obesity include liraglutide 3 mg, naltrexone/bupropion ER, orlistat, and phentermine/topiramate ER (**Table 5**).

Liraglutide 3 mg is a GLP-1r agonist that leads to a reduction in hunger and increase in satiety. This is the only antiobesity medication that the FDA approved for the management in the adolescent population of 12 to 17 years olds with an initial body weight of at least 60 kg and an initial BMI corresponding to 30 kg/m^2 or greater for adults. This medication has a weekly titration to be started at 0.6 mg and titrate up by 0.6 mg weekly until a maximum dose of 3 mg. Long-term efficacy has been shown at 7.4% to 10% reduction in weight for individuals.[27–30] Secondary endpoint improvements have shown reduction in progression of type 2 diabetes for individuals with prediabetes.[27,29] The label states that the medication is to be stopped if an individual does not

Table 5
Food and Drug Administration–approved antiobesity medications for chronic management

Medication	Class/Mechanism of Action	Side Effects	Contraindications/Cautions
Orlistat	Gastrointestinal lipase inhibitor	Oily spotting, cramps, flatus with discharge, fecal incontinence, fecal urgency, fatty oily stool, increased defecation	Chronic malabsorption syndrome, breastfeeding, pregnancy, specific medications (warfarin, levothyroxine, antiepileptic agents, cyclosporine)
Liraglutide 3 mg	Glucagon-like peptide-1 (GLP-1) receptor agonist, improves satiety and reduces hunger	Constipation, nausea, diarrhea, increase in heart rate, hypoglycemia, headache, fatigue, increased lipase, dizziness, abdominal pain	Medullary thyroid cancer history (family and/or self), multiple endocrine neoplasia type 2 history, pregnancy, and breastfeeding. Precaution is noted for individuals with history of pancreatitis
Naltrexone HCL/ Bupropion HCL XR	Opioid receptor antagonist combined with a noradrenaline reuptake inhibitor that helps to reduce cravings	Nausea, constipation, headache, dizziness, headache, vomiting, insomnia, and dry mouth	Seizure disorder, uncontrolled hypertension, anorexia or bulimia, chronic opioid use, MAO inhibitors, drug or alcohol withdrawal, caution with renal/hepatic impairment
Phentermine HCLD/ Topiramate XR	Noradrenergic + GABA-receptor activator, kainite/AMPA glutamate receptor inhibitor that leads to appetite suppression	Dry mouth, memory or cognitive changes, insomnia, constipation, dizziness, taste alterations, paresthesia, elevation in heart rate	Pregnancy and breastfeeding, hyperthyroidism, glaucoma, and use of MAO inhibitors

have at least a 4% reduction in weight 12 weeks after the maximum dose. Contraindications include medullary thyroid cancer history (family and/or self), multiple endocrine neoplasia type 2 history, pregnancy, and breastfeeding. Precaution is noted for individuals with a history of pancreatitis. Common side effects include constipation, nausea, diarrhea, increase in heart rate, hypoglycemia, headache, fatigue, increase lipase, dizziness, and abdominal pain.

Naltrexone/Bupropion ER is an opioid receptor antagonist combined with a noradrenaline reuptake inhibitor that helps to reduce cravings. Studies show an average reduction of weight of 5.4% to 8.2%.[27,29] Secondary endpoint improvements show improvement in cardiometabolic parameters and reduction of HbA$_{1c}$ for individuals with type 2 diabetes.[27,29] Initiation of medication is 1 tablet 8 mg/90 mg with a weekly escalation to target dose of 2 tablets twice a day for a maximum dose of 32 mg/260 mg. The label states to discontinue the medication if the patient does not have a reduction in weight of at least 5% 12 weeks after the maximum dose. Contraindications include seizure disorder, uncontrolled hypertension, anorexia or bulimia, chronic opioid use, MAO inhibitors, drug or alcohol withdrawal, and caution with renal/hepatic impairment. Common side effects include nausea, constipation, headache, dizziness, headache, vomiting, insomnia, and dry mouth.

Orlistat is a pancreatic lipase inhibitor that impairs gastrointestinal energy absorption that leads to an excretion of ~30% of ingested triglycerides in stool. Studies have shown a range of weight reduction from 3.8% to 10.2% with a mean reduction of 6.1%.[27,29] Dosing of Orlistat is 60 mg over the counter, and 120 mg 3 times a day within 1 hour of a fat-containing meal. Secondary endpoint improvements show a reduction in blood pressure and triglycerides, improvement in LDL and fasting glucose, as well as slowing progression of type 2 diabetes.[27,29] Precautions and contraindication are chronic malabsorption syndrome, breastfeeding, pregnancy, specific medications (warfarin, levothyroxine, antiepileptic agents, cyclosporine). Common side effects for Orlistat are oily spotting, cramps, flatus with discharge, fecal incontinence, fecal urgency, fatty oily stool, and increased defecation.

Phentermine/topiramate ER is a noradrenergic agent combined with a GABA-receptor activator, kainite/AMPA glutamate receptor inhibitor that leads to appetite suppression. Studies have shown an average reduction in weight of 10%. Secondary endpoints have shown improvement in cardiometabolic markers and reduction in progression of type 2 diabetes.[27,29,31] The label states to discontinue the medication if the patient does not have a reduction in weight of at least 5% after 12 weeks on maximum dose. Phentermine/topiramate ER dosing is a titrating dose with a 2-week titration dose of 3.75 mg/23 mg; increase to 7.5 mg/46 mg following the 2-week initiation. Escalation of dose to 11.25 mg/69 mg and 15 mg/92 mg is available as clinically necessary. Precautions and contraindications include pregnancy and breastfeeding, hyperthyroidism, glaucoma, and use of MAO inhibitors. Common side effects include dry mouth, memory or cognitive changes, insomnia, constipation, dizziness, taste alterations, paresthesia, and elevation in heart rate. This is a schedule IV medication.

Because of the topiramate component, there is a risk elevation and mitigation strategy, as topiramate can cause cleft palate issues during pregnancy. For women of childbearing age, it is important to have a pregnancy prevention plan while on this medication.

DEVICES

Plenity is a device that can be prescribed. It is a hydrogel matrix of cellulose and citric acid. It is approved for individuals with BMI greater than 25 kg/m^2 to less than 40 kg/m^2.

The mechanism of action is the capsule releases nonaggregating particles that absorb water, thereby increasing the volume and elasticity of the stomach and small intestines. Dosing is to take 3 capsules 20 minutes before lunch and dinner with 16 to 20 ounces of water. Precaution includes individuals with severe reflux or ulcers. Common side effects include abdominal distention, constipation, nausea, diarrhea, and abdominal pain. Of note, the capsule of this device is made from gelatin that is a porcine-derived product so is not considered kosher or likely to be used by a vegan.

Other FDA-approved devices include the intragastric balloons, transpyloric bulb, aspiration therapy, and vagal nerve block therapy, but are beyond the scope of this article.

BARIATRIC SURGERY

Individuals with a BMI $\geq$40 kg/m^2 or BMI $\geq$ 35 kg/m^2 with comorbid conditions are candidates for bariatric surgery. Bariatric surgeries are metabolic procedures that lead to reduction in weight and treatment of obesity by creating a change in microbiome, hunger hormones, and satiety hormones.

Gastric bypass Roux-en-Y is a procedure in which the stomach is stapled to create a 15- to 30-mL pouch. The small bowel is divided at the jejunum. The mechanism of action is a decrease in ghrelin along with an increase in satiety hormones. This procedure has shown a 35% to 45% reduction in total weight.

Vertical sleeve gastrectomy is a procedure in which 75% to 85% of the stomach is removed with no intestinal disruption. The mechanism of action is a reduction in the hunger hormone ghrelin and increase in satiety hormones. A 25% to 35% total reduction in weight has been seen with this procedure.

Duodenal switch is a procedure in which a bypass is created and is the most restrictive of all the procedures and the least commonly completed surgical intervention. The mechanism of action is a decrease in ghrelin and increase in satiety hormones. This procedure has the strongest potential for remission of type 2 diabetes, although it also has the greatest potential for vitamin deficiency. An average 40% reduction in weight has been seen with this procedure.

The adjustable gastric band, commonly known as the LAP band, is a procedure that is uncommonly if ever preformed anymore. It has been shown to have minimal long-term management of obesity along with multiple complications.

Contraindications for bariatric surgery include active substance abuse disorder, active psychiatric disease, and active binging/bulimia. Annual laboratory evaluation is needed for all individuals' status post bariatric surgery. Vitamin supplementation is also needed to help minimize deficiencies. The American Society of Bariatric Surgeons has a guideline to provide the clinician with a process for postbariatric surgery follow-up.

GOALS

Goals for management of obesity go beyond the scale. There are clinically meaningful benefits from a 5% to 10% reduction in weight. Other goals for management include improvement in metabolic markers and a reduction in visceral adiposity measured by a reduction in waist circumference. Reduction of obesity-related complications, reduction in CVD risks, prevention and or delay of T2DM, and improvement in joint disease are other overarching goals as we move to a whole-person care approach with the clinical management of obesity. An improvement of individual health and quality of life becomes the long-term goal and the rewarding aspect to helping patients in the management of preobesity and obesity (**Fig. 4**).

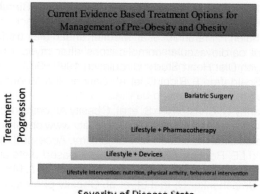

Fig. 4. Obesity management treatment goals.

SUMMARY

Obesity is a complex, chronic, relapsing disease state the requires a comprehensive approach for successful long-term management. The foundation of care includes nutritional education, physical activity progression, and supportive behavioral intervention. For many individuals, intensification of treatment is medically necessary as the disease state progresses. This intensification of management may include pharmacotherapy, devices, and/or surgical interventions for the patient. It is important for HCPs to stay up-to-date with current evidence-based guidelines as the understanding of this complex disease state continues to increase.

CLINICS CARE POINTS

- Best practices around evidence-based management of the chronic disease state of obesity include progressive level of treatment modalities as the disease state progresses, including lifestyle interventions, pharmacotherapy, and bariatric surgery when clinically appropriate.

- Individualizing treatment recommendations is key for long-term, sustainable success with management of obesity using motivational interviewing and shared decision making to create a comprehensive care plan.

- If 1 treatment does not work, try another. Similar to other chronic conditions, not all individuals will respond the same.

DISCLOSURE

Speaker, Novo Nordisk, Obesity and Diabetes.

REFERENCES

1. Gardner CD, Kiazand A, Alhassan S, et al. Comparison of the Atkins, Zone, Ornish, and LEARN diets for change in weight and related risk factors among overweight premenopausal women: the A to Z Weight Loss Study: a randomized trial. JAMA 2007; 297(9):969–77 [published correction appears in JAMA. 2007 Jul 11;298(2):178].
2. Sacks FM, Lichtenstein AH, Wu JHY, et al. Dietary fats and cardiovascular disease: a presidential advisory from the American Heart Association. Circulation

2017;136(3):e1–23 [published correction appears in Circulation. 2017 Sep 5;136(10):e195].

3. de Lorgeril M, Salen P, Martin JL, et al. Mediterranean diet, traditional risk factors, and the rate of cardiovascular complications after myocardial infarction: final report of the Lyon Diet Heart Study. Circulation 1999;99(6):779–85.

4. Mentella MC, Scaldaferri F, Ricci C, et al. Cancer and Mediterranean diet: a review. Nutrients 2019;11(9):2059.

5. Bays HE, McCarthy W, Christensen S, et al. Obesity Algorithm eBook, presented by the Obesity Medicine Association. Available at: www.obesityalgorithm.org.2021 https://obesitymedicine.org/%20obesity-algorithm/. Accessed April 1, 2021.

6. Kim H, Caulfield LE, Rebholz CM. Healthy plant-based diets are associated with lower risk of all-cause mortality in US adults. J Nutr 2018;148(4):624–31.

7. Saunders KH, Umashanker D, Igel LI, et al. Obesity pharmacotherapy. Med Clin North Am 2018;102(1):135–48.

8. Varady KA, Bhutani S, Church EC, et al. Short-term modified alternate-day fasting: a novel dietary strategy for weight loss and cardioprotection in obese adults. Am J Clin Nutr 2009;90(5):1138–43.

9. Mechanick JI, Youdim A, Jones DB, et al. Clinical practice guidelines for the perioperative nutritional, metabolic, and nonsurgical support of the bariatric surgery patient–2013 update: cosponsored by American Association of Clinical Endocrinologists, the Obesity Society, and American Society for Metabolic & Bariatric Surgery. Endocr Pract 2013;19(2):337–72.

10. Patterson RE, Sears DD. Metabolic effects of intermittent fasting. Annu Rev Nutr 2017;37:371–93.

11. Hendricks EJ, Greenway FL, Westman EC, et al. Blood pressure and heart rate effects, weight loss and maintenance during long-term phentermine pharmacotherapy for obesity. Obesity (Silver Spring) 2011;19(12):2351–60.

12. Gonzalez-Campoy JM, St Jeor ST, Castorino K, et al. Clinical practice guidelines for healthy eating for the prevention and treatment of metabolic and endocrine diseases in adults: cosponsored by the American Association of Clinical Endocrinologists/the American College of Endocrinology and the Obesity Society. Endocr Pract 2013;19(Suppl 3):1–82.

13. Leslie WS, Ford I, Sattar N, et al. The Diabetes Remission Clinical Trial (DiRECT): protocol for a cluster randomised trial. BMC Fam Pract 2016;17:20.

14. Hendricks EJ. Off-label drugs for weight management. Diabetes Metab Syndr Obes 2017;10:223–34.

15. Jakicic JM, Davis KK. Obesity and physical activity. Psychiatr Clin North Am 2011;34(4):829–40.

16. Ahmad N, Alfaris N. VLCD for weight loss and remission of type 2 diabetes? Lancet 2018;392(10155):1306–7.

17. Danielsen KK, Svendsen M, Mæhlum S, et al. Changes in body composition, cardiovascular disease risk factors, and eating behavior after an intensive lifestyle intervention with high volume of physical activity in severely obese subjects: a prospective clinical controlled trial. J Obes 2013;2013:325464.

18. Brown T, Avenell A, Edmunds LD, et al. Systematic review of long-term lifestyle interventions to prevent weight gain and morbidity in adults. Obes Rev 2009; 10(6):627–38.

19. Peterson JA. Get moving! Physical activity counseling in primary care. J Am Acad Nurse Pract 2007;19(7):349–57.

20. Bray GA. Why do we need drugs to treat the patient with obesity? Obesity (Silver Spring) 2013;21(5):893–9.

21. Swift DL, Johannsen NM, Lavie CJ, et al. The role of exercise and physical activity in weight loss and maintenance. Prog Cardiovasc Dis 2014;56(4):441–7.

22. Hyde PN, Sapper TN, Crabtree CD, et al. Dietary carbohydrate restriction improves metabolic syndrome independent of weight loss. JCI Insight 2019; 4(12):e128308.

23. Vallis M, Piccinini-Vallis H, Sharma AM, et al. Clinical review: modified 5 As: minimal intervention for obesity counseling in primary care. Can Fam Physician 2013; 59(1):27–31.

24. Apovian CM, Aronne LJ, Bessesen DH, et al. Pharmacological management of obesity: an Endocrine Society Clinical Practice Guideline [published correction appears in J Clin Endocrinol Metab. 2015 May;100(5):2135-6]. J Clin Endocrinol Metab 2015;100(2):342–62.

25. Bushman BA. Determining the I (Intensity) for a FITT-VP aerobic exercise prescription. ACSM's Health Fitness J 2014;18(3):4–7.

26. Garvey WT, Mechanick JI, Brett EM, et al. American Association of Clinical Endocrinologists and American College of Endocrinology comprehensive clinical practice guidelines for medical care of patients with obesity. Endocr Pract 2016;22(Suppl 3):1–203.

27. Kumar RB, Aronne LJ. Efficacy comparison of medications approved for chronic weight management. Obesity (Silver Spring) 2015;23(Suppl 1):S4–7.

28. Borradaile KE, Halpern SD, Wyatt HR, et al. Relationship between treatment preference and weight loss in the context of a randomized controlled trial. Obesity (Silver Spring) 2012;20(6):1218–22.

29. Bray GA, Frühbeck G, Ryan DH, et al. Management of obesity. Lancet 2016; 387(10031):1947–56.

30. Ingersoll A, Christensen S, The Art and Science of Prescribing Anti-Obesity Medications. Lecture Presented at American Academy of Physician Assistant Annual Conference, May 22, 2019, Denver, CO.

31. Bays HE, Gadde KM. Phentermine/topiramate for weight reduction and treatment of adverse metabolic consequences in obesity. Drugs Today (Barc) 2011;47(12): 903–14 [published correction appears in Drugs Today (Barc). 2012 Jan;48(1):95].

The Influence of Obesity on Care of Adults with Cardiovascular Disease

Leslie L. Davis, PhD, RN, ANP-BC, FAAN, FAANP, FACC, FAHA, FPCNA*,
Melissa Z. Nolan, MSN, RN

KEYWORDS

- Obesity • Cardiovascular disease • Hypertension • Heart failure
- Coronary heart disease • Nursing • Physical examination

KEY POINTS

- Obesity is a common precursor to cardiovascular conditions.
- Cardiovascular risk in adults with obesity is directly related to their type of excess body mass and level of cardiorespiratory fitness.
- The presence of excess body mass frequently obscures the physical examination requiring adaptive techniques to be used for patients with obesity.
- Lifestyle modifications are the cornerstone of treatment for improving outcomes In patients with obesity and cardiovascular disease.

INTRODUCTION

The prevalence of obesity has increased in epidemic proportions over the past several decades. According to the 2020 American Heart Association (AHA) statistics, 39.6% of adults in America have obesity, including 7.7% who have severe obesity.[1] Prevalence is even higher in Hispanic and non-Hispanic blacks, as compared to non-Hispanic whites and Asians.[2] Furthermore, obesity is a strong independent predictor of cardiovascular disease (CVD),[2] including common cardiovascular conditions such as hypertension (HTN),[1,3] coronary heart disease (CHD),[1,4] chronic heart failure (HF),[1,5] atrial fibrillation (AFib),[1,6] stroke,[1] and venous thromboembolism.[1] In fact, about 75% of the incidence of HTN is directly related to obesity,[7] which is important because HTN is frequently a precursor to other cardiovascular conditions.

In this article, we briefly review the physiologic effects of obesity on the cardiovascular system. We also discuss how obesity influences assessment (history taking, vital

University of North Carolina at Chapel Hill, School of Nursing, 4007 Carrington Hall, CB # 7460, Chapel Hill, NC 27599-7460, USA
* Corresponding author.
E-mail address: LLDavis@email.unc.edu
Twitter: @LLDavis_UNCCH (L.L.D.)

Nurs Clin N Am 56 (2021) 511–525
https://doi.org/10.1016/j.cnur.2021.07.002
0029-6465/21/© 2021 Elsevier Inc. All rights reserved.

nursing.theclinics.com

signs, physical examination), cardiovascular diagnostic testing, and treatment (pharmacologic and nonpharmacologic) in adults with cardiovascular conditions. We will focus on conditions commonly encountered by nurses in everyday practice, namely HTN, CHD, and HF.

PHYSIOLOGIC EFFECTS OF OBESITY ON THE CV SYSTEM

The pathophysiology of obesity results in insulin resistance, causing the pancreas to secrete too much insulin (hyperinsulinemia).[8] As a result, the sympathetic nervous system (SNS) and the renin-angiotensin-aldosterone system (RAAS) are activated, sodium reabsorption and retention are increased through the kidneys, and circulatory plasma volume and peripheral vascular resistance are increased.[8] Obesity-associated increased SNS activity also occurs due to dysregulation of the baroreceptor reflex (depressing the ability to inhibit the SNS) and increased circulatory amounts of leptin (an adipocyte that regulates appetite suppression).[8] Furthermore, fat deposits that surround the kidneys combined with central adiposity associated with obesity result in an additional increase in sodium reabsorption by the kidneys.[8] Over time, these collective mechanisms have prohypertensive blood pressure (BP) effects, increase the development of hypertrophy, and accelerate the proliferation of vascular smooth muscle.[8] Refer to **Table 1** that summarizes the physiologic effects of obesity on the cardiovascular system and targeted treatment for those effects, categorized by 3 common cardiovascular conditions.

OBESITY PARADOX

Once a patient is diagnosed with CVD, the mechanism of how a higher body mass index (BMI) influences outcomes for patients with CVD is unclear.[2] Often referred to as "the obesity paradox," some cardiovascular patients with higher BMI do better than others.[2] For example, it is well known that obesity increases the risk of developing HF. However, once a patient is diagnosed with HF, regardless of whether the patient has reduced ejection fraction or preserved ejection fraction, outcomes related to BMI vary. Therefore, in addition to BMI being an imprecise measure of nutritional assessment, it is also an imperfect predictor of outcomes.[2] To overcome this challenge, excess body weight is often categorized as *fat-free mass* versus *fat mass*. Fat-free mass consists of lean mass and skeletal muscle mass (typically associated with a more favorable prognosis) as compared to excessive fat mass (typically associated with a negative impact on the cardiovascular system and metabolism).[2] Furthermore, fat mass influences the production of proinflammatory cytokines and adipokines resulting in cardiodepressive effects and proatherosclerotic effects (negatively effecting contractility and plaque stability, respectively).[2] However, *where* fat mass is distributed on the body also matters. For example, if the fat mass is located at the waist area (ie, larger waist circumference), there is a substantially higher cardiometabolic risk for the particular patient. Therefore, it is recommended that waist circumference be measured to help risk stratify patients.

Beyond what makes up the excess weight (fat-free mass vs fat mass), cardiovascular risk is also related to cardiorespiratory fitness. Improvements in cardiorespiratory fitness have been shown to be associated with improved survival in the general population.[2] The association between fitness and survival is even more pronounced in patients with established CVD or with CVD risk factors.[2] In fact, some cardiologists refer to cardiorespiratory fitness as "another vital sign."[2] Studies have also shown that excess lean mass (a type of fat-free mass as opposed to fat mass) associated with improved prognosis in HF and CVD is a result of patients having higher

Table 1 Physiologic effect of obesity on the cardiovascular system		
Cardiovascular Condition	Physiologic Effects of Obesity	Targeted Treatment
HTN	• SNS overactivity (neurohormonal response) → renal vasoconstriction → increased BP • Increased salt sensitivity → volume expansion → increased BP • Increased intraabdominal and intravascular fat mass → increased sodium reabsorption (in kidneys) → increased circulatory plasma volume → increased BP • Increased RAAS (humoral response) → increased adipokine activity → hypertrophy smooth muscle cells → accelerated atherosclerosis → increased peripheral vascular resistance → impaired vasodilation → increased BP • Inflammation, oxidative stress, & insulin resistance → accelerates vascular aging → arterial stiffness → increased BP • Increased free fatty acids → increased alpha-adrenergic tone → increased vascular smooth muscle tone and resistance → vasoconstriction • Increased risk of obstructive sleep apnea (secondary cause of HTN)	Lifestyle: • Sodium restriction • Weight loss (decreases SNS & RAAS response) • Increased water intake • DASH eating plan • Alcohol moderation • Increased physical activity, including muscle strengthening Medications: • RAAS inhibition (decreases humoral response) • Diuretics (addresses salt sensitivity) • Beta-blockers
CHD	• Diet high in fat & carbohydrates → dyslipidemia → increased arterial intima-media thickness → decreased arterial lumen diameter • Increased oxidative stress & proinflammatory cytokines → decreased nitric oxide → vasoconstriction & vascular resistance • Increased ventricular load & decreased diastolic function → less coronary artery filling time • Increased sympathetic tone → increased HR → less coronary artery filling time	Lifestyle: • Caloric restriction • Increased physical activity, including muscle strengthening Medications: • Cholesterol lowering meds (for plaque stabilization) • Antiplatelet therapy (aspirin) • Beta-blockers (increase coronary artery filling time)
HF	• Increased proinflammatory state • Increased preload & stroke volume → compensatory improvement in cardiac output → deteriorates over time • Initially increased LV dilatation → compensatory concentric LV hypertrophy → increased risk of HF • Increased LV end-diastolic pressure, right atrial pressure, pulmonary wedge pressure • Increased arterial HTN	Lifestyle: • Sodium restriction • Fluid restriction for some • Daily weight monitoring Medications: • RAAS inhibition, including aldosterone antagonists • Beta-blockers • Diuretics

Abbreviations: ; DASH, dietary approaches to stop hypertension; HR, heart rate; LV, left ventricular.
Data from Tanaka M. Improving obesity and blood pressure. *Hypertens Res.* 2020;43(2):79-89.

cardiorespiratory fitness levels.[2] However, the exact mechanisms through which increased lean mass may improve cardiorespiratory fitness and prognosis are unclear.[2]

Currently, the most precise way to assess cardiorespiratory fitness is through direct measurement of peak VO_2 collected during a maximal cardiopulmonary exercise test.[2] This test measures patient effort and exercise tolerance. Strategies to increase cardiorespiratory fitness include exercise training (aerobic training combined with resistance training) and structured exercise programs (like cardiac rehabilitation). In addition, weight loss through caloric restriction has demonstrated improvements in both cardiorespiratory fitness and quality of life in patients with obesity and HF, particularly those who have HF with a preserved ejection fraction.[2]

INFLUENCE OF OBESITY ON ASSESSMENT
Vital Signs

Adults with preobesity and obesity are more likely to be deconditioned. Thus, it is prudent to have the patient seated quietly for 15 minutes before checking vital signs to avoid obtaining a falsely elevated heart rate, BP, and/or respiratory rate.

Heart rate

Heart rate, if assessed manually, should be counted for a full minute radially and apically to determine rate and rhythm. As noted, the heart rate may be elevated because of SNS exaggeration, especially if taken immediately after entering the examination room or if the patient is deconditioned. Alternatively, the heart rate may be assessed simultaneously with BP measurement if an automated oscillatory device is used to obtain BP readings. If the heart rate is obtained during oscillatory BP measurement, then the heart rhythm may be assessed during the heart sounds portion of the physical examination.

BP: cuff selection

When measuring BP, it is critical to select the correct cuff size, especially with adults who have obesity. The most frequent error in measuring office BPs is using the wrong size BP cuff, also known as "miscuffing."[9] In adults with obesity, this most often translates to using a cuff that is too small, in which case the BP reading(s) will be falsely elevated. Ideally, the BP cuff bladder length should be 75% to 100% of the patient's measured arm circumference, while the width should be 37% to 50% of the arm circumference, which indicates a length-to-width ratio of 2:1.[9] Generally, in adults with obesity, longer wider cuffs are needed to adequately compress the brachial artery.

Paper measuring tapes are helpful to measure the arm circumference to ensure the correct size cuff is used. Arm circumference should be measured at the midpoint between the acromion process of the shoulder and the elbow.[9] Once the correct size is determined, documentation in the medical record will indicate which size cuff should be used for future patient encounters. If a patient experiences a dramatic weight change, however, reassessment of arm circumference is needed. Relevant to patients with obesity, a large adult cuff should be used for an arm circumference of 35 to 44 cm.[9] Whereas an extra-large adult cuff (also known as a thigh cuff) should be used for an arm circumference measuring 45 to 52 cm.[9]

Upper arm BP measurements (with a properly fitted cuff) are regarded as the gold standard for noninvasive BP measurement.[9,10] However, based on results from a 2016 meta-analysis on BP measurement for diagnosing HTN in adults with obesity, if an extra-large adult size (thigh) cuff is not large enough, a wrist cuff may be used as the next best alternative.[9,10] Notably, wrist measurement has better sensitivity and specificity for diagnosing HTN as compared with the finger measurements (which generally provide falsely lower BP readings).[10] If a wrist BP cuff is used, it is important to place the cuff at the level of the heart. In addition to the upper arm cuff, some clinical settings that specialize in caring for patients with obesity use troncoconical-shaped BP cuffs (in the shape of a cone), which provide a more accurate estimation of BP for individuals with obesity.[9]

BP measurement technique

When measuring BPs, the cuff should be placed on bare skin. Shirt sleeves should not be rolled up because this may create a tourniquet effect (falsely elevating the BP). To correctly position the BP cuff, the midline of the cuff bladder should be positioned over the brachial artery (found by palpating the location in the antecubital fossa). There should be a 2 to 3 cm space between the lower end of the cuff and the antecubital fossa for the stethoscope (if the BP is taken manually). If space is not available for the stethoscope, the patient likely has too small of a cuff being used.

BMI and Waist Circumference

Cardiovascular risk assessment in patients with obesity includes obtaining the patient's BMI and waist circumference. When calculating the BMI, it is important to use a digital scale that measures weight for up to 500 pounds (225 kg).[11] This is especially true for patients with chronic HF, to capture a rise or fall in body weight, as many scales in the home setting have a weight limit of 350 pounds (158 kg).[11]

It is well known that a BMI of >30 kg/m^2 is consistent with obesity. However, there are also subcategories of obesity including class I (30.0–34.9 kg/m^2), class II (35.0–39.9 kg/m^2), and class III ($\geq$40.0 kg/m^2).[12] Notably, lower cut points have been suggested for the Asian population.[12] Awareness of the subcategories of obesity gives clinicians an estimation of the patient's risk for comorbidities. Specifically, class I obesity places a patient at high risk for CVD, whereas classes II and III place patients at very high and extremely high for CVD, respectively.[12] Keep in mind that the largely unexplained obesity paradox (discussed earlier) exists in patients with *existing* CHD and HF with class I obesity; the paradox has not been observed in patients with class II or III obesity.[12]

Waist circumference should be routinely measured during physical assessment for adults who have a BMI of 25 to 39.9 kg/m^2, ideally at each visit.[1] As recommended by the World Health Organization (WHO), waist circumference should be measured with a tape measure placed snuggly (not compressing the skin) horizontally around the waist, *midway* between the lowest ribs and the iliac crest.[13] The measurement should be done while the patient is standing, just after they have exhaled. Waist circumference measured at the midabdomen (WC-mid), as opposed to measuring *at* the superior border of the iliac crest (WC-IC), has been shown to be a better predictor of HTN, diabetes, and metabolic syndrome, particularly in women.[13] Current obesity guidelines define a waist circumference $\geq$ 102 cm (40 inches) for men and $\geq$88 cm (35 inches) for women as the cutoff point that is associated with an increased CVD risk.[1,12] Notably, lower cutoffs are recommended for certain racial/ethnic groups (eg, $\geq$90 cm for Asian men and $\geq$80 cm for Asian women) because of variation in body fat composition.[1,12]

Subjective Assessment

In addition to reviewing past medical and surgical history, current medications (including over-the-counter medications), and family history, it is important to ask patients about current (or past) symptoms that may be suggestive of cardiovascular conditions. Dyspnea at rest or with exertion, including orthopnea (inability to breathe comfortably when lying flat) and paroxysmal nocturnal dyspnea (suddenly waking up short of breath) may be present in patients with obesity, especially in those who are deconditioned. Thus, if any of these symptoms are present, it is important to determine whether the symptoms represent a change from baseline. New or worsened dyspnea could be indicative of CHD (as an anginal equivalent, especially for women, the elderly, and/or those with diabetes) or new-onset or worsened HF. Furthermore, patients with obesity may have comorbid sleep-disordered breathing, placing them at heightened risk for HTN. In fact, a 10% increase in body weight has been shown to be associated with a 6-fold increase in developing obstructive sleep apnea syndrome.[8] This is important because comorbid HTN and obstructive sleep apnea syndrome increase the risk of CHD and stroke.[8] Beyond dyspnea, patients should be asked about the presence of chest pain or pressure; unusual indigestion; neck, jaw, or arm pain/numbness; palpitations, dizziness, or syncope; claudication; and stroke symptoms. As appropriate, patients who have been prescribed nitroglycerin should be asked about recent use (regardless of whether they endorsed chest pain or pressure in the review of symptoms).

CVD Risk

Notably, obesity is not a part of the Atherosclerotic Cardiovascular Disease (ASCVD) risk calculation from the AHA and American College of Cardiology (http://tools.acc.org/ASCVD-Risk-Estimator-Plus/#!/calculate/estimate/). However, several of the components used to calculate 10-year and lifetime ASCVD risk are associated with obesity (namely cholesterol levels, BP, presence of diabetes, treated HTN, and tobacco use).

Physical Examination

Physical examination includes inspection, palpation, auscultation, and percussion—all of which can be obscured by extra viscera and vasculature enclosed in a thick layer of adipose tissue present in patients with obesity.[11] Because of these challenges, the presence of pathologic abnormalities in the structure and function of the heart and vasculature may be underestimated.[11] However, there is limited evidence about best practices to maximize the yield from routine physical examination techniques beyond BP measurement technique when caring for patients with obesity.[11]

Physical examinations (and appointments in general) often take a little more time to complete when caring for patients with obesity. In addition, accommodations to the examination environment are needed including providing chairs without arms, extra-large gowns, and placing reinforced (bolted to the floor) examination tables in their lowest position.[11] For patients with limited mobility, extra time and assistance may be needed to help with undressing and positioning the patient for the examination. Refer to **Table 2** which provides an outline of challenges and suggested accommodations for conducting a focused cardiovascular examination in patients with obesity.[11]

Effect of Obesity on Diagnostic Tests

Common diagnostic tests ordered for patients at risk or with cardiovascular conditions include 12 lead electrocardiogram (ECG), echocardiography, and exercise stress testing—all of which may be confounded by excessive fat mass or the physiologic effects of obesity. Diagnostic testing typically starts with a 12 lead ECG. Testing beyond a 12 lead ECG is determined by risk stratification based on symptoms, risk factors, and functional capacity.

Table 2
Cardiovascular physical examination accommodations for patients with obesity

Body System	Challenge	Accommodation
General	• Patient may be embarrassed to undergo a physical examination or change into a gown	• Use frank, open, respective words to discuss obesity as a medical condition • Provide extra-large gowns • Respectfully ask patient to lift large breasts or abdominal folds as appropriate • Schedule longer appointment if needed
Head and Neck	• Jugular vein pressure difficult to measure • Carotid bruits, if present, may be hard to hear	• Hepatojugular reflex maneuver may help with visualization of jugular veins • Palpate carotid pulse to identify the location of carotid arteries & listen with stethoscope bell while the patient is not breathing
Cardiovascular	• Point of maximal impulse hard to palpate • Right ventricular heave hard to appreciate • Heart sounds may be distant • Murmurs, gallops, rubs hard to discern	• Decrease ambient room noise including conversation during auscultation • Auscultate directly over the skin (not over clothing) • Position stethoscope in optimal ear position of clinician (move head and neck to find the best spot) • Position patient in 2 alternative positions: sitting up and leaning forward or in the left lateral position (both bring heart closer to the chest wall as compared to using the supine position) • Palpate carotid artery when listening to heart sounds (synchronous with S1) to discern S1 vs S2 • Ask patient to stop breathing for a few seconds to listen closely to suspected murmurs, rubs, or gallops. • Ask patient to raise arms above the head when assessing for right ventricular heave to spread out chest wall soft tissue
Respiratory	• Breath sounds may be diminished • Patient may become dyspneic during exam	• Demonstrate mouth breathing for the patient before listening to breath sounds • Have the patient breath in/out as the clinician slowly moves the stethoscope to each position—avoiding rapid shallow breathes

(continued on next page)

Table 2 (continued)		
Body System	Challenge	Accommodation
		• Start at the posterior bases (to detect rales) if the patient tires easily
Abdomen	• Deep structures may be difficult to percuss, palpate, or auscultate for bruits • Presence of ascites may be hidden due to adipose • Bulging flanks not helpful to detect ascites	• Use the "scratch test" to detect the lower liver border (place stethoscope near the umbilicus, costal margin, or liver; lightly and briskly stroke the skin with the finger edge or bristle brush starting at right lower quadrant moving toward right costal margin along the midclavicular line; sound of the scratch first heard through the stethoscope is the liver edge).[14] • Look for ascites using fluid wave or shifting dullness[13] (present if ascitic fluid is > 1500 mL) • If suspect renal artery stenosis, need diagnostic testing
Extremities	• Pulses may be difficult to palpate • Lower extremity edema common and nonspecific	• Use of handheld Doppler to assess peripheral pulses • If suspect fluid overload (especially with heart failure), check for increased weight and S3

Data from Silk AW, McTigue KM. Reexamining the physical examination for obese patients. *JAMA.* 2011;305(2):193 to 194.

There are several changes to the 12 lead ECG that may occur because of obesity. For example, the heart rate is usually about 7 beats per minute higher in adults with obesity versus those with an optimal BMI.[15] Other obesity-associated 12 lead ECG changes may include increased P-wave duration and PR-interval duration (similar to changes seen with atrial enlargement); low QRS voltage especially in the limb leads (due to a thick chest wall); and leftward axis deviation (associated with adipose tissue accumulation around the heart creating a more horizontal position than usual).[15,16] However, leftward axis deviation may also be a result of left ventricular hypertrophy or prolonged QT (or QTc) interval duration (potentially indicating HF and/or CHD).[16,17] Right-sided heart ECG changes, including right axis deviation from ventricular hypertrophy and/or right bundle-branch block, may be indicative of pulmonary HTN.[16] Although nonspecific T wave flattening or inversion may occur, there are usually no ST segment changes associated with obesity.[15] Interestingly, some of these ECG changes are reversible if the patient experiences significant weight loss.[16] Thus, because 12 lead ECGs from patients with obesity often underestimate pathologic abnormalities in structure or function of the heart, it is imperative that prior ECGS (if available) are used for comparison to determine if a change from baseline has occurred.[16]

Echocardiography is helpful in determining if symptoms such as chest pain, dyspnea, and exercise intolerance are cardiac-related. Echocardiography uses high-frequency sound waves (ultrasound) to assess chamber size and function, valve size and function, and wall motion. However, obesity negatively affects echocardiography image quality due to signal attenuation.[18] To overcome this, contrast echocardiography microbubbles may be used to enhance the detection of structural remodeling and left ventricular dysfunction in patients with obesity.[18] In addition, transesophageal echocardiography may be used as an alternative for suboptimal transthoracic echocardiography views.

Stress testing, performed with exercise or pharmacologically, is used to assess for known or suspected cardiac ischemia. However, because exercise performance is inversely related to BMI, many patients with obesity do not have the functional capacity to undergo standard ECG exercise stress testing either due to deconditioning or chronic musculoskeletal pain. Even in the estimated 40% of patients with obesity who can exercise according to the protocol,[19] some exercise bicycles or treadmills have a weight limit. Therefore, stress echocardiography, nuclear stress testing (SPECT or PET), or cardiovascular magnetic resonance imaging provide options for detecting ischemia and assessing right and left ventricular function in patients with obesity. Refer to **Table 3** to review the advantages and disadvantages of each type of noninvasive imaging in patients with obesity.

TREATMENT
Lifestyle Modifications

Lifestyle modifications are the cornerstone of treatment for common cardiovascular conditions, especially for patients with obesity. Specifically, weight reduction, increased physical activity, and dietary modification (including sodium reduction and moderation of alcohol consumption) have all been shown to reduce BP. Furthermore, adopting (and sustaining) a healthy lifestyle, especially one that facilitates weight loss, has been shown to increase the responsiveness to antihypertensive medications and to reduce cardiovascular risk factors.[20]

Weight loss obtained through increased physical activity and dietary modification has been shown to improve survival in patients with CVD.[21-24] Studies have shown a linear relationship between BMI and BP; as BMI increases so does BP.[21] Likewise, with weight loss, there is a reduction in BP (primarily due to a decrease in obesity-associated SNS and RAAS activity).[21] A general rule of thumb is that for every 1 kg of weight loss, there is a 1-point corresponding reduction in systolic BP.[20,21]

Physical activity
Regular physical activity is also an important component of a heart-healthy lifestyle, especially for weight maintenance in those who have been in an active treatment program to reduce weight. In fact, results from meta-analyses have shown that engaging in regular aerobic activity reduces systolic BP as much as ~ 5 mm Hg and diastolic BP ~ 3 mm Hg.[23,25] Therefore, based on the WHO recommendations for physical activity, adults aged 18 years and above (including those with chronic health conditions and/or living with disability, unless contraindicated) should be instructed to engage in at least 150 to 300 minutes of moderate-intensity aerobic physical activity per week (eg, walking briskly at 4 miles/h).[24] This equates to an average of ~30 minutes per day, 5 days a week. Alternatively, if the adult is able to undertake vigorous intensity aerobic activity (eg, jogging at 6 miles/h), the goal is for less accumulative minutes per week (75–100 minutes per week).[24] In addition to the aerobic activity, adults are encouraged to do muscle-strengthening activities that involve all major muscle groups at least 2 or more days per week.[24]

If the patient is not currently meeting the WHO guideline recommendations, it is best to start with small amounts of activity (in duration, frequency, and intensity).[24] A key

Table 3
Noninvasive cardiovascular imaging options for patients with obesity

Type of Imaging	Advantages	Disadvantages
Stress echocardiography (SE)	• More widely available • Portable (can be done at bedside) • Relatively lower cost (compared to other imaging options) • No radiation exposure • Physiologic stress option available (bicycle or treadmill if patient can exercise) • Able to use with patients who have cardiac devices, kidney failure, asthma, or claustrophobia	• Limited by suboptimal image quality (somewhat better with ultrasound enhancing contrast agents) • Requires intravenous access (unless physiologic stress option used)
Single-photon emission computed tomography (SPECT) or positron emission tomography (PET)	• Physiologic stress option available (bicycle or treadmill if patient can exercise) • Able to use for patients who have cardiac devices and kidney failure	• Exposure to ionizing radiation • Excess soft tissue produces artifact which may appear as myocardial perfusion defects (less so with technetium tracers) • Costs more than stress echocardiography • Less available than stress echocardiography • Requires intravenous access (unless physiologic stress option used) • Contraindicated in patients with asthma or those with claustrophobia
Cardiovascular magnetic resonance (CMR)	• Excellent image quality • No exposure to ionizing radiation	• Less available, costs more than stress echocardiography • Requires intravenous access • Requires repeated breath holding for sequence acquisitions • Contraindicated in patients with asthma, kidney failure, or claustrophobia (tight space with loud noise) • Contraindicated in patients with cardiac devices within the past 5 y (pacemakers, implanted defibrillators, or cardiac resynchronization devices)

Data from Shah BN, Senior R. Stress echocardiography in patients with morbid obesity. *Echo Res Pract.* 2016; 3(2):R13-R18.

message to convey to patients is that *some* physical activity is *better than none*.[24] In addition, keep in mind that even low-intensity activity (ie, walking at a comfortable pace) for patients with obesity may result in significant fatigue as it represents a higher level of intensity expended as compared to those who do not have obesity.[22] For example, adults with a normal weight BMI typically use about 35% of aerobic capacity when walking at a comfortable pace as compared to individuals with obesity who expend about 56% or more to match the same demands.[22] Generally, medical clearance is not needed for patients with CVD to begin regular physical activity, especially if they begin with low-level intensity activity.[24] However, referral to physical therapy or cardiac rehabilitation is encouraged for those interested in a supervised exercise program, especially if the patient has been recently hospitalized for HF or CHD.

Dietary modification

For patients with obesity-related HTN, a palatable low sodium diet (eg, the Dietary Approaches to Stop Hypertension [DASH] eating plan) that has been shown to reduce BP is recommended.[20] Endorsed by the National Heart Lung and Blood Institute (https://www.nhlbi.nih.gov/health-topics/dash-eating-plan), the DASH eating plan that is rich in potassium, calcium, magnesium, and fiber; fruits, vegetables, nuts, seeds and legumes; low (or no) fat dairy products; and poultry and fish.[20,25,26] The DASH eating plan discourages sodium, saturated fat and cholesterol, red meats, and sweet foods or sugary beverages.[20,26] In patients with elevated BP and stage I HTN, a combination of the DASH diet and sodium reduction (1150 mg vs 2300 mg/d) has been shown to reduce systolic BP by as much as 20.8 mm Hg (1150 mg sodium/d) and 9.7 mm Hg (2300 mg sodium/d) as compared to a high-sodium (3450 mg/d) control diet ($P < .001$).[26] BP reductions are greatest in those with higher (>140 mm Hg) versus lower (120–139) baseline systolic BPs.[26] This decrease in systolic BP from a combined DASH diet plus sodium reduction is comparable to pharmacologic treatment using angiotensin-converting enzyme inhibitors (ACE-Is), beta-blockers, and calcium-channel blockers (~ 12, ~ 13, and ~ 16 mm Hg, respectively).[26] Beyond treating HTN, the DASH eating plan is also appropriate for patients with CHD and chronic HF. However, if the patient has a history of hyperkalemia, they should be cautioned against ingesting foods high in potassium.

Sodium reduction

Salt sensitivity has been shown to be associated with obesity.[20] Thus, sodium reduction for patients with cardiovascular conditions and obesity is indicated due to the joint benefit gained. The 2018 American College of Cardiology (ACC)/AHA guidelines for HTN indicate an optimal goal of no more than 1500 mg of sodium/d, which can reduce systolic BP as much as 5 to 6 mm Hg.[25] However, because the average adult in American ingests more than twice this amount, a goal of at least a 1000 mg/d reduction may be more desirable for some patients. In the absence of data, these same recommendations are used for patients with CHD or those with symptomatic chronic HF.

Alcohol moderation

Increased alcohol intake has been associated with higher BP and greater long-term weight gain. In fact, research has shown that for every 10 g of alcohol (one standard serving), there is a corresponding increase in systolic BP by 1 mm Hg.[20] Thus, the recommendation for adults with HTN and comorbid obesity is for no more than one serving of alcohol (5 oz of wine, 12 oz of regular beer, 8–9 oz malt liquor/IPA beer, or 1.5 oz of 80 proof liquor) for women and no more than 2 servings per day for men.[25] Moderation of alcohol equates to an approximate 3 to 4 mm Hg reduction in systolic BP.[25]

Smoking cessation

Generally, adults who smoke cigarettes tend to have a lower body weight. However, since unhealthy behaviors tend to cluster together, it is important to assess tobacco use in adults who have comorbid CVD and obesity. Negative effects of smoking include an acute rise in BP and overtime increased arterial stiffness.[20] Because smoking cessation has been shown to be associated with weight gain, pharmacologic treatment for smoking cessation should be accompanied by behavioral counseling.[20]

Pharmacologic Treatment

Patients with comorbid obesity and HTN are more likely to have treatment-resistant BP and higher rates of end-organ damage due to uncontrolled HTN.[21,25] Beyond the adipose tissue mechanism driving higher BP, obesity influences the pharmacokinetics and pharmacodynamics of common cardiovascular medications. For example, alterations in absorption may occur due to polypharmacy (needing more medications to treat BP).[21] Patients with obesity also have an expanded volume of distribution, which could result in greater distribution to lean tissue (in beta-blockers for example) indicating that starting dosage should be based on lean tissue, not BMI.[27] Hepatic metabolism may also be delayed in patients with obesity, most commonly due to nonalcoholic fatty liver disease.[21] Impairments in renal clearance may also occur due to obesity-associated glomerular hyperfiltration or comorbid chronic kidney disease, both resulting in delayed clearance.[21]

First-line treatment for HTN includes RAAS blockers (ACE-Is or ARBs), calcium channel blockers (dihydropyridines [eg, amlodipine] or nondihydropyridines [eg, verapamil or diltiazem]), and/or thiazide or thiazide-like diuretics (chlorthalidone is preferred due to its prolonged half-life).[25] Refer to the ACC/AHA 2018 HTN treatment guidelines for more details.[25] A BP target of less than 130/80 mm Hg is recommended; treatment goals do not differ for patients with obesity.[25]

Pharmacologic treatment for chronic HF with reduced ejection fraction includes baseline therapy with target doses of an RAAS blocker (ACE-I, ARB, or angiotensin receptor neprilysin inhibitor [ARNI]), beta-blocker (only those approved for HF), diuretic (generally a loop due to co-morbid kidney disease), and an aldosterone antagonist.[28] Target doses of each of these medication classes do not differ for patients with obesity other than for carvedilol; the target dose is higher (50 mg twice daily) for patients who weigh $\geq$ 85 kg.[28]

Pharmacologic treatment for CHD includes antiplatelet agents (daily aspirin), beta-blockers, statins, and RAAS blockers (especially if the patient has left ventricular dysfunction).[29] Anti-ischemic medications (eg, nitrates, calcium channel blockers, and ranolazine) may be considered for patients as appropriate. As with HTN, treatment goals (or medication doses) do not differ for patients with obesity. Selection of which beta-blocker to prescribe should be carefully considered as the majority are obesogenic and could worsen obesity for a patient with CHD.

Antiobesity Treatment

Historically, antiobesity medications have been used cautiously with patients who have CVD. Two antiobesity medications, fenfluramine and sibutramine, that were previously FDA approved for weight loss in the United States were removed from the market because of serious cardiac adverse effects.[30] Currently, there are several options to choose from that may be used in patients with cardiovascular conditions (phentermine, orlistat, liraglutide, lorcaserin, phentermine/topiramate, and naltrexone/bupropion).[30] Many of these agents have pleiotropic (added beneficial) effects beyond weight loss for patients with CVD, such as modest reductions in BP, LDL cholesterol, and blood glucose.[30] However, although HTN and dyslipidemia are common comorbid conditions in patients that are prescribed these agents, some agents (eg, phentermine) are contraindicated in patients with uncontrolled HTN, CHD, HF, and/or arrhythmias. Thus, providers should refer to the latest packet insert for antiobesity medications to confirm the indications/contraindications for specific patients to determine risk/benefit.

Bariatric surgery may be considered for patients with obesity that have severe disease. Beneficial effects of bariatric surgery on cardiovascular conditions include long-term and short-term reduction in HTN and cardiovascular risk reduction of diabetes, HF, and AFib.[7,31] The most common types of bariatric surgery include laparoscopic-adjustable gastric banding, roux-en-Y gastric bypass, and sleeve gastrectomy.[7,31] Generally, patients are referred to bariatric programs to discuss options, to determine if there is an FDA indication for the particular procedure, and to arrange nutritional counseling before and after the procedure to obtain and maintain the desired weight loss.

SUMMARY

In everyday clinical practice, nurses frequently encounter adults who have obesity and comorbid cardiovascular conditions. Physical assessment techniques, including attainment of vital signs, should be adapted to accommodate patients with obesity to ensure findings are accurate. Nurses should also be mindful of how CVD risk increases with co-occurring obesity to inform patient education regarding lifestyle modifications. Finally, although the obesity paradox exists, nurses should continue to work with patients to aim for an appropriate BMI while taking into consideration cardiorespiratory fitness.

CLINICS CARE POINTS

- Accurate blood pressure measurement in adults with obesity is dependent on using an appropriately sized blood pressure cuff.
- Physical examination techniques should be accommodated for patients with obesity.
- It is essential to develop treatment plans to address obesity in the context of cardiovascular conditions.
- Lifestyle modifications are a vital part of the treatment plan for patients with comorbid obesity and cardiovascular conditions.

DISCLOSURE

The authors have nothing to disclose.

REFERENCES

1. Virani SS, Alonso A, Benjamin EJ, et al. Heart disease and stroke statistics-2020 update: a report from the American Heart Association. Circulation 2020;141(9): e139–596.
2. Carbone S, Canada JM, Billingsley HE, et al. Obesity paradox in cardiovascular disease: where do we stand? Vasc Health Risk Manag 2019;15:89–100.
3. Jayedi A, Shab-Bidar S. Nonlinear dose-response association between body mass index and risk of all-cause and cardiovascular mortality in patients with hypertension: a meta-analysis. Obes Res Clin Pract 2018;12(1):16–28.

4. Lavie CJ, De Schutter A, Parto P, et al. Obesity and prevalence of cardiovascular diseases and prognosis-the obesity paradox updated. Prog Cardiovasc Dis 2016;58(5):537–47.
5. Carbone S, Lavie CJ, Arena R. Obesity and heart failure: focus on the obesity paradox. Mayo Clin Proc 2017;92(2):266–79.
6. Sandhu RK, Ezekowitz J, Andersson U, et al. The 'obesity paradox' in atrial fibrillation: observations from the ARISTOTLE (Apixaban for Reduction in Stroke and Other Thromboembolic Events in Atrial Fibrillation) trial. Eur Heart J 2016;37(38): 2869–78.
7. Landsberg L, Aronne LJ, Beilin LJ, et al. Obesity-related hypertension: pathogenesis, cardiovascular risk, and treatment: a position paper of The Obesity Society and the American Society of Hypertension. J Clin Hypertens (Greenwich) 2013; 15(1):14–33.
8. Tanaka M. Improving obesity and blood pressure. Hypertens Res 2020;43(2): 79–89.
9. Muntner P, Shimbo D, Carey RM, et al. Measurement of blood pressure in humans: a scientific statement from the American Heart Association. Hypertension 2019;73(5):e35–66.
10. Irving G, Holden J, Stevens R, et al. Which cuff should I use? Indirect blood pressure measurement for the diagnosis of hypertension in patients with obesity: a diagnostic accuracy review. BMJ Open 2016;6(11):e012429.
11. Silk AW, McTigue KM. Reexamining the physical examination for obese patients. JAMA 2011;305(2):193–4.
12. Kushner RF. Clinical assessment and management of adult obesity. Circulation 2012;126(24):2870–7.
13. Ma WY, Yang CY, Shih SR, et al. Measurement of waist circumference: midabdominal or iliac crest? Diabetes Care 2013;36(6):1660–6.
14. Gupta K, Dhawan A, Abel C, et al. A re-evaluation of the scratch test for locating the liver edge. BMC Gastroenterol 2013;13:35.
15. Blackstone RP. The assessment of the adult patient with overweight and obesity. In: Blackstone RP, editor. Obesity: the medical practitioner's essential guide. Cham: Springer; 2016. p. 193–229. Available at: https://link.springer.com/book/ 10.1007%2F978-3-319-39409-1. Accessed April 9, 2021.
16. Hassing GJ, van der Wall HEC, van Westen GJP, et al. Body mass index related electrocardiographic findings in healthy young individuals with a normal body mass index. Neth Heart J 2019;27(10):506–12.
17. Kurisu S, Ikenaga H, Watanabe N, et al. Electrocardiographic characteristics in the underweight and obese in accordance with the World Health Organization classification. IJC Metab Endocr 2015;9:61–5.
18. El Hajj MC, Litwin SE. Echocardiography in the era of obesity. J Am Soc Echocardiogr 2020;33(7):779–87.
19. Shah BN, Senior R. Stress echocardiography in patients with morbid obesity. Echo Res Pract 2016;3(2):R13–8.
20. Leggio M, Lombardi M, Caldarone E, et al. The relationship between obesity and hypertension: an updated comprehensive overview on vicious twins. Hypertens Res 2017;40(12):947–63.
21. Cohen JB, Gadde KM. Weight loss medications in the treatment of obesity and hypertension. Curr Hypertens Rep 2019;21(2):16.
22. Poirier P, Alpert MA, Fleisher LA, et al. Cardiovascular evaluation and management of severely obese patients undergoing surgery: a science advisory from the American Heart Association. Circulation 2009;120(1):86–95.

23. Akyuz A. Exercise and coronary heart disease. Adv Exp Med Biol 2020;1228: 169–79.
24. Bull FC, Al-Ansari SS, Biddle S, et al. World Health Organization 2020 guidelines on physical activity and sedentary behaviour. Br J Sports Med 2020;54(24): 1451–62.
25. Whelton PK, Carey RM, Aronow WS, et al. 2017 ACC/AHA/AAPA/ABC/ACPM/ AGS/APhA/ASH/ASPC/NMA/PCNA guideline for the prevention, detection, evaluation, and management of high blood pressure in adults: a report of the American College of Cardiology/American Heart Association task force on clinical practice guidelines. Hypertension 2018;71(6):e13–115.
26. Juraschek SP, Miller ER 3rd, Weaver CM, et al. Effects of sodium reduction and the DASH diet in relation to baseline blood pressure. J Am Coll Cardiol 2017; 70(23):2841–8.
27. Sankaralingam S, Kim RB, Padwal RS. The impact of obesity on the pharmacology of medications used for cardiovascular risk factor control. Can J Cardiol 2015;31(2):167–76.
28. Maddox TM, Januzzi JL Jr, Allen LA, et al. 2021 Update to the 2017 ACC expert consensus decision pathway for optimization of heart failure treatment: answers to 10 pivotal issues about heart failure with reduced ejection fraction: a report of the American College of Cardiology solution set oversight committee. J Am Coll Cardiol 2021;77(6):772–810.
29. Amsterdam EA, Wenger NK, Brindis RG, et al. 2014 AHA/ACC guideline for the management of patients with non-ST-elevation acute coronary syndromes: a report of the American College of Cardiology/American Heart Association task force on practice guidelines. J Am Coll Cardiol 2014;64(24):e139–228.
30. Kushner RF. Weight loss strategies for treatment of obesity: lifestyle management and pharmacotherapy. Prog Cardiovasc Dis 2018;61(2):246–52.
31. Jensen MD, Ryan DH, Apovian CM, et al. 2013 AHA/ACC/TOS guideline for the management of overweight and obesity in adults: a report of the American College of Cardiology/American Heart Association Task Force on Practice Guidelines and The Obesity Society. Circulation 2014;129(25 Suppl 2):S102–38.

Obesity and Diabetes

Mohini Aras, MD*, Beverly G. Tchang, MD,
Joy Pape, MSN, RN, FNP-C, CDCES, CFCN, FADCES

KEYWORDS

- Type 2 diabetes • Overweight and obesity • Intensive lifestyle modification
- Weight centric approach to the treatment of diabetes
- Antihyperglycemic pharmacotherapy • Antiobesity pharmacotherapy
- Surgical treatment for obesity and diabetes

KEY POINTS

- Obesity and type 2 diabetes are inextricably linked and their pathophysiologies overlap in such a way that treatment of one often results in improvement in the other.
- One in 5 adults with obesity also has type 2 diabetes.
- Adopting a weight-centric approach to the treatment of diabetes is imperative with a focus on selecting weight-reducing antihyperglycemic medications including metformin, glucagon-like peptide 1RA, and sodium-glucose transporter 2 inhibitor.
- Metabolic surgery is the most effective intervention for both weight loss and improved glycemia in patients with diabetes and a body mass index of 35 kg/m^2 or greater.

DEFINITIONS

Obesity is a state of energy dysregulation characterized by impaired appetitive hormone signaling and excess adiposity. Body mass index (BMI) classifies obesity based on severity (**Table 1**).[1,2] *Type 2 diabetes* (T2D) is a state of relative insulin insufficiency and peripheral insulin resistance resulting in hyperglycemia.[3]

EPIDEMIOLOGY

From 2013 to 2016, the prevalence of adult obesity (age $\geq$20 years) was 38.8%.[4] The prevalence of T2D was 14.0%,[5] and 1 in 5 adults with obesity also had T2D[5] (**Fig. 1**). Populations models predict that 1 out of every 2 adults in the United States will have obesity by 2030.[6] The risk of incident T2D increases with higher BMI,[7] with greater risk conferred by earlier weight gain.[8]

Division of Endocrinology at Weill Cornell Medicine, Comprehensive Weight Control Center, 1165 York Avenue, New York, NY 10021, USA
* Corresponding author.
E-mail address: moa9031@med.cornell.edu

Nurs Clin N Am 56 (2021) 527–541
https://doi.org/10.1016/j.cnur.2021.07.008
0029-6465/21/© 2021 Elsevier Inc. All rights reserved.

Table 1 BMI thresholds		
BMI (kg/m²)	Non-Asian	Asian
Normal weight	18.0–24.9	18.5–22.9
Overweight	25.0–29.9	23.0–27.4
Obesity		>27.5
Class I	30.0–34.9	
Class II	35.0–39.9	
Class III	>40	

ECONOMIC BURDEN

The economic costs of obesity or diabetes encompass direct medical costs as well as indirect costs related to losses in productivity caused by premature mortality, disability, and absenteeism. Costs of obesity were predicted to double every decade reaching $860 to 956 billion by 2030.[9] A 1.0 kg/m² increase above normal BMI conferred a 7% increase in direct, personal health costs.[10] Individuals with diabetes incurred an average $16,750 of medical expenditures per year, about 2.3 times higher than individuals without diabetes.[11]

PATHOPHYSIOLOGY

The relationship between obesity and T2D is complex. The prevailing model of "diabesity" begins with overnutrition and associated leptin resistance (**Fig. 2**). The impaired leptin action results in the accumulation of fat in nonadipose tissues, such as the pancreas and skeletal muscle, where excess free fatty acids induce a state of peripheral insulin resistance and pancreatic β-cell apoptosis, a process defined as "lipotoxicity".[12] Because insulin is an anorexigenic hormone, the impaired insulin secretion and peripheral insulin resistance that characterize T2D stimulates food intake.[13] If beta cell function is relatively preserved, as in the early stages of T2D, hyperinsulinemia suppresses lipolysis, resulting in increased adiposity.[14]

SCREENING

All adults should be screened for obesity at every clinic visit with height and weight measurements to calculate the BMI.[15] Screening for T2D is recommended by the

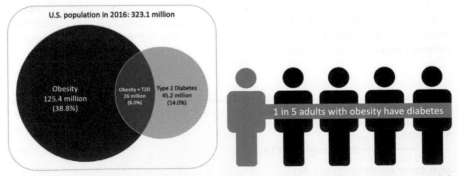

Fig. 1. Prevalence of obesity and T2D in US adults from 2013 to 2016. (*Data from*: Mendola et al.[5])

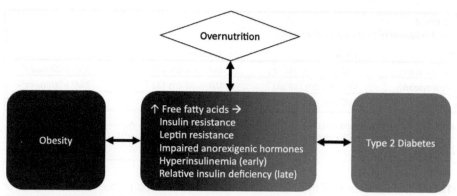

Fig. 2. The pathophysiology of the "diabesity" model to explain the complex relationship between obesity and T2D.[12–14]

American Diabetes Association (ADA) starting at age 45, with specific considerations for special populations (**Table 2**).[3]

DIAGNOSIS

The diagnosis of obesity is confirmed with a BMI of 30 kg/m² or greater in the non-Asian individual or a BMI of 27.5 kg/m² or greater in a person of Asian descent. Other criteria, such as waist circumference, have been recommended to diagnose abdominal obesity specifically because visceral adiposity confers greater risk of cardiometabolic diseases than other adiposity distributions (**Table 3**).[16] The diagnosis of T2D is made through 2 abnormal test results in the absence of hyperglycemic crisis

Table 2	
Screening recommendations for T2D	
Population	**Screening Recommendation**
Age ≥45 without risk factors	Every ≤3 y if asymptomatic and initial screening test is normal
Age <45, BMI ≥25 kg/m², ≥1 risk factor,[a] non-Asian descent	
Age <45, BMI ≥23 kg/m², ≥1 risk factor,[a] Asian descent	
All adults with history of GDM	
All adults with prediabetes	Annually
All adults with HIV	Screen with a fasting glucose test before starting ART, at the time of switching ART, and 3–6 mo after starting or switching ART. If initial screening results are normal, fasting glucose should be checked annually

Abbreviations: ART, antiretroviral therapy; GDM, gestational diabetes mellitus; HIV, human immunodeficiency virus.

[a] Risk factors include a first-degree relative with diabetes, high-risk race/ethnicity (eg, African American, Latino, Native American, Asian American, Pacific Islander), history of cardiovascular disease, hypertension (blood pressure ≥140/90 mm Hg or on antihypertensive medications), high-density lipoprotein cholesterol of <35 mg/dL or triglycerides of >250 mg/dL; polycystic ovarian syndrome, physical inactivity, signs of insulin resistance (eg, acanthosis nigricans, abdominal obesity).

Table 3
Anthropometric measures of obesity

	Men	Women	All
American	WC >102 cm (40 in)	WC >88 cm (35 in)	BMI >30 kg/m²
European	WC >94 cm (37 in)	WC >80 cm (32 in)	BMI >30 kg/m²
Asian	WC >90 cm (35 in)	WC >80 cm (32 in)	BMI >27.5 kg/m²

Abbreviations: WC, waist circumference.
  Source from: Waist Circumference and Waist-Hip Ratio, World Health Organization, Geneva, 2008.[16]

(**Table 4**) or symptoms of hyperglycemia with random blood glucose of 200 mg/dL or greater.[3]

  The choice of laboratory test should be informed by clinical reasoning and practical considerations. Although hemoglobin A1c (HbA1c) is preferred by many because it provides a 3-month estimate of glucose excursions, an A1c of 6.5% or greater misses 30% of T2D diagnosed by fasting plasma glucose or impaired glucose tolerance.[3] HbA1c can be inaccurate in patients with altered red blood cell turnover, altered glycation rate, or hemoglobin variants (**Table 5**). In these patients, fasting plasma glucose or impaired glucose tolerance diagnostic criteria should be used.

TREATMENT OF OBESITY AND TYPE 2 DIABETES

The glycemic targets for an individual with T2D may vary. In general, the ADA recommends a HbA1c goal for nonpregnant adults of less than 7% (53 mmol/mol) and a less strict goal of less than 8% (64 mmol/mol) in older adults or patients with limited life expectancy[19] to decrease the risk of microvascular and macrovascular complications of T2D. The treatment goal for obesity is clinically significant weight loss defined as 5% or more of total body weight, which significantly improves insulin resistance, beta cell function, and cardiometabolic parameters.[20] This degree of weight loss renders clinically significant improvements in blood pressure, glycemia, and lipids, thus decreasing the risk of progression to diabetes.[21] Achieving this clinically meaningful

Table 4
Diagnostic criteria for T2D in adults

Laboratory Diagnosis
Two of 3:
Fasting plasma glucose >126 mg/dL
2-h postprandial glucose >200 mg/dL
Hemoglobin A1c ≥ 6.5%
Clinical Diagnosis
Random blood glucose ≥200 mg/dL plus any of the following:
Polyuria
Polydipsia
Unintentional weight loss
Increased thirst
Fatigue
Diabetic ketoacidosis

Table 5
Conditions that may affect accuracy of HbA1c in the diagnosis of T2D

Increased HbAlc	Decreased HbAlc
Iron deficiency anemia	Iron repletion
Vitamin B_{12} deficiency	Vitamin B_{12} repletion
High-dose aspirin	Aspirin, vitamin C, vitamin E
Chronic kidney disease	Hemodialysis
Alcoholism	Chronic liver disease
Splenomegaly	Splenectomy
Some antiretroviral treatments	Erythropoietin therapy
Rheumatoid arthritis	Blood transfusion
Hemoglobinopathies	Hemoglobinopathies
Genetic variants	Genetic variants

Data from: Gallagher et al.[17] National Institutes of Diabetes Digestive and Kidney Diseases.[18]

weight loss and improved glycemic control requires a multidisciplinary approach focused on lifestyle interventions, including behavioral changes, nutrition, and physical activity, in addition to pharmacotherapy and possible endobariatric or other surgical management (**Table 6**).[22,23]

LIFESTYLE MODIFICATION

Lifestyle modification, which includes behavioral counseling, nutritional changes and exercise, is the cornerstone to both weight and diabetes management. The Look Action for Health and Diabetes (AHEAD) trial[24] randomized 5145 patients with T2D (average baseline A1c of 7.25%) and overweight or obesity to an intensive lifestyle modification program or a standard diabetes support and education group. For the duration of the study, with a median follow-up of 9.6 years, there was a significantly greater decrease in weight (8.6% vs 0.7% from baseline at 1 year and 6.0% vs 3.5% at the end of the study) and significantly greater reduction in HbA1c in the intensive group by −0.22% at 1 year compared with standard diabetes education. Although the incidence of cardiovascular events were similar in both groups, the intensive lifestyle modification group required fewer medications and reported improved quality of life.[24]

Nutrition

Nutritional interventions of various eating patterns have been shown to have significant improvements in glycemia with decrease in HbA1c by up to 2%.[25] No one diet,

Table 6
Treatment options recommended in patients with T2D and overweight or obesity according to BMI categories

	BMI Category (kg/m²)			
	25.0–26.9	27.0–29.9	30.0–34.9	>35.0
Lifestyle modification	x	x	x	
Pharmacotherapy		x	x	
Endobariatric procedures			x	x
Metabolic surgery				x

Data from: American Diabetes Association[22] and Sharaiha et al.[23]

eating pattern, or macronutrient breakdown is applicable to all individuals with diabetes and obesity. The ADA recommends that nutritional counseling should be focused on incorporating nonstarchy vegetables, minimizing added sugar and refined grains, and avoidance of highly processed foods.[25] The chosen diet must establish a calorie deficit to induce weight loss. The Obesity Society guidelines recommend 1200 to 1500 kcal/d for women and 1500 to 1800 kcal/d for men or decreasing daily caloric intake by 500 to 750 kcal, but recommendations should always be tailored to patients' goals.[21,26]

Physical Activity and Exercise

In addition to nutrition, increased physical activity is necessary for comprehensive management of both obesity and diabetes. Physical activity is associated with improvements in cardiovascular mortality, insulin resistance, glycemia, blood pressure, and lipid parameters.[27,28] The ADA recommends at least 150 minutes per week of moderate-to-vigorous intensity aerobic activity weekly in addition to 2 to 3 sessions per week of resistance exercise.[28,29]

PHARMACOTHERAPY

For many patients with obesity and T2D, intensive lifestyle modification is not sufficient to achieve and maintain weight loss and glucose control. Pharmacotherapy is an adjunct to intensive lifestyle modification and is the next step for the treatment of obesity in an individual with T2D. The Endocrine Society guidelines recommend consideration of pharmacotherapy in individuals with a BMI of 30 kg/m^2 or greater or a BMI of 27 kg/m^2 or greater with at least 1 obesity-related comorbidity; examples include T2D, hypertension, hyperlipidemia, or obstructive sleep apnea.[30] The purpose of pharmacotherapy is to strengthen adherence to behavioral modifications and to address comorbidities and pathophysiologic mechanisms that cause weight gain.[31]

Antihyperglycemic Medications

The primary goal of antihyperglycemic medications in T2D is achieving improved glucose control; however, practitioners should be mindful in their selection of these medications because many conventional antihyperglycemic medications contribute to weight gain (**Table 7**).[32] To limit the use of insulin or other obesogenic antihyperglycemic medications, practitioners should maximize the use of weight-reducing or weight-neutral antihyperglycemic medications.

Metformin

Metformin is the first-line pharmacologic agent for the treatment of T2D because it is effective, safe, and inexpensive.[33] It is generally well-tolerated; common side effects are nausea, bloating, abdominal discomfort, and diarrhea or constipation. Metformin increases insulin sensitivity by improving peripheral glucose uptake, decreases intestinal glucose absorption, and decreases gluconeogenesis. It also may have anorectic effects directly[34] or indirectly through its effect on glucagon-like peptide-1 (GLP-1)[35] or growth/differentiation factor-15.[36] Metformin is associated with a 2% long-term average weight loss in clinical trials[37] and about 7% average weight loss has been observed in clinical practice.[38] Metformin should be continued as long as it is tolerated and not contraindicated. Unfortunately, because T2D is a progressive disease, monotherapy with metformin plus intensive lifestyle modification may not be sufficient in achieving glycemic goals and, thus, combination therapy may be required. The selection of the next antihyperglycemic agent for improved glycemic control in patients with

Table 7
The effects of glucose-lowering therapies on weight

Weight Gain	Weight Neutral	Weight Loss
Insulin	α- Glucosidase inhibitors (acarbose, miglitol)	Biguanides (metformin)
SUs (glipizide, glimepiride, gliclazide)	DPP4i (sitagliptin, saxagliptin, linagliptin, alogliptin)	GLP-1RA (exenatide, lixisenatide, liraglutide, dulaglutide, semaglutide)
Meglitinides (repaglinide, nateglinide)	–	SGLT-2i (dapagliflozin, canagliflozin, empagliflozin, ertugliflozin)
TZDs (rosiglitazone, pioglitazone)	–	Amylin analogs (pramlintide)

Abbreviations: DPP4i, Dipeptidyl peptidase 4 inhibitors; GLP-1RA, glucagon-like peptide 1 receptor agonists; SGLT-2i, sodium-glucose cotransporter 2 inhibitors; SU, sulfonylureas; TZD, thiazolidinediones.
Data from: Van Gaal L et al.[32]

overweight or obesity is a GLP-1 receptor agonist (GLP-1RA) or sodium-glucose transporter-2 inhibitor (SGLT-2i).[33]

Glucagon-like peptide-1R agonists

GLP-1 is an endogenous peptide hormone that is secreted by the gut in response to the ingestion of food. GLP-1RA improve glycemia by increasing glucose-dependent insulin secretion and decreasing glucagon secretion.[32,39] GLP-1RA promote weight loss by decreasing gastric emptying to increase satiety[40] and through their actions in the central nervous system to increase satiety and decrease appetite.[41] GLP-1RA are a class of medications that include 5 GLP-1RAs (exenatide, liraglutide 1.8 mg, dulaglutide, lixisenatide, and semaglutide) that are approved by the US Food and Drug Administration for T2D and 1 (liraglutide 3.0 mg) that is approved for obesity. Phase III clinical trials show average HbA1c decreases of 1.0% to 1.5% and average weight losses of 2 to 6 kg.[39] This class of medications has been shown to be safe and to reduce macrovascular complications of T2D in cardiovascular outcomes trials.[42] Dulaglutide is the only GLP-1RA approved for the primary prevention of cardiovascular disease; dulaglutide, liraglutide, and subcutaneous semaglutide are all approved for the secondary prevention of cardiovascular disease. GLP-1RA are generally well-tolerated and the most common side effects include nausea, vomiting, and diarrhea.[39] The effects of GLP-1RA are glucose dependent and thus unlikely to cause hypoglycemia, but the risk is higher in individuals on insulin or insulin secretagogues. Practitioners should plan a 20% decrease in the basal insulin dose when GLP-1RA is initiated[43] and a 30% to 40% decrease in prandial insulin.[44] Caution is recommended in patients with a history of pancreatitis or retinopathy; lipase and amylase levels are not predictive of pancreatitis and regular monitoring is not recommended. GLP-1RAs are contraindicated in the setting of a personal or family history of medullary thyroid carcinoma or in patients with multiple endocrine neoplasia syndrome type 2, but the mechanism by which it causes cancer has been found to be specific only to rodents.[45] Most GLP-1RA are subcutaneous injectables with varying frequency from twice daily to once weekly. Oral semaglutide is the only noninjectable GLP-1RA, which could be preferable to some patients.

Sodium-glucose transporter-2 inhibitors

SGLT-2 inhibitors induce glucosuria by preventing the reabsorption of glucose at the sodium-glucose cotransporter 2 in the proximal tubular cells of the kidney. SGLT-2i decrease both blood glucose and body weight through the same mechanism of increasing renal glucose excretion to about 90 g of glucose per day or about 360 kcal/d.[46] SGLT-2 inhibitors currently approved for T2D are canagliflozin, dapagliflozin, empagliflozin, and ertugliflozin. This class of medications has been shown to decrease HbA1c levels by approximately −0.61% when added to metformin and are associated with about −2 kg of weight loss.[47] Cardiovascular outcomes trials including EMPA-REG OUTCOME, CANVAS, and CREDENCE have shown a decrease in the rates of cardiovascular events and slowed progression the of diabetic kidney disease.[42] SGLT-2i are generally well-tolerated, and the most common side effects include an increased risk of genitourinary infections and volume depletion.[33] Rare adverse events include euglycemic diabetic ketoacidosis and Fournier's gangrene.[33] Similar to GLP-1RA, expect insulin requirements to decrease and plan to decrease insulin regimens by up to 20% to avoid hypoglycemia.[48]

ANTIOBESITY MEDICATIONS

Metformin, GLP-1RA, and SGLT-2i are the preferred antihyperglycemic agents used to concurrently treat both T2D and overweight or obesity. However, if these agents are not tolerated, contraindicated, or result in a persistent BMI of 27 kg/m^2 or more despite maximal use, antiobesity medications should be considered to facilitate weight loss and thereby further improve glycemic and cardiovascular risk factors. There are 4 medications approved by the US Food and Drug Administration for the long-term treatment of obesity, which have all been shown to be safe and effective in patients with diabetes (**Table 8**).[49–57] Details on treatment of obesity are discussed elsewhere in this issue (3: Current Evidence-based Treatment of Obesity). Treatment of obesity in patients with T2D is particularly challenging as patients with both obesity and T2D lose about 25% less weight than those with obesity alone.[46]

METABOLIC SURGERY

Metabolic surgery is the most effective intervention for achieving and maintaining weight loss and improved glycemic control in patients with T2D and obesity. It is currently recommended for patients with a BMI of 35 kg/m^2 or greater and T2D.[26] The ADA further recommends consideration of metabolic surgery in patients with T2D and a BMI as low as 30.0 kg/m^2 who do not achieve control of hyperglycemia despite maximal medical management.[22] In the United States, the most common procedures include sleeve gastrectomy, Roux-en-Y gastric bypass, and less commonly laparoscopic adjustable gastric band and biliopancreatic diversion with duodenal switch (**Table 9**).[58–61]

In the STAMPEDE trial, bariatric surgery was shown to decrease HbA1c levels by 2.1% versus 0.3% through medical management alone at 5 years.[59] At 10 years of follow-up, Mingrone and colleagues[62] demonstrated T2D remission rates of 37.5% in the bariatric surgery group (Roux-en-Y gastric bypass and biliopancreatic diversion with duodenal switch) versus 5.5% in the medical therapy group. Last, the Swedish Obese Subjects study recently reported that the adjusted mean life expectancy in the surgery group was 3 years longer than for the control group.[63] Complication and mortality rates for metabolic surgeries are 1.4% and 0.04%, respectively.[64] Postoperatively, there is an increase in satiety hormones, decrease in hunger, and increase in insulin sensitivity, leading to rapid improvements in glucose levels even before

Table 8
One-year weight loss and HbAlc outcomes in double-blinded randomized controlled trials utilizing pharmacotherapy for obesity in patients with T2D

	Trial	Intervention Groups	Weight Loss % (Drug vs Placebo)	Decrease in HbA1c (drug vs Placebo)
Orlistat	Hollander et al,[49] 1998	120 mg TID vs placebo	6.2 vs 4.3 at 57 wk	0.28 vs 0.18
Orlistat	Kelley et al,[50] 2002	120 mg TID vs placebo	3.89 vs 1.27 at 48 wk	0.62 vs 0.27
Orlistat	Miles et al,[51] 2002	120 mg TID vs placebo	4.6 vs 1.7 at 48 wk	0.90 vs 0.61
Orlistat	Hanefeld et al,[52] 2002	120 mg TID vs placebo	5.4 vs 3.6 at 48 wk	0.9 vs 0.4
Orlistat	Berne et al,[53] 2005	120 mg TID vs placebo	5.0 vs 1.8 at 52 wk	1.1 vs 0.2
Phentermine/ topiramate ER	OB-202/DM-230[54]	15 mg/92 mg vs placebo	9.4 vs 2.7 at 56 wk	1.6 vs 1.2
Phentermine/ topiramate ER	[a]CONQUER[55]	15/92 mg vs 7.5/46 mg vs placebo	[a]8.8 vs 6.8 vs 1.9 at 56 wk	[a]0.4 vs 0.4 vs 0.1
Naltrexone SR/ bupropion SR	COR-Diabetes[56]	32 mg/360 mg vs placebo	5.0 vs 1.8 at 56 wk	0.6 vs 0.1
Liraglutide	SCALE- Diabetes[57]	3.0 mg vs 1.8 mg vs placebo	6.0 vs 4.7 vs 2.0 at 56 wk	1.3 vs 1.1 vs 0.3

Abbreviations: ER, extended release; SR, sustained release; TID, 3 times a day.
[a] 15.6% of patients in CONQUER had T2D and results reported here represent only this population.

Table 9
Available bariatric procedures, target weight loss and diabetes remission rates

Procedure	Target Weight Loss (% of Initial Weight)	Diabetes Remission Rate at 5 y (%)
LAGB	20–25	19[58]
SG	25–30	23.4[59]
RYGB	30–35	28.6[59]
BPD/DS	35–45	37[60]

Abbreviations: BPD/DS, biliopancreatic diversion with duodenal switch; LAGB, laparoscopic adjustable gastric band; RYGB, Roux-en-Y gastric bypass; SG, sleeve gastrectomy.
    Diabetes remission defined as HbA1c of $\leq$6.5%[58] or $\leq$6%.[59,60]
    Data from: Courcoulas AP et al.[58], Schauer PR et al.,[59] Mingrone G et al.,[60] and Mechanick JI et al.[61]

significant weight loss.[65] Perioperatively in the hospital, decrease or hold oral antihyperglycemic medications and monitor glucose levels every 4 to 6 hours targeting a goal of 140 to 180 mg/dL[66] using rapid or short-acting insulin for correction (sliding scale). On the day of surgery, decrease basal insulin by 50% and continue after surgery.[65] Reincorporate oral antihyperglycemic medications as needed; continuous adjustment and weaning will be necessary up to 1 year from the date of surgery.[65] For long-term follow-up, obtain annual laboratory tests for micronutrient and vitamin deficiencies[61] focusing on B_{12} deficiency in patients with T2D who have a history of metformin use, because the long-term use of metformin has been associated with vitamin B_{12} deficiency.[67] Bariatric surgery is a means to obtaining dramatic and durable weight loss, improvement and possible remission of T2D, and decreased mortality.

SUMMARY

Obesity and T2D are becoming exceedingly common as the worldwide prevalence continue to increase to epidemic proportions. These chronic diseases inflict enormous individual and community burden with poorer quality of life, shortened life expectancy, and socioeconomic pressure. The comanagement of obesity and T2D requires a comprehensive medical approach that includes lifestyle modification, pharmacotherapy and possible surgical management.

Practitioners should adopt a weight-centric approach to the treatment of T2D by optimizing weight-reducing antihyperglycemic medications including metformin, GLP-1RA, and SGLT-2i while avoiding or decreasing the use of obesogenic antihyperglycemic medications including insulin, sulfonylureas, and thiazolidinediones. Antiobesity medications are safe in patients with diabetes, and weight loss of 5% or more renders improvements in glycemic control and cardiometabolic parameters. Medical devices and endobariatric procedures are novel and are not currently considered to be part of the standard of care for patients with obesity and T2D. Finally, metabolic surgery is available for persistently uncontrolled diabetes and obesity and results in significant and sustained weight loss with improvement and possible remission of T2D. Many effective treatment pathways are available to nurses and other practitioners to concurrently treat obesity and T2D.

CLINICS CARE POINTS

- A weight loss of 5% or greater is associated with improvements in glycemic control and other cardiometabolic parameters

- Nutrition and physical activity are the cornerstone of weight and diabetes management. Expert guidelines recommend any nutritional plan with a calorie deficit of at least 500 kcal/d and 150 minutes of moderate to vigorous exercise per week with 2 to 3 sessions of resistance training weekly.

- In patients with obesity and T2D who have preexisting cardiovascular disease or high cardiovascular disease risk, add a GLP-1RA to first-line metformin.

- In patients with obesity and T2D who have congestive heart failure, chronic kidney disease, or cardiovascular disease, add an SGLT-2i to first-line metformin.

- Antiobesity medications have proven long-term benefit and safety in patients with obesity and T2D.

- Metabolic surgery is a safe and effective option for patients with BMI of greater than 30 to 35 kg/m^2 who desire T2D remission.

DISCLOSURE

B.G. Tchang is a consultant for Novo Nordisk. J. Pape is a consultant for Novo Nordisk, MannKind, and Gelesis. All other authors have nothing to disclose.

ACKNOWLEDGMENTS

The authors thank Laura Boyer, FNP-C, for her insight and expertise in metabolic surgery.

REFERENCES

1. World Health Organization (WHO). Physical status: the use and interpretation of anthropometry. Report of a WHO Expert Committee. World Health Organ Tech Rep Ser 1995;854:1–452.
2. World Health Organization (WHO). Appropriate body-mass index for Asian populations and its implications for policy and intervention strategies. Lancet Jan 2004;363(9403):157–63.
3. American Diabetes Association (ADA). Classification and diagnosis of diabetes: standards of medical care in diabetes—2021. Diabetes Care 2021; 44(Supplement 1):S15–33.
4. Centers for Disease Control and Prevention (CDC). Overweight & obesity: adult obesity facts. Available at: https://www.cdc.gov/obesity/data/adult.html. Accessed February 1, 2021.
5. Mendola ND, Chen TC, Gu Q, et al. Prevalence of total, diagnosed, and undiagnosed diabetes among adults: United States, 2013-2016. NCHS Data Brief 2018;(319):1–8.
6. Ward ZJ, Bleich SN, Cradock AL, et al. Projected U.S. state-level prevalence of adult obesity and severe obesity. N Engl J Med 2019;381(25):2440–50.
7. Abdullah A, Peeters A, de Courten M, et al. The magnitude of association between overweight and obesity and the risk of diabetes: a meta-analysis of prospective cohort studies. Diabetes Res Clin Pract Sep 2010;89(3):309–19.
8. Kodama S, Horikawa C, Fujihara K, et al. Quantitative relationship between body weight gain in adulthood and incident type 2 diabetes: a meta-analysis. Obes Rev Mar 2014;15(3):202–14.
9. Wang Y, Beydoun MA, Liang L, et al. Will all Americans become overweight or obese? Estimating the progression and cost of the US obesity epidemic. Obesity 2008;16(10):2323–30.

10. Wang F, McDonald T, Bender J, et al. Association of healthcare costs with per unit body mass index increase. J Occup Environ Med 2006;48(7):668–74.

11. American Diabetes Association (ADA). Economic costs of diabetes in the U.S. in 2017. Diabetes Care 2018;41(5):917–28.

12. Unger RH. Lipotoxicity in the pathogenesis of obesity-dependent NIDDM. Diabetes 1995;44:863–70.

13. Kahn SE, Hull RL, Utzschneider KM. Mechanisms linking obesity to insulin resistance and type 2 diabetes. Nature 2006;444(7121):840–6.

14. Ludwig DS, Ebbeling CB. The carbohydrate-insulin model of obesity: beyond "calories in, calories out". JAMA Intern Med 2018;178(8):1098–103.

15. Moyer VA. Screening for and management of obesity in adults: U.S. Preventive Services Task Force recommendation statement. Ann Intern Med 2012;157(5): 373–8.

16. World Health Organization (WHO). Waist circumference and waist–hip ratio: report of a WHO expert consultation. WHO Libr 2008;(1):1–47.

17. Gallagher EJ, Le Roith D, Bloomgarden Z. Review of hemoglobin A1c in the management of diabetes. J Diabetes 2009;1(1):9–17.

18. National Institute of Diabetes and Digestive and Kidney Diseases (NIDDK). Sickle cell trait & other hemoglobinopathies & diabetes. Bethesda, MD: National Institutes of Health; 2020.

19. American Diabetes Association. 6. Glycemic targets: standards of medical care in diabetes-2021. Diabetes Care 2021;44(Suppl 1):S73–84.

20. Magkos F, Fraterrigo G, Yoshino J, et al. Effects of moderate and subsequent progressive weight loss on metabolic function and adipose tissue biology in humans with obesity. Cell Metab 2016;23(4):591–601.

21. Bray GA, Frühbeck G, Ryan DH, et al. Management of obesity. Lancet 2016; 387(10031):1947–56.

22. American Diabetes Association. 8. Obesity management for the treatment of type 2 diabetes: standards of medical care in diabetes-2021. Diabetes Care 2021; 44(Suppl 1):S100–10.

23. Sharaiha R. Managing obesity with endoscopic sleeve gastroplasty. Gastroenterol Hepatol (N Y) 2017;13(9):547–9.

24. Look AHEAD Research Group, Wing RR, Bolin P, et al. Cardiovascular effects of intensive lifestyle intervention in type 2 diabetes. N Engl J Med 2013;369(2): 145–54 [published correction appears in N Engl J Med. 2014 May 8;370(19): 1866].

25. Evert AB, Dennison M, Gardner CD, et al. Nutrition therapy for adults with diabetes or prediabetes: a consensus report. Diabetes Care 2019;42(5):731–54.

26. Jensen MD, Ryan DH, Apovian CM, et al. 2013 AHA/ACC/TOS guideline for the management of overweight and obesity in adults: a report of the American College of Cardiology/American Heart Association Task Force on Practice Guidelines and The Obesity Society. Circulation 2014;129(25 Suppl 2):S102–38 [published correction appears in Circulation. 2014 Jun 24;129(25 Suppl 2): S139-40].

27. Snowling NJ, Hopkins WG. Effects of different modes of exercise training on glucose control and risk factors for complications in type 2 diabetic patients: a meta-analysis. Diabetes Care 2006;29:2518–27.

28. Piercy KL, Troiano RP. Physical activity guidelines for Americans from the US Department of Health and Human Services. Circ Cardiovasc Qual Outcomes 2018;11(11):e005263.

29. Colberg SR, Sigal RJ, Yardley JE, et al. Physical activity/exercise and diabetes: a position statement of the American Diabetes Association. Diabetes Care 2016; 39(11):2065–79.

30. Apovian CM, Aronne LJ, Bessesen DH, et al. Pharmacological management of obesity: an endocrine Society clinical practice guideline [published correction appears in J Clin Endocrinol Metab. 2015 May;100(5):2135-6]. J Clin Endocrinol Metab 2015;100(2):342–62.

31. Tchang BG, Saunders KH, Igel LI. Best practices in the management of overweight and obesity. Med Clin North Am 2021;105(1):149–74.

32. Van Gaal L, Scheen A. Weight management in type 2 diabetes: current and emerging approaches to treatment. Diabetes Care 2015;38(6):1161–72.

33. American Diabetes Association. 9. Pharmacologic approaches to glycemic treatment: standards of medical care in diabetes-2021. Diabetes Care 2021;44(Suppl 1):S111–24.

34. Lv WS, Wen JP, Li L, et al. The effect of metformin on food intake and its potential role in hypothalamic regulation in obese diabetic rats. Brain Res 2012;1444:11–9.

35. Preiss D, Dawed A, Welsh P, et al. Sustained influence of metformin therapy on circulating glucagon-like peptide-1 levels in individuals with and without type 2 diabetes. Diabetes Obes Metab 2017;19(3):356–63.

36. Coll AP, Chen M, Taskar P, et al. GDF15 mediates the effects of metformin on body weight and energy balance. Nature 2020;578(7795):444–8 [published correction appears in Nature. 2020 Feb 13].

37. Diabetes Prevention Program Research Group, Knowler WC, Fowler SE, et al. 10-year follow-up of diabetes incidence and weight loss in the Diabetes Prevention Program Outcomes Study. Lancet 2009;374(9702):1677–86 [published correction appears in Lancet. 2009 Dec 19;374(9707):2054].

38. Chukir T, Mandel L, Tchang BG, et al. Metformin-induced weight loss in patients with or without type 2 diabetes/prediabetes: a retrospective cohort study. Obes Res Clin Pract 2021;15(1):64–8.

39. Chun JH, Butts A. Long-acting GLP-1RAs: an overview of efficacy, safety, and their role in type 2 diabetes management. JAAPA 2020;33(8):3–18.

40. Willms B, Werner J, Holst JJ, et al. Gastric emptying, glucose responses, and insulin secretion after a liquid test meal: effects of exogenous glucagon-like peptide-1 (GLP-1)-(7-36) amide in type 2 (noninsulin-dependent) diabetic patients. J Clin Endocrinol Metab 1996;81(1):327–32.

41. Toft-Nielsen MB, Madsbad S, Holst JJ. Continuous subcutaneous infusion of glucagon-like peptide 1 lowers plasma glucose and reduces appetite in type 2 diabetic patients. Diabetes Care 1999;22(7):1137–43.

42. North EJ, Newman JD. Review of cardiovascular outcomes trials of sodium-glucose cotransporter-2 inhibitors and glucagon-like peptide-1 receptor agonists. Curr Opin Cardiol 2019;34(6):687–92.

43. Anderson SL, Trujillo JM. Basal insulin use with GLP-1 receptor agonists. Diabetes Spectr 2016;29(3):152–60.

44. Artigas CF, Stokes V, Tan GD, et al. Insulin dose adjustments with add-on glucagon-like peptide-1 receptor (GLP-1R) agonists in clinical practice. Expert Opin Pharmacother 2015;16(10):1417–21.

45. Nauck MA, Friedrich N. Do GLP-1-based therapies increase cancer risk? Diabetes Care 2013;36(Supplement_2):S245–52.

46. Kahan S, Fujioka K. Obesity pharmacotherapy in patients with type 2 diabetes. Diabetes Spectr 2017;30(4):250–7.

47. Mikhail N. Place of sodium-glucose co-transporter type 2 inhibitors for treatment of type 2 diabetes. World J Diabetes 2014;5(6):854–9.
48. Gomez-Peralta F, Abreu C, Lecube A, et al. Practical approach to initiating SGLT2 inhibitors in type 2 diabetes [published correction appears in Diabetes Ther. 2017 Aug 23;:]. Diabetes Ther 2017;8(5):953–62.
49. Hollander PA, Elbein SC, Hirsch IB, et al. Role of orlistat in the treatment of obese patients with type 2 diabetes. A 1-year randomized double-blind study. Diabetes Care 1998;21(8):1288–94.
50. Kelley DE, Bray GA, Pi-Sunyer FX, et al. Clinical efficacy of orlistat therapy in overweight and obese patients with insulin-treated type 2 diabetes: a 1-year randomized controlled trial. Diabetes Care 2002;25(6):1033–41 [published correction appears in Diabetes Care. 2003 Mar;26(3):971.].
51. Miles JM, Leiter L, Hollander P, et al. Effect of orlistat in overweight and obese patients with type 2 diabetes treated with metformin. Diabetes Care 2002; 25(7):1123–8 [published correction appears in Diabetes Care. 2002 Sep;25(9): 1671.].
52. Hanefeld M, Sachse G. The effects of orlistat on body weight and glycaemic control in overweight patients with type 2 diabetes: a randomized, placebo-controlled trial. Diabetes Obes Metab 2002;4(6):415–23.
53. Berne C, Orlistat Swedish Type 2 diabetes Study Group. A randomized study of orlistat in combination with a weight management programme in obese patients with type 2 diabetes treated with metformin. Diabet Med 2005;22(5):612–8.
54. Garvey WT, Ryan DH, Bohannon NJ, et al. Weight-loss therapy in type 2 diabetes: effects of phentermine and topiramate extended release. Diabetes Care 2014; 37(12):3309–16.
55. Gadde KM, Allison DB, Ryan DH, et al. Effects of low-dose, controlled-release, phentermine plus topiramate combination on weight and associated comorbidities in overweight and obese adults (CONQUER): a randomised, placebo-controlled, phase 3 trial. Lancet 2011;377(9774):1341–52 [published correction appears in Lancet. 2011 Apr 30;377(9776):1494].
56. Hollander P, Gupta AK, Plodkowski R, et al. Effects of naltrexone sustained-release/bupropion sustained-release combination therapy on body weight and glycemic parameters in overweight and obese patients with type 2 diabetes. Diabetes Care 2013;36(12):4022–9 [published correction appears in Diabetes Care. 2014 Feb;37(2):587].
57. Davies MJ, Bergenstal R, Bode B, et al. Efficacy of liraglutide for weight loss among patients with type 2 diabetes: the SCALE Diabetes Randomized Clinical Trial [published correction appears in JAMA. 2016 Jan 5;315(1):90]. JAMA 2015;314(7):687–99.
58. Courcoulas AP, Gallagher JW, Neiberg RH, et al. Bariatric surgery vs lifestyle intervention for diabetes treatment: 5-year outcomes from a randomized trial. J Clin Endocrinol Metab 2020;105(3):866–76.
59. Schauer PR, Bhatt DL, Kirwan JP, et al. Bariatric surgery versus intensive medical therapy for diabetes - 5-year outcomes. N Engl J Med 2017;376(7):641–51.
60. Mingrone G, Panunzi S, De Gaetano A, et al. Bariatric-metabolic surgery versus conventional medical treatment in obese patients with type 2 diabetes: 5 year follow-up of an open-label, single-centre, randomised controlled trial. Lancet 2015;386(9997):964–73.
61. Mechanick JI, Apovian C, Brethauer S, et al. Clinical practice guidelines for the perioperative nutrition, metabolic, and nonsurgical support of patients undergoing bariatric procedures - 2019 update: cosponsored by American Association

of Clinical Endocrinologists/American College of Endocrinology, The Obesity Society, American Society for Metabolic & Bariatric Surgery, Obesity Medicine Association, and American Society of Anesthesiologists. Surg Obes Relat Dis 2020;16(2):175–247.

62. Mingrone G, Panunzi S, De Gaetano A, et al. Metabolic surgery versus conventional medical therapy in patients with type 2 diabetes: 10-year follow-up of an open-label, single-centre, randomised controlled trial. Lancet 2021;397(10271): 293–304.

63. Carlsson LMS, Sjöholm K, Jacobson P, et al. Life expectancy after bariatric surgery in the Swedish Obese Subjects Study. N Engl J Med 2020;383(16):1535–43.

64. Campos GM, Khoraki J, Browning MG, et al. Changes in utilization of bariatric surgery in the United States From 1993 to 2016. Ann Surg 2020;271(2):201–9.

65. Kheniser KG, Kashyap SR. Diabetes management before, during, and after bariatric and metabolic surgery. J Diabetes Complications 2018;32(9):870–5.

66. NICE-SUGAR Study Investigators for the Australian and New Zealand Intensive Care Society Clinical Trials Group and the Canadian Critical Care Trials Group, Finfer S, Chittock D, et al. Intensive versus conventional glucose control in critically ill patients with traumatic brain injury: long-term follow-up of a subgroup of patients from the NICE-SUGAR study. Intensive Care Med 2015;41(6): 1037–47.

67. Aroda VR, Edelstein SL, Goldberg RB, et al. Long-term metformin use and vitamin B12 deficiency in the Diabetes Prevention Program Outcomes Study. J Clin Endocrinol Metab 2016;101(4):1754–61.

Obesity and Nonalcoholic Fatty Liver Disease

Amanda Chaney, DNP, APRN, AF-AASLD

KEYWORDS

- Fatty liver disease • NASH • NAFLD • Obesity

KEY POINTS

- Obesity and nonalcoholic fatty liver disease (NAFLD) have a significant global impact.
- Complications of NAFLD are life threatening and most commonly related to cardiovascular disease.
- Lifestyle modifications are the mainstay of treatment and include a plan to eat, move, and change behavior.

INTRODUCTION

Obesity is an increasing health concern worldwide, impacting more than 200 million adults and more than 40 million children (**Fig. 1**).[1] There are many complications of obesity, including hypertension, hyperlipidemia, cardiovascular disease (CVD), chronic kidney disease, type 2 diabetes mellitus (T2DM), obstructive sleep apnea, osteoarthritis, certain types of cancers (ie, prostate, breast, colon), and nonalcoholic fatty liver disease (NAFLD).[1] The health care burden of obesity is significant and increases when complications of obesity are present.[2] This article focuses on NAFLD and obesity and reviews the background, prevalence of NAFLD, pathogenesis of NAFLD and nonalcoholic steatohepatitis (NASH), the clinical presentation and diagnostic criteria of NAFLD, and management recommendations according to current practice guidelines.

BACKGROUND OF NONALCOHOLIC FATTY LIVER DISEASE

NAFLD is increasing in prevalence, with of a global impact of around 25%.[3] Prevalence depends on population and is higher in patients of Hispanic ethnicity and occurs in more than 85% of patients undergoing bariatric surgery.[1,3,4] It is estimated that by 2030, 27% of NAFLD will become NASH, or the more advanced stage of fatty liver disease.[3] In fact, NASH is one of the most common reasons for liver transplant (LT) and is the third most common cause of hepatocellular carcinoma (HCC).[3] NAFLD is

Department of Transplant, Mayo Clinic College of Medicine, Mayo Clinic, 4500 San Pablo Road, Jacksonville, FL 32224, USA
E-mail address: CHANEY.AMANDA@MAYO.EDU
Twitter: @AmandachaneyNp (A.C.)

Nurs Clin N Am 56 (2021) 543–552
https://doi.org/10.1016/j.cnur.2021.07.009
0029-6465/21/© 2021 Elsevier Inc. All rights reserved.

Lifestyle Therapy

Plan to Eat	Movement	Behaviors
• Reduced calories (500 calorie per day reduction) • Individualized plan[a] • Options: Mediterranean, DASH, high-protein, low-carb • Meal replacements	• Aerobic exercise 3–5x/w (goal = 150 min/wk) • Resistance training 2–3x/w • Individualized plan[b]	• SMART goals • Education (nutrition, activity, stress reduction) • Support groups • Self-monitoring • Motivational Interviewing

Fig. 1. Lifestyle therapy recommendations for NAFLD.[21] [a]Based on religious/cultural preferences. [b]Based on physical limitations. SMART, specific, measurable, achievable, relevant, timely. (*Adapted from* Ryan DH, Kahan S. Guideline Recommendations for Obesity Management. Med Clin North Am. 2018;102(1):49-63.)

associated with a significant economic impact costing more than $292 billion in the United States each year.[5] In addition, NALFD is associated with increased CVD and chronic kidney disease risk.[6] Long-term mortality is associated with more advanced fibrosis.[3]

There are several definitions that the clinician should be familiar with when discussing NAFLD. NAFLD is a spectrum of disease and includes nonalcoholic fatty liver (NAFL) or simple steatosis (ie, fat in the hepatocytes) without inflammation, and NASH (or steatosis with inflammatory changes).[1,3,7] This inflammation can progress to fibrosis, cirrhosis, and/or HCC.[1] The existence of primary hepatic steatosis seen on histology or imaging, and exclusion of other causes of secondary hepatic steatosis are required to make the diagnosis of NAFLD.[7] In most patients, primary hepatic steatosis occurs because of metabolic factors, including dyslipidemia, insulin resistance, and obesity.[7]

Several experts have recently discussed the possibility of changing the NAFLD nomenclature to metabolic (dysfunction)-associated fatty liver disease (MAFLD).[6,8] It was thought that there was too much emphasis on the "nonalcoholic" term when the emphasis should be applied to the metabolic components of the disease.[8] In contrast to the definition above of NAFLD, MAFLD would be distinct in that hepatic steatosis is present plus presence of overweight or obesity or T2DM or at least 2 metabolic risk factors (high weight circumference, high triglyceride levels, low high-density lipoprotein levels, hypertension, prediabetes, insulin resistance, elevated high-sensitivity C-reactive protein levels).[9] There are still varied opinions on this topic, and more work must be done to further define and characterize subtypes.

PATHOPHYSIOLOGY OF NONALCOHOLIC FATTY LIVER DISEASE

As discussed above, simple steatosis is the early stage of NAFLD. It is thought that more fat (in the form of triglycerides) accumulates in the hepatocytes because of insulin resistance, obesity, unhealthy lifestyle (diet high in fat and carbohydrates), gut microbiota, and/or genetic predisposition.[6] The patient with obesity may not only have a part in the development NAFL, but also in the evolution to NASH.[1] If left untreated, the increased fat in the hepatocytes causes cellular damage and inflammation (ie, NASH). This occurs more easily if insulin resistance is present. Leptin, released by adipose tissue, contributes to free fatty acid oxidation and glucose update; in addition, it avoids buildup of lipids in the liver.[6] Leptin is directly related to worsening NAFLD.[6] There is also an alteration in the liver's ability to process dietary lipids, an increase in the liver's production of lipids, and a reduced ability to remove lipids from the hepatocytes.[1,7] Early explanations of this process was called the "two-hit hypothesis," with the "first-hit" being the increase in fat (in the form of triglycerides) in the hepatocytes,[10] or hepatic steatosis. The "second hit" was defined as additional inflammation caused by a disparity of anti-inflammatory and proinflammatory factors,[7,10] therefore resulting in instability of the cellular wall. An immune response led by the dendritic cells, hepatic stellate cells, and Kupffer cells within the liver is activated.[1,6] The entire liver becomes enlarged, greasy, and yellow. Once inflammation is present (plus simple steatosis), the patient has diagnostic criteria of NASH. If this process continues, the structure of the liver is compromised, and the liver can no longer regenerate. Scar tissue forms, and the liver becomes fibrotic, then cirrhotic, and sometimes develops into HCC.[6] Newer explanations state that rather than "two-hits," there is a "parallel, multiple-hit" process that occurs taking into account the multiple factors of genetics, sedentary lifestyle, obesity, insulin resistance, gut microbiota, and a diet rich in fat and carbohydrates.[6]

DIAGNOSIS AND SCREENING RECOMMENDATIONS

Clinical presentation for the patient with NAFLD is typically asymptomatic.[7] When symptoms do present, characteristically symptoms are vague and include fatigue and mild right upper quadrant abdominal pain.[7] Despite the increasing prevalence of NAFLD and its increasing economic burden, there is no routine screening process that is recommended in the United Stated by professional organizations.[11] The European Association for the Study of Liver Disease (EASL) recommends screening by laboratory testing and/or ultrasound for NAFLD for patients with metabolic syndrome or obesity.[11] Practice guidelines mention family screening; however, screening is not recommended for family members unless there is a genetic disorder present (ie, lysosomal acid lipase deficiency). Liver biopsy is the gold standard if advanced liver disease is suspected.[12] Pandyarajan and colleagues[11] recommend that primary care providers (PCP) should be aware of high-risk patients (ie, those with metabolic syndrome, and/or >50 years of age with diabetes) that may develop NAFLD. It is argued that with the increasing prevalence and severe effects (ie, cirrhosis and/or HCC), if left untreated, routine screening is logical for those high-risk patients.[11] Godoy-Matos and colleagues[13] include overweight/obesity as one of the high-risk metabolic criteria.[13] In a study done by Blais and colleagues,[14] only 39.4% of patients had a formal diagnosis of NAFLD, and only 14.7% received lifestyle management counseling.[14] This brings concerns to light that diagnosis of NAFLD is grossly underestimated and undertreated, especially when in the setting of obesity as well.

Not only is NAFLD underdiagnosed but also weight and lifestyle changes are typically avoided as a topic of conversation during PCP visits. Less than 5% of PCP visits are for management of weight.[15] However, more than 70% of adults in the United States have a body mass index (BMI) of greater than 25.3, and 90% of patients with a BMI of 30 to 35 do not have a diagnosis of obesity documented in their medical record. Medicare covers behavioral therapy for obesity; however, less than 1% of eligible patients receive this benefit.[15]

If NAFLD is considered for a patient, the first step for diagnosis is imaging by an abdominal ultrasound and laboratory testing (specifically alanine aminotransferase

[ALT]), with repeat testing annually.[11] In approximately 50% of patients with NAFL, there will be elevation of transaminases (ALT and aspartate-aminotransferase [AST]).[7] Other imaging, such as magnetic resonance (MR) and computed tomography, are acceptable modalities, but ultrasound is the most cost-effective.[11] The next step is to determine severity of disease. This can be accomplished in several ways (**Table 1**), including laboratory calculations and/or transient elastography.[7,11] The gold standard remains liver biopsy; however, this comes with significant risk and expense.[7,11]

If advanced fibrosis or cirrhosis is identified, the patient should be referred to a specialist for further evaluation, management, and possible LT evaluation (if concern for HCC or decompensated cirrhosis). If advance fibrosis is not present, lifestyle changes should be recommended.[11] There is consensus among several professional organizations that lifestyle changes that lead to weight loss targeted to 7% to 10% of body weight is the mainstay of treatment for NAFLD.[11,16–18] For the patient with obesity, obesity management (including lifestyle changes, antiobesity medications, and/or bariatric surgery) is the mainstay of treatment.[13,19]

TREATMENT OF NONALCOHOLIC FATTY LIVER DISEASE AND OBESITY

Lifestyle management is the current treatment for NAFLD. It is important to discuss with patients that treatment includes changing their life in multiple ways, from food, to exercise, possibly to work-related changes. This will not be a "quick fix," but a long process. Food choices should be aimed at more fruits and vegetables and lean protein sources.[3,20] To meet appropriate amounts of daily protein intake (which has been shown to be beneficial to remove fat from the liver),[20] protein with each meal should be planned. Patients should review amount and reduce the number of carbohydrates consumed, as more carbohydrates will convert to fat and more fat will be deposited in the liver.[20] This can lead to more inflammation. Also, high-fructose corn syrup is brought to the liver without being processed and damages the hepatocytes and thus should be avoided.[20] Patients should also avoid all alcohol consumption, as alcohol

Table 1
Assessment of nonalcoholic fatty liver disease severity of disease

Scoring Tools	Imaging/Procedures
Enhanced liver fibrosis test (ELF)[a] • Commercial panel • Markers include hyaluronic acid, aminoterminal propeptide of type III procollagen, metalloproteinase-1	Transient Elastography • Noninvasive • Vibration-controlled transient elastography (VCTE), approved by FDA • MR (can be done/expensive)
Fibrosis-4 score • AST • ALT • Platelet count • Age	Liver biopsy • Gold standard for confirmation of fibrosis/cirrhosis
Nonalcoholic fatty liver disease fibrosis (NFS) • Albumin • AST/ALT ratio • Platelet count • Age • Body mass index • Fasting blood glucose	

[a] Not available in the United States.

can cause more inflammation and injury to the hepatocytes.[3] Nutrition strategies should be individualized and include cultural and religious considerations. Initially, a calorie reduction of 500 calories per day should be recommended.[3,20] Common recommended nutrition plans are the Mediterranean, DASH, high-protein, low-carbohydrate diets.[20] Open communication and a partnership with the patient through regular visits to check in on their progress is essential for success. In addition, providers should recommend support groups, a nutritionist, as well as behavioral counseling to assist the patient in building a network to empower them to success on their obesity treatment journey.[21]

Several studies have been performed that show benefit with aerobic exercise and anaerobic resistance training.[3] Like the nutrition plan, exercise programs should be individualized for the patient, taking into consideration any mobility limitations or other comorbidities.[21] Partnership with an exercise group can provide motivation to establish behavioral changes. Setting small, reasonable goals that are realistic can assist with making impactful changes. Stress reduction support groups and motivational interviewing techniques are proven to be beneficial in treatment.[15]

The Society of Behavioral Medicine recommends the 5 A's counseling framework for obesity management and primary care.[22] This is a very well-accepted approach for behavioral counseling and has important implications for NAFLD treatment. Consensus statements by the American Heart Association, the Obesity Society, and the US Preventative Services Task Force recommend routine screening for overweight and obesity, and if present, behavioral counseling for those with CVD risk.[22] The American Association of Clinical Endocrinologists and American College of Endocrinology recommend for those in the overweight disease stage to engage in lifestyle therapy, which would include behavioral therapy.[19] The Centers for Medicare and Medicaid Services will reimburse PCP for providing this behavioral therapy for patients with obesity.[23] It is known that this is only done less than 30% of the time.[24] The 5 A's framework includes the following: Assess, Advise, Agree, Assist, and Arrange.[22] Utilization of this technique, along with a multidisciplinary approach, can maximize long-term success as part of a treatment plan for obesity.[22]

There are no approved pharmacologic treatments for NAFLD currently. There are many research trials, with more than 50 interventional studies ongoing.[25] Treatments are focused on prioritizing patients who are at high risk for progression of fibrosis and cirrhosis. The goals are to improve liver-related outcomes and reduce morbidity and mortality (specifically looking cardiovascular risk reduction). Because of the complex pathophysiology of the development of NAFLD, there are several drug classes that are under investigation for management (either monotherapy or in combination), including chemokine inhibitors, farnesoid X receptor agonists, fibroblast growth factor 21, peroxisome proliferator-activated receptors, glucagon-like peptide-1 (GLP-1), thyroid hormone receptor beta agonists, mitochondria pyruvate carrier inhibitors, sodium/glucose transport protein 2 inhibitors, and metabolic enzyme inhibitors.[25]

Several medications that have been approved for obesity management have been studied in patients with NAFLD. One is liraglutide, which is a GLP-1 class medication. Liraglutide has shown benefit to stimulate weight loss, stimulate insulin production, and contribute to production of proinflammatory cytokines.[1] There is another GLP-1 medication, called semaglutide, that is being investigated in fibrosis regression and resolution of NASH.[26] The phase 2 trial showed that patients with NASH who were given subcutaneous semaglutide once a week for 72 weeks showed more resolution of NASH (43%) than those patients treated with placebo (33%).[26] Orlistat has been shown to improve hepatic fat content and decrease transaminases (ALT/AST).[13]

As mentioned above, most patients undergoing bariatric surgery have some degree of NAFLD present.[3] Bariatric surgery is not a recommended treatment for NASH. However, there are several promising studies.[27,28] One study by Lassailly and colleagues[27] followed 180 patients with obesity and NASH, who underwent bariatric surgery, for 5 years.[27] In 84% of patients, NASH was resolved.[27] In 70% of patients with severe obesity and biopsy-proven NASH, there was a reduction in fibrosis.[27] In a meta-analysis by Lee and colleagues,[28] 32 cohort studies were analyzed. Results showed that in most patients (66%), hepatic steatosis was resolved after bariatric surgery, and fibrosis resolved in 40% of patients. In another study done by Zamora-Valdes and colleagues,[29] a select group of patients with obesity and NASH underwent a combined LT and sleeve gastrectomy simultaneously. Outcomes after 3 years showed that this population showed significant weight loss, reduction in hypertension, insulin resistance, and hyperlipidemia, as well as a reduction in hepatic steatosis.[29]

MANAGEMENT OF OTHER COMORBIDITIES ASSOCIATED WITH NONALCOHOLIC FATTY LIVER DISEASE

As mentioned above, NASH is an independent risk factor for CVD.[3] Knowing this, providers must be vigilant in optimization of risk factors. Dyslipidemia should be treated per practice guidelines with statin therapy (except patients with decompensated cirrhosis).[3,30] Omega-3 fatty acids have been shown to have some benefit.[3] For those with hypertriglyceridemia, fibrates may be given.[3,30] Hypertension management for the patient with NAFLD is the same as the general population.[3] Angiotensin converting enzyme inhibitors and angiotensin receptor blockers may play a role in decreasing hepatic fibrosis.[30,31] The presence of obstructive sleep apnea by increased risk of metabolic syndrome, CVD, and sudden death.[3,7] Diagnosis of OSA with a formal sleep study is important, and if present, then management with continuous positive airway pressure, weight loss, and possibly a dental appliance (if indicated), is required. For those patients with diabetes mellitus, providers should aim for a HbA_{1c} goal of less than 6.5%.[3] Chronic kidney disease is commonly present in patients with obesity, diabetes, and NAFLD.[32,33] Careful considerations of appropriate dosing of medications and avoidance of nephrotoxic medications are important.[3]

Not all patients that have a diagnosis of NAFLD will develop end-stage liver disease. Approximately 30% of patients with hepatic steatosis will progress to NASH.[7] Progression to fibrosis and cirrhosis occurs in roughly 40% of patients with NASH.[7] In recent years, the prevalence of NASH-related cirrhosis has doubled.[1] If cirrhosis is confirmed, providers must determine if the patient has compensated or decompensated cirrhosis. Decompensated cirrhosis develops when one or more complications of cirrhosis occur (**Box 1**). Once a patient has moved from a state of compensated cirrhosis to decompensated cirrhosis, LT evaluation is recommended.[32] The American Association for the Study of Liver Disease recommends regular surveillance with screening endoscopy when the diagnosis of cirrhosis is made, again every 2 to 3 years for compensated cirrhosis without varices, and every year for those with decompensated cirrhosis.[34]

Obesity can trigger chronic inflammation of the hepatocytes, and development of HCC could be more likely.[35] NASH-associated HCC is more common in patients with obesity and diabetes.[1] Because patients with cirrhosis and NAFLD have a higher prevalence for the development of HCC, screening with ultrasound with or without alpha-fetoprotein is recommended every 6 months.[36]

Patients with obesity will need close follow-up and regular nutrition counseling before LT.[32] It is a relative contraindication to proceed with LT for the patient with a

---

Box 1
Common complications of cirrhosis[32]

Ascites

Hepatic hydrothorax

Spontaneous bacterial peritonitis

Gastrointestinal bleeding (esophageal/gastric varices)

Hepatorenal syndrome

Renal impairment (Acute kidney injury in patients with cirrhosis)

Hepatic encephalopathy

Not all inclusive.

BMI of greater than 40. There are some promising studies mentioned above that report the option of bariatric surgery at the time of LT.[29] Posttransplant nutrition consideration should continue. More than 50% of patients will have some degree of steatosis postoperatively.[32,37] There are several medications that are required in the posttransplant setting that can further cause insulin resistance and hypertension, both of which can worsen metabolic syndrome.[37] Berkovic and colleagues[38] propose utilization of GLP-1 and sodium-glucose cotransporter-2 inhibitors optimizing diabetes and avoidance of NAFLD recurrence in the posttransplant setting.[38] Providers should be aware of these factors and adjust medications appropriately to optimize risk factors.

Given the global pandemic in the year 2020, it is important to discuss guidelines published that review patients with NAFLD and the novel coronavirus disease 2019. The EASL and the European Society of Clinical Microbiology and Infectious Diseases developed a position statement in 2020 that emphasized the importance of social distancing, early diagnosis (by PCR testing) and treatment/hospitalization for all patients with liver disease and nutritional advice, tight diabetes control, and obesity treatment specifically for those patients with NAFLD.[39–41]

SUMMARY

Obesity and NAFLD commonly go together and have a significant global impact. NAFLD is a broad spectrum of disease ranging from hepatic steatosis to NASH; progression of disease can move to fibrosis, cirrhosis, and HCC. In addition, complications across organ systems are life threatening, particularly for CVD. Many times, patients are asymptomatic, so it is important for other causes of liver disease to be ruled out. Lifestyle modifications are the mainstay of treatment and include a plan to eat, move, and change behavior. Antiobesity medications and bariatric surgery are options that should be considered. The future holds potential for new drug therapies in treating NAFLD. Providers can assist patients with NAFLD and obesity to a new path to health and vitality.

CLINICS CARE POINTS

- The development of nonalcoholic fatty liver disease is the result of multiple factors (ie, genetics, sedentary lifestyle, obesity, insulin resistance, gut microbiota, and diet); therefore, a multifaceted approach to treatment is required.

- Symptoms of nonalcoholic fatty liver disease range from none to vague symptoms of fatigue and mild right upper quadrant abdominal pain.
- When nonalcoholic fatty liver disease is considered as a diagnosis, abdominal ultrasound and laboratory testing including a hepatic panel should be ordered with repeating of testing annually.
- Reduction of cardiovascular risk is paramount to reducing mortality in this patient population.
- Partnership between patient and provider is essential to success of patient outcomes and treatment response. Trust and rapport can develop over time.

DISCLOSURE

The authors have nothing to disclose.

REFERENCES

1. Polyzos SA, Kountouras J, Mantzoros CS. Obesity and nonalcoholic fatty liver disease: from pathophysiology to therapeutics. Metabolism 2019;92:82–97.
2. Tremmel M, Gerdtham UG, Nilsson PM, et al. Economic burden of obesity: a systematic literature review. Int J Environ Res Public Health 2017;14(4):435.
3. Chalasani N, Younossi Z, Lavine JE, et al. The diagnosis and management of nonalcoholic fatty liver disease: practice guidance from the American Association for the Study of Liver Diseases. Hepatology (Baltimore, Md) 2018;67(1):328–57.
4. Berzigotti A, Garcia-Tsao G, Bosch J, et al. Obesity is an independent risk factor for clinical decompensation in patients with cirrhosis. Hepatology (Baltimore, Md) 2011;54(2):555–61.
5. Perumpail BJ, Khan MA, Yoo ER, et al. Clinical epidemiology and disease burden of nonalcoholic fatty liver disease. World J Gastroenterol 2017;23(47):8263–76.
6. Makri E, Goulas A, Polyzos SA. Epidemiology, pathogenesis, diagnosis and emerging treatment of nonalcoholic fatty liver disease. Arch Med Res 2021; 52(1):25–37.
7. Dietrich P, Hellerbrand C. Non-alcoholic fatty liver disease, obesity and the metabolic syndrome. Best Pract Res Clin Gastroenterol 2014;28(4):637–53.
8. Eslam M, Sanyal AJ, George J, et al. MAFLD: a consensus-driven proposed nomenclature for metabolic associated fatty liver disease. Gastroenterology 2020;158(7):1999–2014.e1.
9. Eslam M, Newsome PN, Sarin SK, et al. A new definition for metabolic dysfunction-associated fatty liver disease: an international expert consensus statement. J Hepatol 2020;73(1):202–9.
10. Day CP, James OF. Steatohepatitis: a tale of two "hits"? Gastroenterology 1998; 114(4):842–5.
11. Pandyarajan V, Gish RG, Alkhouri N, et al. Screening for nonalcoholic fatty liver disease in the primary care clinic. Gastroenterol Hepatol (N Y) 2019;15(7): 357–65.
12. European Association for the Study of the L, European Association for the Study of D, European Association for the Study of O. EASL-EASD-EASO Clinical Practice Guidelines for the management of non-alcoholic fatty liver disease. J Hepatol 2016;64(6):1388–402.
13. Godoy-Matos AF, Silva WS, Valerio CM. NAFLD as a continuum: from obesity to metabolic syndrome and diabetes. Diabetol Metab Syndr 2020;12(1).

14. Blais P, Husain N, Kramer JR, et al. Nonalcoholic fatty liver disease is underrecognized in the primary care setting. Am J Gastroenterol 2015;110(1):10–4.

15. Kahan S, Manson JE. Obesity treatment, beyond the guidelines: practical suggestions for clinical practice. JAMA 2019;321(14):1349–50.

16. Lazo M, Solga SF, Horska A, et al. Effect of a 12-month intensive lifestyle intervention on hepatic steatosis in adults with type 2 diabetes. Diabetes Care 2010; 33(10):2156–63.

17. Vilar-Gomez E, Martinez-Perez Y, Calzadilla-Bertot L, et al. Weight loss through lifestyle modification significantly reduces features of nonalcoholic steatohepatitis. Gastroenterology 2015;149(2):367–78.e5 [quiz: e314–5].

18. Hannah WN Jr, Harrison SA. Effect of weight loss, diet, exercise, and bariatric surgery on nonalcoholic fatty liver disease. Clin Liver Dis 2016;20(2):339–50.

19. Garvey WT, Mechanick JI, Brett EM, et al. American Association of Clinical Endocrinologists and American College of Endocrinology Comprehensive Clinical Practice Guidelines for Medical Care of Patients with Obesity. Endocr Pract 2016;22(7):842–84.

20. Neuschwander-Tetri BA. Non-alcoholic fatty liver disease. BMC Med 2017; 15(1):45.

21. Ryan DH, Kahan S. Guideline recommendations for obesity management. Med Clin North Am 2018;102(1):49–63.

22. Fitzpatrick SL, Wischenka D, Appelhans BM, et al. An evidence-based guide for obesity treatment in primary care. Am J Med 2016;129(1):115 e111–117.

23. Centers of Medicare and Medicaid Services. Intensive behavioral therapy (IBT) for obesity. Medicare Learning Network Web site. 2012. Available at: https://www.cms.gov/medicare-coverage-database/details/nca-decision-memo.aspx?&NcaName=Intensive%20Behavioral%20Therapy%20for%20Obesity&bc=ACAAAAAAIAAA&NCAId=253&. Accessed June 5, 2021.

24. Kraschnewski JL, Sciamanna CN, Stuckey HL, et al. A silent response to the obesity epidemic: decline in US physician weight counseling. Med Care 2013; 51(2):186–92.

25. Dufour JF, Caussy C, Loomba R. Combination therapy for non-alcoholic steatohepatitis: rationale, opportunities and challenges. Gut 2020;69(10):1877–84.

26. Newsome PN, Buchholtz K, Cusi K, et al. A placebo-controlled trial of subcutaneous semaglutide in nonalcoholic steatohepatitis. N Engl J Med 2021;384(12): 1113–24.

27. Lassailly G, Caiazzo R, Ntandja-Wandji LC, et al. Bariatric surgery provides long-term resolution of nonalcoholic steatohepatitis and regression of fibrosis. Gastroenterology 2020;159(4):1290–301.e5.

28. Lee Y, Doumouras AG, Yu J, et al. Complete resolution of nonalcoholic fatty liver disease after bariatric surgery: a systematic review and meta-analysis. Clin Gastroenterol Hepatol 2019;17(6):1040–60.e1.

29. Zamora-Valdes D, Watt KD, Kellogg TA, et al. Long-term outcomes of patients undergoing simultaneous liver transplantation and sleeve gastrectomy. Hepatology (Baltimore, Md) 2018;68(2):485–95.

30. Corey KE, Gawrieh S, deLemos AS, et al. Risk factors for hepatocellular carcinoma in cirrhosis due to nonalcoholic fatty liver disease: a multicenter, case-control study. World J Hepatol 2017;9(7):385–90.

31. Shim KY, Eom YW, Kim MY, et al. Role of the renin-angiotensin system in hepatic fibrosis and portal hypertension. Korean J Intern Med 2018;33(3):453–61.

32. Martin P, DiMartini A, Feng S, et al. Evaluation for liver transplantation in adults: 2013 practice guideline by the American Association for the Study of Liver

Diseases and the American Society of Transplantation. Hepatology (Baltimore, Md) 2014;59(3):1144–65.

33. Bonora E, Targher G. Increased risk of cardiovascular disease and chronic kidney disease in NAFLD. Nat Rev Gastroenterol Hepatol 2012;9(7):372–81.

34. Garcia-Tsao G, Abraldes JG, Berzigotti A, et al. Portal hypertensive bleeding in cirrhosis: risk stratification, diagnosis, and management: 2016 practice guidance by the American Association for the Study of Liver Diseases. Hepatology (Baltimore, Md) 2017;65(1):310–35.

35. Luo Y, Lin H. Inflammation initiates a vicious cycle between obesity and nonalcoholic fatty liver disease. Immun Inflamm Dis 2021;9(1):59–73.

36. Heimbach JK, Kulik LM, Finn RS, et al. AASLD guidelines for the treatment of hepatocellular carcinoma. Hepatology (Baltimore, Md) 2018;67(1):358–80.

37. Yalamanchili K, Saadeh S, Klintmalm GB, et al. Nonalcoholic fatty liver disease after liver transplantation for cryptogenic cirrhosis or nonalcoholic fatty liver disease. Liver Transplant 2010;16(4):431–9.

38. Berkovic MC, Virovic-Jukic L, Bilic-Curcic I, et al. Post-transplant diabetes mellitus and preexisting liver disease-a bidirectional relationship affecting treatment and management. World J Gastroenterol 2020;26(21):2740–57.

39. Ghoneim S, Butt MU, Hamid O, et al. The incidence of COVID-19 in patients with metabolic syndrome and non-alcoholic steatohepatitis: a population-based study. Metabol Open 2020;8:100057.

40. Boettler T, Newsome PN, Mondelli MU, et al. Care of patients with liver disease during the COVID-19 pandemic: EASL-ESCMID position paper. JHEP Rep 2020;2(3):100113.

41. Boettler T, Marjot T, Newsome PN, et al. Impact of COVID-19 on the care of patients with liver disease: EASL-ESCMID position paper after 6 months of the pandemic. JHEP Rep 2020;2(5):100169.

Obesity and Psychiatric Disorders

Christy Perry, DNP, PMHNP, ANP[a], Twila Sterling Guillory, PhD, FNP-BC[b], Sattaria S. Dilks, DNP, PMHNP-BC[b],*

KEYWORDS

- Obesity • Mental illness • Stigma • Depression • Anxiety

KEY POINTS

- Psychiatric illnesses and treatment can influence weight and possibly cause obesity.
- Psychiatric illnesses can possibly interfere with the treatment of obesity.
- Patients with obesity should be screened for psychiatric illnesses.
- Destigmatizing both obesity and mental illness could enhance the ability to intervene and treat each of them.

Obesity is defined as body mass index (BMI) >30 kg/m².[1] The prevalence of persons diagnosed having overweight and obesity has steadily risen over recent decades and now affects more than 2 billion people or 30% of the world's population and is a global public health challenge.[2] The old proverb, "which came first the chicken or the egg," applies to the issue of obesity and mental illness. It is important to examine the correlation between obesity and mental illnesses as both impact the other presenting an important focus of treatment. Failure to address either of them may result in a worsening of both.

OVERVIEW

Many psychiatric disorders are associated with obesity and include mood disorders, anxiety disorders, personality disorders, attention deficit hyperactivity disorder, binge eating disorders, trauma, bipolar disorder, and schizophrenia. Depression and anxiety have the highest percentage coupled with obesity and serious mental illnesses and obesity may be linked more to a genetic tendency along with the medications used.[3]

According to National Obesity Observatory, there is evidence that both obesity and mental health disorders take up a significant portion of the global burden of disease.[4]

[a] Southeastern Louisiana University, School of Nursing, 4849 Essen Lane, Baton Rouge, LA 70809, USA; [b] Graduate Nursing McNeese State University, 550 Sale Road, Lake Charles, LA 70605, USA
* Corresponding author.
E-mail address: tdilks@mcneese.edu

Nurs Clin N Am 56 (2021) 553–563
https://doi.org/10.1016/j.cnur.2021.07.010
0029-6465/21/© 2021 Elsevier Inc. All rights reserved.

The World Health Organization estimates that 40% of adults who have obesity have a well-established relationship between medical illnesses and obesity. What is less studied has been the psychiatric sequelae of the interaction between obesity and certain mental illnesses.[5] Numerous studies have identified a high association between psychiatric symptoms and obesity. The relationship between BMI and lifetime prevalence of mental disorders indicates that in individuals with a BMI more than 30 kg/m², there is a prevalence rate of 56.7% for all mental illnesses, anxiety disorders 50%, disorders of childhood 16.7%, and affective disorders 20%. In comparison, the prevalence rates of disorders with a BMI less than 19 kg/m² are 44.8% for all mental disorders, 31% for anxiety disorders, 14% affective disorders, and 9.8% for childhood disorders.[6] (Table 1).

Strong evidence suggests a relationship between obesity and poor mental health, especially in teenagers and adults. It appears that the perception of having obesity is more predictive of mental disorders than actual obesity and is unconnected to age. Mediation factors between the 2 conditions in adults include things like stigma, lower self-esteem, weight cycling, hormones, and medications.[4]

There are alarming rates of 45% to 55% cardiometabolic health issues and type 2 diabetes rates of 10% to 15% in patients with psychiatric disorders. This is up to 4 times higher than in the general population of comparable age. Several factors can contribute to the link between obesity and psychiatric disorders such as genetic factors, environmental factors, the mental illness itself, and the effect of medications coupled with an unhealthy lifestyle.[7] Environmental factors include not having access to healthy food options or not having the financial resources for healthy options.

It is thought that lifestyle risk factors and psychopharmacological treatments may be some causal factors to obesity. Lifestyle factors include diets that are high in fats and low in fiber, and a higher percentage of individuals who smoke, which is especially true in those with severe mental illnesses. Risk factors include gender, socioeconomic status, level of education, the severity of obesity, age, and ethnicity.[4]

PATHOPHYSIOLOGY

Many neurotransmitters affect mental status, but they can also affect appetite and food intake. Dopamine can be downregulated in patients with obesity, which decreases the reward and may lead to increased intake. Dopamine is increased when a high fat/high cholesterol diet is consumed, and it can have a rewarding effect. The intake may need to increase to have the same effect. Dysregulation of this reward can lead to overeating.[3]

The patient with a psychiatric illness is at a higher risk because of symptoms of the illness such as depressive symptoms that can lead to disinterest and a lower level of

Table 1		
Prevalence rates of psychiatric disorders in comparison to BMI		
	BMI <19 kg/m²	BMI >30 kg/m²
All mental health disorders	44.8%	56.7%
Anxiety	30%	50%
Affective disorders	14%	20%
Childhood disorders	9.8%	16.7%

autonomous motivation toward physical activity, their treatment (antipsychotic medication, other psychotropic medications, inadequate somatic treatment) and lifestyle factors (eg, lack of exercise, unhealthy diet, smoking).[8]

Adults with obesity that have diminished cognitive function have been associated with some structural brain changes. Reduced hippocampal volume, compromised white matter microstructural integrity, cerebral atrophy, and an increase in spinal fluid volume have been noted in these adults.[9]

Obesity is also associated with a decrease in cognitive function globally. The neural circuitry attached to cognitive functioning appears to be altered in a certain subset of individuals, which may be indicative of obesity being neurotoxic in susceptible individuals.[9]

There is some research to support a gut-brain connection. Gastrointestinal flora is affected by stress and high-fat diets, which can affect neurotransmitters that can lead to fluctuations in mood.[10]

Weight gain can be multifactorial for individuals with mental illness. Weight fluctuation that patients experience may be associated with psychological factors including mood states, eating distress, or hormonal changes, or other medical conditions.

BIAS

The destigmatization of both obesity and mental health disorders could enhance the ability to intervene. It has been suggested that there is a relationship between socio-economic status and level of education as potential risk factors, but the relationship is a bit unclear.

The stigma around mental illness is well known. What is not as well studied is the bias regarding mental health nursing. Mental health nurses' contributions are often discredited because of negative and stigmatizing beliefs, but more importantly, it discredits the needs of the patient population they serve.[11]

According to the American Nurses Associations' code of ethics, nurses are required to use evidence-based practices and current research in the treatment of obesity and mental illness.[12] The myth that generally surrounds obesity is that these persons have a choice in consuming more calories than they expend. Part of relieving the stigma associated with obesity is recognizing that there is a complex interaction, which includes genetic predisposition, affording and finding nutritious food, environmental chemicals, and gut bacteria.

It is incumbent upon nurses to recognize their own biases that if only people would eat less and exercise more, they would decrease their BMI. Obesity is far more complex than this paradigm. Implicit biases exist including the feeling that individuals with obesity must be lazy, unintelligent, and gluttonous. Nurses need to assess if the patient is ready to discuss weight loss and avoid using terms just as "ideal weight."[12]

AGE AND GENDER

Younger women appear to be at greater risk for developing obesity and mental illness.[3] There is evidence to suggest that older people may be at a higher risk because of health problems associated with aging, which might cause weight gain and depression or anxiety. Midlife central obesity has demonstrated an increased risk of dementia, which is independent of BMI, demographics, and additional comorbidities.

Epidemiologic studies indicate that maternal prepregnancy obesity is associated with a higher risk of their children developing autism spectrum disorders, attention deficit hyperactivity disorders, and cognitive dysfunction.[13] There is also an increased risk of developmental delay, lower IQs, poor motor spatial and verbal skills, and emotional\behavioral problems in women with prepregnancy obesity. Maternal obesity and diabetes together increase the risk for autistic spectrum disorder as opposed to either one alone.[13]

Women appeared to be at greater risk for obesity and mental health disorders than men. There is strong evidence to suggest that the bidirectional effect is present by adolescent ages with development of low self-esteem and impaired quality of life in individuals with overweight or obesity.[4]

DEPRESSION AND ANXIETY

Obesity can be a result of the mental disorder itself or the medications used to treat the illness. Intervention strategies have been recommended for providers to monitor the weight of patients with depression and conversely to monitor depression in patients who have obesity. Early identification of these problems may lead to early interventions resulting in better outcomes.[3]

There is strong evidence for the bidirectional nature of obesity and mental health issues, particularly depression and anxiety.[5,7] Symptoms associated with major depressive disorder (MDD) and bipolar disorder impact appetite, energy, sleep, cognitive functions, and/or motivation. Individuals with mood disorders have a twofold risk of developing obesity as compared to the general population.[4]

The level of obesity is a risk factor for mental health disorders with suggestions that severe obesity puts individuals at a greater risk to develop a mental health disorder, especially for depression. The amount of stigma may vary across culture, age, and ethnic groups.[3]

Depression and anxiety are the most studied mental illnesses in relation to obesity.[6] Depression has the strongest evidence of the bidirectional nature of obesity. Anxiety has a more modest link to evidence of co-occurrence with individuals with obesity. That said, there appear to be higher odds of lifetime panic disorders and agoraphobia in individuals with obesity and anxiety.[5,14] A study of people over 50 indicated that there was an increased risk of developing depression associated with 5 or more years of obesity.[15]

Adolescents with depression have a 70% higher risk of being diagnosed with obesity or overweight, older women with obesity have a 38% higher risk for the development of depression, and 10% of persons with depression have a higher risk of being diagnosed with overweight or obesity. This supports the notion of the bidirectional relationship between obesity and depression in particular.[5] There may be a gender bias toward women and the severity of the obesity may mediate the level of depression particularly in women. This relationship is greater in adolescent females and may be associated with hormonal changes and social pressures.[5] Interestingly, the relationship between depression and obesity is inversely related in adolescent males.[6] Depression was also significantly associated with metabolic parameters such as high triglycerides, low-density lipoprotein, very-low-density lipoprotein, and a weaker association with very-low-density lipoprotein.[16]

Obesity itself is one of the most prevalent somatic comorbidities with MDD. Individuals with MDD and bipolar disorder tend to have greater centra adiposity compared to those without these disorders. Persons with depression have changes in the hippocampus and the HPA axis, the same is true for obesity, which has low-grade inflammation as a part of its underlying pathophysiology that creates a dysregulation of the HPA axis, demonstrating the bidirectional effect of depression and obesity.[3] Dysregulation of cortisol is also indicative of the interaction between mood and weight.

Depression in adolescence is a significant predictor of an increase in BMI in adulthood. Persons who have obesity have an increased lifetime risk for depression 42.6% and somatoform indicators at 14.9%.[17]

SEVERE MENTAL ILLNESS

There appears to be a pathophysiological link between severe mental illnesses such as schizophrenia and bipolar disorders and particular metabolic conditions including obesity. Persons with severe mental illness generally have more central adiposity and it is postulated that there may be a genetic tendency to accumulate abdominal tissue.[7] Lifestyle and many psychopharmacological treatments can cause weight gain and disturb carbohydrate metabolism. Unhealthy lifestyles in persons with severe mental illness include poor diet, less physical activity compared to the general population, smoking (70%), and obesity.[7] The stigma around mental illness is well known. What is not as well studied is the bias regarding mental health nursing. Mental health nurses' contributions are often discredited because of negative and stigmatizing beliefs, but more importantly, it discredits the needs of the patient population they serve.[11]

Severe mental illness can create financial problems because of difficulties associated with sustainable work and problems with quality interaction in family as well as other interpersonal relationships. Access to medical care is often compromised in these individuals in part because of the illnesses themselves and in part due to stigma.[15]

Drug naive patients with schizophrenia had a higher level of abdominal adiposity suggestive of a genetic tendency toward overweight or obesity before being treated with neuroleptics. It is noted that persons with schizophrenia had metabolic issues before the development of neuroleptic medications.[15] In one study of adults with severe mental illness, 59% had obesity, 25% had diabetes, and 19% had both.[18] Another study found nearly 80% of 10,000 persons with schizophrenia in the study had overweight or obesity.[7]

Some symptoms of mental illness may affect what the person chooses to eat. Persons diagnosed with schizophrenia may have delusional thinking that could interfere with their food choices.[15] These symptoms may also interfere with obtaining proper medical care, which can result in not identifying or treating metabolic issues.[7] Psychopharmacological regimens for mood disorders, especially bipolar disorder, may affect weight gain through increasing appetite and sedation.[3]

ACES AND PTSD

Traumatic childhood experiences as noted within the adverse childhood experiences study (ACES) show there is a relationship of the development of obesity in adulthood related to the severity of the traumatic experiences.[12] Studies have indicated that 60% of women and 33% of men with obesity have identified a problem with post-traumatic stress disorder (PTSD) linked to the development of obesity.[3] Traumatic experiences combined with depression can increase the likelihood of developing obesity. Women with PTSD report greater levels of depression. In men, PTSD is associated more strongly with anxiety disorders. Early life trauma may increase the susceptibility of developing obesity, particularly with severe forms of abuse or abuse that occurs more frequently, especially recurrent sexual abuse. Food may be used as a soothing strategy and enhance coping. This temporarily will elevate mood and improve coping. PTSD may cause dysregulation of neuroendocrine functioning including an enhancement of negative feedback sensitivity to glucocorticoid receptors, a blunting of cortisol levels, and exaggeration in catecholamine responses to trauma mediated stimuli. High levels of stress may also contribute to the development of central adiposity.[3]

SUD

There is evidence of a link between binge eating disorder and substance use disorders and obesity.[3,14] Substance use disorder may include food consumption with a compulsive pattern of use even when faced with negative consequences. Tolerance may develop over time to food similar to developing a tolerance to drugs creating the necessity of higher amounts to maintain intoxication or satiety. In this context, withdrawal effects from food while dieting may occur. Specific areas in the mesolimbic system such as the caudate nucleus, hippocampus, and insula are activated by both food and drugs. Sweet foods specifically activate the endogenous opiate system and contribute to reward activation.[3]

ADHD

Children with attention-deficit hyperactive disorder (ADHD) who are not medicated have a 1.5-fold risk of having overweight when compared with controls.[3] Studies show a higher rate of ADHD in persons who seek obesity treatment. Persons with ADHD often have difficulty with organizing their lives, which may include intake of food that can include impulsive eating and these persons may participate less in organized sports both of which can affect weight. It is estimated that up to 60% of children with ADHD have symptoms that continue into adulthood. Symptoms such as disorganization and impulsivity may contribute to the link between adult ADHD and obesity.[3,13] There is a strong correlation between impulsivity and obesity whether or not psychotropic medications are used, with overlapping areas of neurobiology in both. The biological underpinnings are not well understood but may manifest with a low intrinsic dopamine activity that attempts to increase the reward areas of the brain. Attempt to stimulate the reward areas may use compensatory behaviors including an increase in food consumption.[3,13]

MEDICATIONS

Some psychotropic medications can also cause significant weight gain. A strong predictor of the development of metabolic syndrome related to psychotropic medications is a weight gain of greater than 5% in the first month of taking the medications.[6]

Weight gain is also an adverse effect of psychotropic medication.[19] According to Joao and colleagues, pharmacologic agents affecting weight gain have been identified mainly as atypical antipsychotics, mood stabilizers, and antidepressants.[20]

Weight gain is a well-established side effect of almost all antipsychotics. Antipsychotic medications differ in their weight gain liability. Second-generation antipsychotics (SGAs), clozapine and olanzapine, appear to have the greatest potential to induce weight gain. Quetiapine, risperidone, and iloperidone are associated with a moderate risk for weight gain. Aripiprazole, amisulpride, ziprasidone, asenapine, and lurasidone have less or little effect on body weight. Among the first-generation antipsychotics (FGAs), chlorpromazine and thioridazine are reported to induce more weight gain than haloperidol. No antipsychotic should be considered weight neutral as most all antipsychotics cause weight gain after prolonged use compared to placebo.[21] Evidence-based options for the management of antipsychotic-induced weight gain include individual lifestyle counseling, exercise interventions, psychoeducation, and augmentation with metformin, aripiprazole, or topiramate.[21,22]

Owing to the propensity of different antipsychotic inducing weight gain, switching to an antipsychotic with less gain would be a sensible approach. Few studies have reported switching from olanzapine to aripiprazole or quetiapine may be beneficial. However, the switch should consider the risk of a deterioration in mental health. Starting metformin with an antipsychotic can assist with the insulin resistance caused by the medication and provide modest weight loss or at least mitigation. Adding aripiprazole to clozapine or olanzapine has been shown to result in a modest weight reduction.[2] Weight gain has been reported when using antidepressants to treat MDD, especially with long-term use (>6 months) and polypharmacy of antidepressants. Tricyclic antidepressant (TCA) amitriptyline, the tetracyclic, mirtazapine, and the selective serotonin reuptake inhibitor (SSRI) paroxetine have been associated with a weight gain of up to 2.7 kg. Bupropion is more likely to cause weight loss than gain (−1.9 kg).[2]

There has been significant weight gain reported with the use of mood stabilizers to treat bipolar disorder, but it can be less than the antipsychotic medications. Weight gain is more frequent with lithium than placebo. Antiepileptic mood stabilizers, such as valproate is associated with weight gain in up to 50% of patients. Carbamazepine has a lower risk for weight gain and lamotrigine at higher doses and topiramate are associated with weight loss[23] (**Table 2**).

CLINICAL IMPLICATIONS

Psychiatric patients pose unique challenges for obesity management. Behaviors associated with psychiatric illness and the use of certain psychotropic medications contribute to weight gain. In addition, the symptoms and cognitive deficits associated with mental illness can be a barrier to participation in behavioral weight-loss interventions. Treatment of a psychiatric illness needs to include obesity management strategies and a greater integration of behavioral and medical care. When treating this population, clinicians can help improve outcomes by maintaining a focus on both the psychiatric condition and obesity. This can be accomplished by regular monitoring of psychiatric symptoms as well as monitoring of weight, BMI, vital signs, metabolic laboratories (eg, lipids and glucose), binge eating, or any other eating disorder.[1]

Weight gain can be a frequent issue for patients with psychiatric disorders. The weight gain is often not addressed in their treatment plan. Several nonpharmacologic

Table 2
Medications causing weight gain and weight loss

Weight Gain (Great Risk)	Weight Gain (Moderate Risk)	Weight Gain (Less Risk)	Weight Loss
Antipsychotics (SGAs)	Antipsychotics (SGAs)	Antipsychotics (SGAs)	Antidepressant
Clozapine	Quetiapine	Aripiprazole	Bupropion
Olanzapine	Risperidone	Amisulpride	Mood Stabilizers
Antipsychotics (FGAs)	Iloperidone	Ziprasidone	Lamotrigine
Chlorpromazine	Mood Stabilizer	Asenapine	Topiramate
Thioridazine	Lithium	Lurasidone	
Antidepressants		Antipsychotics (FGAs)	
Amitriptyline (TCA)		Haloperidol	
Mirtazapine		Mood Stabilizer	
Paroxetine (SSRI)		Carbamazepine	
Mood Stabilizers			
Valproate (antiepileptic)			

interventions have demonstrated positive results. These interventions include diet/nutritional counseling, exercise, cognitive-behavioral therapy, and psychoeducation. Patients with psychiatric diagnoses may have difficulty implementing nonpharmacologic interventions and the extent of weight loss achieved is modest. Combining both pharmacologic and nonpharmacologic interventions may offer additive benefits to the weight loss treatment in the psychiatric patient with severe mental illness and other psychiatric diagnoses.[20]

Behavioral therapy strategies that enhance individual behavioral change include improving self-management skills such as tailoring information to the individual, identify (lifestyle) areas for improvement goal-setting make action plans, giving personalized feedback to reinforce new behaviors, and using social and environmental strategies to support change. Most of these techniques have a limited effect unless the patient is motivated.[8]

OBESITY TREATMENT

Weight loss itself in adults with obesity or overweight had an association with a reduction of cardiometabolic risk but had no psychological benefit in one prospective cohort study of 1.979 adults. This infers that weight loss strategies themselves may not improve the mental health of individuals. Both weight reduction and mental health treatment should be considered concomitantly.[24]

There is a high prevalence of psychiatric disorders in those seeking bariatric surgery. One study showed that a quarter of the people seeking surgical intervention for obesity had evidence of borderline personality disorder.[3,14] Most studies focus on the immediate aftermath of the surgery in terms of evaluating psychological conditions. Despite undisputed significant weight loss and improvement in medical comorbidities, there is literature suggesting ongoing or worsening psychological outcomes like depression as compared to a control group.[22] Some studies note an improvement in depression after the surgery 6 to 12 months out and some longer-term studies have indicated the depression returns.[25,26] The few long-term studies that have been done suggest minimal improvements in mental health and psychosocial well-being two-plus years after the surgery in a subgroup of patients.[25] The American Society for Metabolic and Bariatric Surgery has published guidelines recommending follow-ups up to year 5.[27] Some studies have indicated that higher than expected suicide rates occur 2 to 8 years after surgery with suicide rates in bariatric patients being 4 times higher than in the general population. It appears that the postoperative improvement in mental health occurs during the first 2 years and begins to dissipate around year 3. Although many patients kept a weight of less than 75% of their preoperative weight, the general mental health showed significant deterioration in neuroticism, sense of control, and fear of intimacy at 10 years follow-up.[25] There is a supposition that individuals experiencing substantial weight loss will experience increased social acceptance. These individuals, however, must develop new social skills with this level of social acceptance. In addition, there is a suggestion that longstanding personality disturbances which were covered up by excessive eating are uncovered by the weight loss. These types of studies highlight the need for long-term follow-up and need to be routinely evaluated at visits up to 10 years.[27]

For patients who are unmotivated or patients who are not ready to change yet, the motivational interviewing (MI) approach by Miller and Rollnick combined with the stages of change from the transtheoretical modal of Prochaska and DiClemente can be beneficial. MI is a counseling approach that is patient-centered and targets the behavior change by addressing intrinsic motivation. MI seems more effective than traditional methods in targeting lifestyle change. It has been shown to be effective in improving weight status BMI, and cholesterol levels of overweight and individuals with obesity. With the transtheoretical model, the stages of change, patient's level of motivation, and self-efficacy to change are reflected in 1 of the 5 stages of changes. These stages are precontemplation, contemplation, preparation, action, or maintenance stage, ranging from no intention to change till the motivation to maintain behavior change.[8]

A combination of action planning with feedback and motivational stages-of-change approach is believed to be effective in behavioral change in patients. Also, peer and family support are considered an essential component for successful intervention implementation. Knowing the disturbingly high levels of cardiometabolic disease in patients, it is of high importance to develop lifestyle interventions. Changing the lifestyle behaviors can be difficult, but combining several successful components (eg, MI, stage-of-change, objective monitoring, self-management, support of peers and family, etc.) into one multidimensional intervention may lead to successful and sustainable lifestyle changes.[8]

SUMMARY

A marked reduction in life expectancy is contributed directly and indirectly to higher rates of obesity. Obesity has been associated with a more severe course of psychiatric illness, lower health-related quality of life, poor self-esteem, stigma, and discrimination. The long-term management is required for obesity and mental illness because both are complex chronic conditions. Psychiatric illness and obesity must be targets for treatment to achieve optimal outcomes for psychiatric patients with comorbid obesity or overweight diagnosis.[1]

Screening, assessments, and management of metabolic aspects in patients with psychiatric disorders remain poor. It is imperative that mental health providers, physical health specialists, and general practitioners are aware of the interaction between psychiatric disorders, psychotropics, and metabolic abnormalities. There needs to be a collaboration with integrated care for these patients so that they can receive optimal treatment.[23]

CLINICS CARE POINTS

- Individuals who have overweight or obesity should be screened for mental illness, especially depression and anxiety.
- Persons with mental illnesses should be monitored regularly for metabolic parameters, including BMI, waist circumference, lipids, hypertension, and diabetes.
- Adolescents who have overweight or obesity are at greater risk for developing mental illness and should be screened regularly.
- It is important that nurses work toward the destigmatization of both mental illness and obesity and be sensitive to the power of words that may be stigmatizing, for instance, "ideal weight."

DISCLOSURE

Dr S.S. Dilks has been a paid speaker for Otsuka and Lundbeck. Dr T.S. Guillory and C. Perry have nothing to disclose.

REFERENCES

1. Lindner center of HOPE. Lindnercenterofhope.org. 2019. Available at: http://lindnercenterofhope.org. Accessed March 31, 2021.
2. Holt RIG. The management of obesity in people with severe mental illness: An unresolved conundrum. Psychother Psychosom 2019;88(6):327–32.
3. Avila C, Holloway AC, Hahn MK, et al. An overview of links between obesity and mental health. Curr Obes Rep 2015;4(3):303–10.
4. Obesity and Mental Health. In: National Obesity Observatory. ; 2011.
5. Rajan TM, Menon V. Psychiatric disorders and obesity: A review of association studies. J Postgrad Med 2017;63(3):182–90.
6. Becker ES, Margraf J, Türke V, et al. Obesity and mental illness in a representative sample of young women. Int J Obes Relat Metab Disord 2001;25(Suppl 1):S5–9.
7. Bradshaw T, Mairs H. Obesity and serious mental ill health: A critical review of the literature. Healthcare (Basel) 2014;2(2):166–82.
8. Looijmans A, Jörg F, Bruggeman R, et al. Design of the Lifestyle Interventions for severe mentally ill Outpatients in the Netherlands (LION) trial; a cluster randomised controlled study of a multidimensional web tool intervention to improve cardiometabolic health in patients with severe mental illness. BMC Psychiatry 2017; 17(1). https://doi.org/10.1186/s12888-017-1265-7.
9. McIntyre RS, Cha DS, Jerrell JM, et al. Obesity and mental illness: implications for cognitive functioning. Adv Ther 2013;30(6):577–88.
10. Sfera A, Osorio C, Inderias LA, et al. The obesity-impulsivity axis: Potential metabolic interventions in chronic psychiatric patients. Front Psychiatry 2017;8:20.
11. Gouthro TJ. Recognizing and addressing the stigma associated with mental health nursing: A critical perspective. Issues Ment Health Nurs 2009;30(11): 669–76.
12. Colbert A, Kalarchian M. Obesity, ethics, and healthcare: A patient-centered approach: A patient-centered approach. Nursing 2019;49(7):20–2.
13. Kong L, Chen X, Gissler M, et al. Relationship of prenatal maternal obesity and diabetes to offspring neurodevelopmental and psychiatric disorders: a narrative review. Int J Obes (Lond) 2020;44(10):1981–2000.
14. Lin H-Y, Huang C-K, Tai C-M, et al. Psychiatric disorders of patients seeking obesity treatment. BMC Psychiatry 2013;13:1.
15. Lopuszanska U. Are metabolic disorders part of a severe mental illness? Historical and current perspective. J Educ Health Sport 2020;10(10):102.
16. Anithakumari A, Midhun S, Biju G, et al. Psychiatric morbidity and lipid profile in patients with obesity. J Obes Metab Res 2015;2(2):74.
17. Strassnig M, Kotov R, Cornaccio D, et al. Twenty-year progression of body mass index in a county-wide cohort of people with schizophrenia and bipolar disorder identified at their first episode of psychosis. Bipolar Disord 2017;19(5):336–43.
18. Cook JA, Razzano L, Jonikas JA, et al. Correlates of co-occurring diabetes and obesity among community mental health program members with serious mental illnesses. Psychiatr Serv 2016;67(11):1269–71.
19. Tham M, Chong TWH, Jenkins ZM, et al. The use of anti-obesity medications in people with mental illness as an adjunct to lifestyle interventions - Effectiveness, tolerability and impact on eating behaviours: A 52-week observational study. Obes Res Clin Pract 2021;15(1):49–57.
20. Hiluy JC, Nazar BP, Gonçalves WS, et al. Effectiveness of pharmacologic interventions in the management of weight gain in patients with severe mental illness: A systematic review and meta-analysis: A systematic review and meta-analysis.

Prim Care Companion CNS Disord 2019;21(6). https://doi.org/10.4088/PCC. 19r02483.

21. Jackson SE, Steptoe A, Beeken RJ, et al. Psychological changes following weight loss in overweight and obese adults: a prospective cohort study. PLoS One 2014; 9(8):e104552.

22. de Silva VA, Suraweera C, Ratnatunga SS, et al. Metformin in prevention and treatment of antipsychotic induced weight gain: a systematic review and meta-analysis. BMC Psychiatry 2016;16(1):341.

23. Mazereel V, Detraux J, Vancampfort D, et al. Impact of psychotropic medication effects on obesity and the metabolic syndrome in people with serious mental illness. Front Endocrinol (Lausanne) 2020;11:573479.

24. Luo C, Wang X, Huang H, et al. Effect of metformin on antipsychotic-induced metabolic dysfunction: The potential role of gut-brain axis. Front Pharmacol 2019;10:371.

25. Jumbe S, Hamlet C, Meyrick J. Psychological aspects of bariatric surgery as a treatment for obesity. Curr Obes Rep 2017;6(1):71–8.

26. Dawes AJ, Maggard-Gibbons M, Maher AR, et al. Mental health conditions among patients seeking and undergoing bariatric surgery: A meta-analysis. JAMA 2016;315(2):150.

27. Canetti L, Bachar E, Bonne O. Deterioration of mental health in bariatric surgery after 10 years despite successful weight loss. Eur J Clin Nutr 2016;70(1):17–22.

Obesity and Sleep

Craig Primack, MD, FOMA*

KEYWORDS

- Obesity • Sleep • Leptin • Ghrelin • Obstructive sleep apnea
- Restless leg syndrome

KEY POINTS

- If you sleep less than 7 hours, you are more likely to have overweight or obesity. If you sleep more than 7 hours, you are less likely to have overweight or obesity.
- A reduction of 1 hour of sleep is associated with a 0.35 increase in body mass index.
- Comparing 8.5-hour sleepers with 5.5-hour sleepers, metabolism decreases by 400 calories a day. As a result of trying to be successful with weight loss, you initially cut back on calories, you begin exercise, and unfortunately because of this metabolism drop, you do not see the results you expect.

WHAT IS HAPPENING IN THE UNITED STATES WITH SLEEP?

In 1998, now 20 years ago, the number of American adults who slept 8 hours was 35%.[1] Therefore, about 1 of every 3 adults slept 8 hours. By 2005, the number of American adults sleeping 8 hours was down to 26% (so only 1 of 4 slept 8 hours). A 2021 sleep survey reported 37% to 40% of adults have shortened sleep duration.[2]

Overall Sleep Duration Is Falling

In the United States, in 1960, the average sleep duration was 8 to 9 hours per night.[3] Statistics by the Centers for Disease Control and Prevention in 2014 demonstrated 35.2% of adults in the United States report sleeping less than 7 hours per night on the average.[4] A percentage of 32.6 of working adults report sleeping less than 6 hours most nights in 2017.[5]

Why do we not sleep?
A questionnaire[6] asked participants 2 questions:

- How much psychological distress do you have? This was defined as 3 things: how much anxiety, how much depression, and how much overall stress over ordinary do you have?

Scottsdale Weight Loss Center, 9989 North 95th Street, Scottsdale, AZ 85258, USA
* Corresponding author.
E-mail address: Drprimack@scottsdaleweightloss.com

Nurs Clin N Am 56 (2021) 565–572
https://doi.org/10.1016/j.cnur.2021.07.012
0029-6465/21/© 2021 Elsevier Inc. All rights reserved.

- What is your self-perceived health status? (excellent health, very good health, and so forth)

The results of the survey demonstrated that answering excellent or very good health, and low distress, correlated with sleeping well. Only 5% of these participants slept less than 6 hours whereas another 20% slept 6 to 7 hours. Seventy-five percent of people sleeping 7 to 8 hours per night on average answered low psychological distress and pretty good health. Participants with answers of more than low distress and not good health had a correlation with poor sleep. The study found one exception; people who exercise a lot. The participants who reported 7 or more hours per week of vigorous leisure activity, or 3 or more strength training sessions per week, described sleeping less than 6 hours.

Insufficient Sleep, Obesity, and Poor Health

Insufficient sleep is associated with many adverse health outcomes,[7] including obesity, type 2 diabetes, coronary heart disease, hypertension, premature death, abnormal immune function, and an increase in cancers associated with obesity. The immune dysfunction may allow cancers to grow faster.

There are several metabolic and endocrine manifestations of insufficient sleep that contribute to obesity and poor health.[8] Decreased glucose tolerance leads to diabetes, decreased insulin sensitivity, increased evening cortisol, increased ghrelin, decreased leptin and increased hunger and appetite with the result, all contributing to weight gain and finally obesity when progressed far enough.

In normal weight individuals, when leptin (from adipose tissue) is high, it signals that the body is "full," on the other hand when ghrelin is low, it cannot signal hunger. Right before a meal, ghrelin level increases, now signaling hunger, and after eating a meal, the ghrelin level goes back down to baseline.

With significant amounts of fat loss, there is less leptin, and therefore increase in hunger and/or less satiated. This change in hormones results in a regain of weight, the body's counterregulatory system kicking in. With insufficient sleep, leptin decreases and ghrelin increases, causing an increased hunger drive and a decreased satiety signal, ultimately potentially increasing the occurrence of obesity in the individual.

Sleep facts: kids
Children who sleep less than 10 hours are at 89% greater risk than their peers to have obesity.[8]

The Obesity and Sleep Connection

Adults sleeping less than 5 hours are 40% more likely to have obesity than those sleeping greater than 5 hours. It was found that a reduction of 1 hour of sleep is associated with a 0.35 increase in body mass index (BMI).[9]

Late sleepers, those whose midpoint of sleep is equal to or later than 5:30 AM, eat 248 more calories per day on average.[10] Late sleepers eat more calories at dinner and after 8 PM, eat more fast food, full-calorie soda, and have lower fruit and vegetable consumption.[10] This may be associated with circadian rhythm signals at a time when people should be awake versus asleep.

Beyond signals from daylight and typical hour of sleep, food helps reset the circadian rhythm. Feeding at "nonstandard" times, may set the whole homeostatic feeding cycle off kilter.

Sleep restriction decreases morning resting metabolic rate in healthy adults, suggesting that sleep loss leads to metabolic changes aimed at conserving energy.[10]

Sleep and Feeding Behavior

Insufficient sleep causes the upregulation of the appetite-stimulating hormone ghrelin, creating a hungrier state.[11] These hormone changes may also affect food choices during times of sleep deprivation, with foods that have fat, sugar, and salt seeming more appetizing.

Total sleep deprivation and restriction demonstrate a metabolism decrease by 135 kcal per day and 100 kcal per day, respectively.[11] Beyond the slowing of metabolism there is an additional intake of 500 calories.[12] The hypothesis as to why this occurs is that sleep restriction produces weight gain due to the overcompensation of neuroendocrine, metabolic, and behavioral responses aimed to increase energy intake and conserve energy in order to counteract the additional energy requirement associated with extended wakefulness. As a result, subjects consumed 35% more calories than needed during sleep restriction.[12]

Leptin Abnormalities

Spaeth and colleagues demonstrated that with 2 nights of 4 hours of sleep (vs 10 hours) there is an average 18% decrease in circulating leptin and an 28% increase in ghrelin.[13] Both these changes cause increased hunger and appetite. Leptin is usually elevated during sleep, yet it was found leptin decreased with sleep restriction.[14] Leptin levels were 19% lower with short versus long sleep. Leptin is usually inhibited via the sympathetic nervous system and has been found to mirror cortisol. When cortisol is high, leptin is typically low. When stress goes high, therefore fullness goes down. Six days of 4 hours of sleep decrease maximum leptin levels by 26%. With 2 days of sleep restriction by 4 hours versus extending sleep by 4 hours, leptin was decreased 18%, ghrelin was increased 28%, and hunger increased proportionately about 24%.[15]

Type 2 Diabetes, Obesity, and Sleep

Type 2 diabetes incidence is inversely correlated very strongly with sleep and directly correlated with increasing weight.[16] The incidence of type 2 diabetes in the United States is 760 for every 100,000 persons. There is an increase of 68 cases of diabetes for every 100,000 persons, for each 1 hour of reduction of sleep less than 7 hours, that is, 9% more diabetes in the United States because of lack of sleep.

Compared with 7 hours, a 1-hour decrease in sleep increased type 2 diabetes by 9% and a 1-hour increase in sleep increased type 2 diabetes by 14%. Men who reported sleeping less than 5 hours were 2 times likely to develop type 2 diabetes as those sleeping 7 hours.[17]

Sleep Disorders

The obesity and sleep apnea connection

In the United States, 24% to 25% of men and 9% women have sleep apnea.[18] For those with severe obesity (class 3 or above), obstructive sleep apnea (OSA) is seen in 93.6% of men and 73.55% of women.[19] With a 10% weight gain, apnea-hypopnea index (AHI) increases by 30% with a 6-time increase in moderate to severe OSA.[14] With a 10% weight loss there is a 26% decrease in AHI.[20] One unit less BMI correlates to 2.3 points less AHI.[21] A meta-analysis showed that a loss of 17.9 BMI points resulted in AHI falling by 38.2.[21]

After 2 consecutive days of Continuous Positive Airway Pressure (CPAP) therapy, Romero-Coral and colleagues indicated a decrease in ghrelin levels (hunger), although no change was seen in leptin or adiponectin.[21] Having obesity increases the risk of developing symptomatic OSA about 10x. Baseline is about 2% to 4% in the general middle-age population, up to 20% to 40% with a BMI greater than 30 kg/m^2.[22]

Obstructive sleep apnea

Sleep apnea is a temporary stop or decrease in breathing during sleep. Apnea is a complete stoppage of breathing. Hypopnea is an incomplete stoppage of breathing with a partial obstruction of oxygen flow. During sleep, apneic patients are also breathing against a closed glottis and see nonsleep arousals. Oxygen saturation decreases by at least 3%, and it lasts a minimum of 10 seconds. In a positive test sleep study, there is an average of 15 or more events per hour.

AHI is defined as the number of apneas and hypopneas per hour. An AHI of 15 is diagnostic of OSA, unless a person has a lot of other health concerns, and then sensitivity increases, and an AHI of 5 can be positive.

OSA is predicted by loud snoring. Other common predictors: gasping, having overweight and obesity, and an increased neck circumference. The higher the neck circumference, the greater the incidence of OSA. Neck circumference of 16 inches or more relates to a higher risk of OSA. Screening for sleep apnea can be completed with STOP BANG questionnaire tool (**Box 1**). The elbow sign (**Box 2**) is another screening tool.

Nocturnal polysomnography is the formal name for a sleep study. Formal sleep studies take place in a specially designed laboratory and are the best way to determine if a pathologic sleep problem exists. Home sleep tests, which unfortunately a lot of insurances mandate as the first testing step, are not as accurate as a laboratory-based full nocturnal polysomnogram. Home-based tests can more often diagnose sleep apnea but less sensitivity for ruling out sleep apnea. Home testing is not indicated with several conditions including congestive heart failure, chronic lung disease, and other neurologic conditions with a lot of associated movement. Treatments of sleep apnea is important. Sleeping supine doubles snoring and the AHI versus side sleeping. Treatments of sleep apnea include mandibular advancement devices, uvulopalatopharyngoplasty (a surgical procedure to remove the palate and uvula), and a newly approved device that provides neurostimulation to the hypoglossal

---

Box 1
The STOP bang questionnaire[22]

This is probably the best of the questionnaires to screen if someone has sleep apnea.

It consists of 8 questions (answered yes or no):

1. Do you snore loudly?
2. Tiredness (Do you feel fatigued, tired, or sleepy during the daytime?)
3. Observed apnea (Has anyone observed that you stop breathing or choke or gasp during your sleep?)
4. High blood pressure (Do you have or are you being treated for high blood pressure?)
5. BMI (Is your BMI more than 35?)
6. Age (Are you older than 50 years?)
7. Neck circumference (Is your neck circumference >15.75 inches?)
8. Gender (Are you male?)

Scoring: 0 to 2 = low risk, 3 to 4 = intermediate risk, and greater than 5 = high risk.

> **Box 2**
> **The elbow sign[22]**
>
> The elbow sign is literally being elbowed in the night by the person you share your bed with. It suggests sleep apnea. Being elbowed by one's bed partner is seen in 97% of people who have a positive sleep study.

nerve, to help tighten up the loose muscles. The gold standard of treatment is positive airway pressure therapy.[22]

Positive Airway Pressure Therapy

Two pressure devices are used for treatment: CPAP and Bilevel Positive Airway Pressure (BiPAP). These work by sending air through a mask via pressure. CPAP uses continuous pressure whereas BiPAP delivers an inhalation pressure and an exhalation pressure. Both devices reduce daytime sleepiness, improve quality of life, lower blood pressure, improve glycemic control and insulin sensitivity, and reduce visceral fat.[23]

Sleep Apnea Is Connected to High Blood Pressure

Blood pressure normally goes down during sleep. Sympathetic activity, the amount of muscle activation stress goes down during sleep, but this does not occur in a person with OSA untreated. Blood pressure in this study maxed out during an apnea with a systolic blood pressure of 240 mm Hg over diastolic blood pressure of 130 mm Hg.[10,24] Sympathetic activity increased with apnea 125% +/- 9% versus wakefulness. On positive airway pressure treatment, O2 saturation increased by 20% and was never less than 90%. The incidence of mortality and morbidity is significantly reduced by using positive airway pressure treatment.

Does Sleep Help Obesity Treatment?

One study showed similar weight loss at 8.5 hours versus 5.5 hours of sleep but unfortunately only 25% of weight loss at 5.5 hours of sleep was adipose tissue. There was a decrease of 55% and an increase in free fat mass loss by 60%. Five and a half hours of sleep versus eight and a half hours also showed a lower resting metabolic rate, and a baseline metabolism was 400 less calories, on average, in a 24-hour period.

People who sleep 8.5 hours burn more fat.[10] An hour after a meal subjects burn more carbohydrate. Then as those nutrients get used/digested, the body starts drawing on fat stores again, and fat burning increases. People who sleep 3 hours less burn less fat over time.

Sleep hygiene

Sleep hygiene is one facet of treatment of obesity. Following are teaching points for improving sleep[25]:

- Avoid light for 30 minutes before bedtime.
  - Blue light: especially, turns off melatonin. Blue light comes from "screens." Apple products have Night Shift, which takes out blue light or try an app called f.lux.
  - Clocks with lit screens can be removed from bedrooms, turned toward the wall, or cover with a little towel.
- Temperature: the optimum temperature for sleep is somewhere between 60° and 67° Fahrenheit.

- Sound: sounds can interrupt sleep
  - White noise machines work very well to help with unfamiliar sounds and inconsistent sounds such as a bed partner snoring
  - Ear plugs
  - Sleep in a different room
- Scents: lavender essential oil has studies on advantages for sleep[19]
- Caffeine: stop caffeine by noon especially for an hour of sleep of 10 PM, as caffeine interferes with deep restorative sleep
- Alcohol: avoid alcohol, especially before bed. Alcohol is known to suppress REM sleep[26]
- Night showers or baths: heating the body temperature and then cooling off, helps sleep onset.
- Meditation: meditation allows the brain to provide better sleep onset.
- Set an alarm for sleep. Sleep onset should occur within 30 minutes and if not get up for stretches, reading, calming in low light, and restarting the sleep schedule preparation program after 30 minutes.
- Sleep schedule routine—30 minutes[20]
  - Section one: wind down time: finish the day's tasks (packing lunches, self-care)
  - Section 2: dim lights, unplug electronics, relaxation (meditation, yoga, progressive relaxation)
  - Section 3: close eyes and sleep

Hormones and Sleep

Melatonin is a hormone that naturally comes from the pineal gland. Although awake, during the normal part of the day, melatonin[27] level is about 1 pg/mg, which is very low. Fifteen hours later, melatonin increases to 10 pg/mL. About 2 hours before going to sleep, it increases further to prepare for sleep. Melatonin peaks at 60 to 70 pg/mL, at about 3:00 AM In the morning, with the absorption of daylight into retinas, melatonin production stops and the levels decrease again. Another hormone that affects sleep/wake is adenosine. It increases with wakefulness. Melatonin works on 2 aspects of the brain involved with sleep. In the first part, melatonin is considered a weak hypnotic. Hypnotics are medicines that initiate sleep or work directly on the sleep process. Melatonin works on a system called the adenosine system. Adenosine needs to be higher for sleep initiation and is the reason to not nap for the most part. Napping can lower the level of adenosine, causing difficulty with sleep initiation in the late evening. The second function of melatonin is as a chronobiotic. It helps to reset the internal circadian clock, to "tell" the body that it is bedtime.

Melatonin Supplementation

The correct dose of melatonin is important. A physiologic blood level of melatonin is 0.3 mg. The correct oral dose is therefore only 0.5 to 3 mg. The best time to take melatonin is 9 hours after rising or 7 hours before sleep.[28]

SUMMARY

The World Health Organization and the Centers for Disease Control and recommend seven to 8 hours of sleep per night. Sleep is intertwined with weight. Treating obesity requires evaluating a patients sleep, possible need for referral for sleep evaluation, and helping patients have better quality and quantity of sleep. The average sleep efficiency is about 90%. To get 8 hours, need 8.5 hours in bed. Obesity is a multifactorial disease process, and sleep is a part of the cause and successful treatment.

Remember "*Sleep is the most sedentary activity. Yet maybe our only sedentary activity that protects you from weight gain and improves your health.*[6]"

CLINICS CARE POINTS

- Insufficient sleep worsens the disease of obesity and make treatment more difficult.
- Insufficient sleep creates a decrease in leptin and an increase in ghrelin, causing increased hunger, so assure your patients are consistently getting a good night's sleep.
- Ask your patients if they are being elbowed at night by their bed partner; this could be a sign they need to get evaluated for sleep apnea.
- Sleep disorders including obstructive sleep apnea and restless leg syndrome lead to difficulty losing weight and worsening of other health conditions; consider screening for both conditions in all patients with obesity.

DISCLOSURE

1. Speakers Bureau and Ad Board—Currax Pharmaceuticals. 2. Ad Board—Gelesis. 3. Consulting agreement—Nestle Nutrition. 4. Consultant: Phenomix.

REFERENCES

1. Patel SR, Hu FB. Short Sleep Duration and Weight Gain: A Systematic Review. Obesity 2008;16:643–53.
2. Sleep statistics 2021. Singlecare.com. Available at: https://www.singlecare.com/blog/news/sleep-statistics/. Accessed May 25, 2021.
3. Brondel L, Romer M. Acute partial sleep deprivation increases food intake in healthy men. Am J Clin Nutr 2010;91(6):1550–9.
4. Data and Statistics. CDC.gov. 2017. Available at: https://www.cdc.gov/sleep/data_statistics.html. Accessed May 25, 2021.
5. MMWR QuickStats. CDC.gov. 2020. Available at: https://www.cdc.gov/mmwr/volumes/69/wr/mm6916a5.htm. Accessed May 25, 2021.
6. Liang W, Chikritzhs T. Sleep Duration and Its Links to Psychological Distress, Health Status, Physical Activity and Body Mass Index among a Large Representative General Population Sample. Int J Clin Med 2013;4(1):45–51.
7. Johnson E. People Need at least 8.5 hours of Sleep Because of Social Media and Cellphones. Available at: www.Techtimes.com. Accessed January 30, 2019.
8. Chaput JP, Tremblay A. Insufficient Sleep as a Contributor to Weight Gain: An Update. Curr Obes Rep 2012;245–56.
9. Cooper CB, Neufeld EV, Dolezal BA, et al. Sleep deprivation and obesity in adults: a brief narrative review. BMJ Open Sport Exerc Med 2018;4(1):e000392.
10. Beccuti G, Pannain S. Sleep and obesity. Curr Opin Clin Nutr Metab Care 2011;14(4):402–12.
11. Spaeth AM, Dinges DF, Goel N. Resting metabolic rate varies by race and by sleep duration. Obesity 2015;23:2349–56.
12. Baron KG, Reid KJ, Kern AS, et al. Role of Sleep Timing in Caloric Intake and BMI. Obesity 2011;19:1374–81.
13. Shan Z, Ma H, Xie M, et al. Sleep duration and risk of type 2 diabetes: a meta-analysis of prospective studies. Diabetes Care 2015;38(3):529–37.

14. McMullan CJ, Schernhammer ES, Rimm EB, et al. Melatonin secretion and the incidence of type 2 diabetes. J Am Med Assoc 2013;309(13):1388–96.
15. Knutson KL, Van Cauter E. Associations between sleep loss and increased risk of obesity and diabetes. Ann N Y Acad Sci 2008;1129:287–304.
16. Chorostowska-Wynimko J, Plywaczewski R, Jonczak J, et al. Leptin measurement in urine is a reliable method of monitoring its secretion in patients with obstructive sleep apnea syndrome. J Physiol Pharmacol 2007;58(5).
17. Spiegel K, Leproult R, L'hermite-Balériaux M, et al. Leptin levels are dependent on sleep duration: relationships with sympathovagal balance, carbohydrate regulation, cortisol, and thyrotropin. J Clin Endocrinol Metab 2004;89(11):5762–71.
18. Nedeltcheva AV, Kilkus JM, Imperial J, et al. Insufficient sleep undermines dietary efforts to reduce adiposity. Ann Intern Med 2010;153(7):435–41.
19. Jehan S, Zizi F, Pandi-Perumal SR, et al. Obstructive Sleep Apnea and Obesity: Implications for Public Health. Sleep Med Disord 2017;1(4):00019.
20. Foster GD, Borradaile KE, Sanders MH, et al. A randomized study on the effect of weight loss on obstructive sleep apnea among obese patients with type 2 diabetes: the Sleep AHEAD study. Arch Intern Med 2009;169(17):1619–26.
21. Romero-Corral A, Caples SM, Lopez-Jimenez F, et al. Interactions between obesity and obstructive sleep apnea: implications for treatment. Chest 2010; 137(3):711–9.
22. Semelka M, Wilson J, Floyd R. Diagnosis and Treatment of Obstructive Sleep Apnea in Adults. Am Fam Physician 2016;94(5):355–60.
23. Borel AL. Sleep Apnea and Sleep Habits: Relationships with Metabolic Syndrome. Nutrients 2019;11(11):2628.
24. Lillehei AS, Halcón LL, Savik K, et al. Effect of Inhaled Lavender and Sleep Hygiene on Self-Reported Sleep Issues: A Randomized Controlled Trial. J Altern Complement Med 2015;21(7):430–8.
25. Sleep Hygiene. Sleepfoundation.org. 2020. Available at: https://www.sleepfoundation.org/sleep-hygiene. Accessed May 25, 2021.
26. Sleep Hygiene. Sleepfoundation.org. 2020. Available at: https://www.sleepfoundation.org/nutrition/alcohol-and-sleep. Accessed May 25, 2021.
27. Zisapel N. New perspectives on the role of melatonin in human sleep, circadian rhythms and their regulation. Br J Pharmacol 2018;175(16):3190–9.
28. Sleep Hygiene. Sleepfoundation.org. 2020. Available at: https://www.sleepfoundation.org/melatonin. Accessed May 25, 2021.

Obesity in the Critical Care Setting

Candice Falls, PhD, ACNP-BC*, Sheila Melander, PhD, ACNP-BC, FCCM, FAANP, FAAN

KEYWORDS

- Obesity • Critical care • Obesity paradox

KEY POINTS

- The obesity paradox encompasses a protective factor for obese patients in the critical care setting and is linked to decreased mortality.
- Obese critically ill patients face many challenges, including sepsis, infection, and respiratory failure.
- Obese patients with coronavirus disease 2019 have worse outcomes, including infection and respiratory failure.
- Obesity can affect pharmacokinetics and pharmacodynamics based on the pharmacochemistry of the drug.
- Obese patients have a decreased response to vaccinations.

Obesity, as defined by the World Health Organization, is an abnormal or excessive fat accumulation that presents a risk to health.[1] A body mass index (BMI) greater than 25 is considered overweight or preobesity, and a BMI over 30 is considered obese.[1–3] There are many causes of obesity, including hereditary or inherited risk factors, as well as those that combine with environmental factors that interact with personal diet and exercise patterns. The prevalence of obesity is on the increase in the United States as well as in the acute and critically ill patient population, with more than 30% of adults and more than one-third of patients in the critical care setting having obesity.[1,2,4–6] Obesity places those at risk for high blood pressure, diabetes, heart disease, and certain types of cancers and has been linked to increased side effects or adverse events associated with different treatment regimens.[1,4,5,7]

Although obesity in the general population is associated with increased morbidity and mortality, recent data in hospitalized patients have shown conflicting outcomes that demonstrate improved outcomes in patients with obesity compared with those with a normal BMI.[6] This phenomenon, known as the "obesity paradox," is not fully understood but involves several mechanisms, including hemodynamic stability, anti-oxidation of muscle mass, protective cytokine profiles, more advantageous fat

University of Kentucky, College of Nursing, 751 Rose Street, Lexington, KY 40536, USA
* Corresponding author.
E-mail address: cdharvo@uky.edu

Nurs Clin N Am 56 (2021) 573–581
https://doi.org/10.1016/j.cnur.2021.08.002
0029-6465/21/© 2021 Elsevier Inc. All rights reserved.

nursing.theclinics.com

distribution, and lipoprotein defense against endotoxins, that demonstrate why obesity may have a "protective" factor against mortality.[1,4,5,7,8] The association of obesity (although not severe obesity) with increased survival has been observed in patients with heart failure, chronic obstructive pulmonary disease, coronary artery disease, end-stage kidney disease, diabetes, as well as in patients who are critically ill.[1,4,9] Regardless of the mortality benefit in hospitalized patients, management of patients with obesity poses many challenges, including but not limited to drug metabolism, ventilation, and infections.[1,9] The purpose of this review is to further discuss these challenges and their association to obesity in critically ill patients, including a focus on patients with COVID-19.

PATHOPHYSIOLOGY OF OBESITY IN THE CRITICALLY ILL

The association between obesity and chronic conditions is well known, but the relationship of obesity and mortality of those that are critically ill remains contradictory. Several researchers have documented worse mortality in patients with obesity in the critical care setting, but newer researchers have contradictory findings supporting better survival. Chronic comorbidities are thought to be a major culprit to these differences in addition to nutritional status.[4,6,10] In the general population, comorbidities, such as diabetes, cardiovascular disease, and chronic renal insufficiency, place a patient at higher risk of mortality and worse outcomes because of eliciting immune and inflammatory responses.[1,6] In addition, malnutrition is more prominent in the critically ill general population and may contribute to worse outcomes. Critically ill patients with obesity are thought to have better nutritional status before hospitalization compared with patients without obesity, which leads to a protective factor against adverse outcomes.[4] The importance of nutrition is well established in critically ill patients.[4] Regardless of these factors, evidence supports that obesity is associated with a higher rate and severity of infections, poorer prognosis, and more complications, which may be attributed to altered metabolic states.

The pathophysiology of obesity is complex and multifactorial, involving genetic factors, the central nervous system, and the endocrine system.[6] Genetic factors can lead to obesity by causing genetic syndromes. In addition, the central nervous system regulates energy balance and signals satiety and adiposity hormones regarding metabolic needs based on the information it receives from organs in the body and adipose tissue.[6] Patients with obesity show a proinflammatory state with altered immune surveillance. A chronic, low-grade inflammatory state alters circulating hormones and nutrients at a systemic level and in adipose tissue.[1,6,11]

Adipose tissue is involved in several physiologic mechanisms, including lipid metabolism, endocrine, and immunologic responses.[11] Adipose tissue is composed of adipocytes, which are highly metabolic and inflammatory. Adipocytes play an active role in homeostasis through coordination of physiologic functions involving inflammatory cytokines and hormonal factors that are linked to insulin resistance and chronic inflammation.[1,11,12] In addition, immune cells reside within adipose tissue, which also exerts effects on metabolism and endocrine functions. Obesity and comorbid conditions result in adipose tissues eliciting a systemic response, resulting in an increase of macrophage accumulation, leading to increased cytokine release, decreased insulin sensitivity, and increased lipolysis, altering metabolic, immune, and endocrine function.[12,13] As a result, obesity is interlinked with conditions such as sepsis and infection.

SEPSIS

Obesity is a risk factor for the development of sepsis. Patients with obesity admitted to critical care units often suffer from more comorbidities than patients without obesity, leading to physiologic changes, such as increased blood volume, altered cardiac output, changes to volume distribution, changes to vascular tone, and altered response to pharmacodynamics.[1] In turn, this leads to longer lengths of intensive care unit stay. Contrary to expectations, obesity is associated with lower mortality in patients with sepsis when assessing 30 day and 1-year mortality.[14]

Septic shock usually occurs from a failure to meet hemodynamic demands, resulting in oxygen impairment, organ failure, and mortality. Fluid resuscitation and vasopressor support are often needed to maintain hemodynamic compromise. Patients with obesity often require less volume of fluid resuscitation and lower vasopressor support to maintain hemodynamic goals.[4,10,15] Normally, fluid resuscitation is based indexed to BMI to account for circulating blood volume. In patients with obesity, circulating blood volume increases in a nonlinear fashion and plateaus as BMI increases. This leads to administering lower fluid volumes with respect to blood volume.[16] In addition, the amount of vasopressors used per weight is less than in patients with normal weight, resulting in a decreased amount of vasopressors used per weight. Patients with obesity and septic shock require less weight-based doses of norepinephrine compared with patients without obesity.[17] This in turn leads to a decreased need for additional agents for support and a decreased risk of developing adverse effects from higher doses of medications and additional agents.

INFECTIONS

Obesity is an independent risk factor for increased intensive care unit length of stay and the development of infections.[9,18] Obesity is associated with a 50% increased rate of hospital infections, including subcutaneous tissue, nosocomial infection, such as pneumonia, *Clostridium difficile*, colitis, and sepsis, and other infections (**Box 1**).[12,19] Patients with obesity have more than a twofold increase in the risk of a bacteremia, respiratory infection, or urinary tract infection compared with patients with normal weight.[20]

The exact mechanism between obesity and infections is not clear, but dysregulation of the immune system, increased inflammatory mediators, decreased cell-mediated immune response, and respiratory dysfunction are contributing factors.[20,21] The downregulation and decreased effectiveness of the immune system create an environment conducive for infection. Women with obesity are at a 45% greater risk of a urinary tract infection than those without obesity.[22] In addition, several other risk factors, including increased risk of invasive procedures, changes in gut microbiota, altered pharmacokinetics, and comorbidities, place critically ill patients with obesity at increased risk of infection.[21] Some comorbidities, such as chronic obstructive pulmonary disease, increase the risk of patients developing pneumonia because of persistent mucus production and pathogenic bacteria in the airways.[23]

Although evidence supports that critically ill patients with obesity are at higher risk of developing postoperative infections, bloodstream infections, increased risk of pneumonia, and urinary infections, it is important to mention that obesity is not associated with increased mortality.[18] Critically ill patients with obesity have better 30-day and 60-day mortality than patients with normal weight.[4,17] This is attributed to the metabolic syndrome and attenuated inflammatory response found in patients with obesity.[12,18,21]

RESPIRATORY

Severe obesity increases the risk of respiratory failure owing to anatomic and physiologic changes to the respiratory system.[24,25] The excess cervical adipose tissue

---

Box 1
Obesity increases the risk of infection[12,19]

Subcutaneous tissue infection

Bacteremia

Urinary tract infection

Respiratory infections
  Pneumonia
  Coronavirus disease 2019

Clostridium difficile

Colitis

Sepsis

---

causes increased neck circumference, leading to upper airway collapse. In addition, the adipose tissue makes it difficult to identify landmarks and results in complications for bag-mask ventilation and placement of an airway.[6,26] Obesity also leads to decreased lung volumes effecting expiratory reserve volume, functional capacity, and functional residual volume.[6,24–26] In addition, there is increased airway resistance and decreased lung compliance, which results in alveolar collapse leading to ventilation-perfusion mismatch and intrapulmonary shunting. Decreased chest wall compliance also occurs because of increased adipose tissue around the abdomen and rib cage.[6,24] These physiologic changes that worsen with the greater the severity of the disease of obesity and results in an increase work of breathing eventually lead to hypoxia.[6,26]

Along with anatomic changes to the respiratory system, additional physiologic changes occur. Obesity increases the need for oxygen consumption, leading to decreased oxygenation.[26–28] Oxygen consumption in patients with obesity is 1.5 times higher than in patients without obesity.[27] This results in an increase in the work of breathing and excess production of carbon dioxide.[26–28] This eventually leads to hypoventilation syndrome and decreases respiratory drive, leading to the need for respiratory support, including noninvasive and mechanical ventilation.[26,27]

Mechanical ventilation in patients with obesity can be challenging. If inappropriate ventilator settings are applied, respiratory and hemodynamic deterioration may occur.[23,26] After mechanical ventilation is initiated, low tidal volume, moderate to high positive end-expiratory pressure, and recruitment maneuvers should be applied to avoid barotrauma and ventilator-induced lung injury.[26,27]

Evidence supports that patients with obesity admitted to a critical care setting have longer duration of mechanical ventilation compared with individuals without obesity.[18] In addition, critically ill patients with obesity are associated with higher rate of respiratory infections, such as pneumonia. Patients with obesity are also at higher risk of obstructive sleep apnea. The changes to the pulmonary system, such as pulmonary inflammation, restricted lung volumes, and lung compliance, are contributing factors that place these patients at higher risk.[18,29,30]

Despite the increased risk of developing respiratory infections, evidence supports that there is a negative relationship between respiratory infections and mortality. Studies support a protective association between obesity and mortality from pneumonia and other respiratory infections.[23] The association of lower mortality and obesity is influenced by underlying conditions, such as emphysema, nutritional status, and other types of infections, such as catheter infection.[29] In addition, insulin resistance and diabetes are known to impair host defenses and are linked to not only nosocomial infections and skin infections but also higher rates of respiratory infections, including pneumonia and influenza.[29]

CORONAVIRUS DISEASE 2019

With the effects that obesity has on the respiratory system and infections, it should come as no surprise that there is an association between obesity and coronavirus disease 2019. Patients with obesity and comorbidities, such as diabetes, renal dysfunction, underlying respiratory conditions, and cardiovascular disease, had a higher rate of mortality compared with patients with normal weight.[22,31,32] Mortality at 90 days was 31% higher in older patients with obesity and other comorbidities than those without baseline comorbidities.[33] In addition, comorbidities, such as diabetes, hypertension, and cardiovascular disease, place patients at higher risk of severe disease, and obesity may pose an additional risk.[34–37]

Patients with obesity and coronavirus disease 2019 have worse outcomes, including infection and respiratory failure.[38] Evidence supports that in hospitalized, critically ill patients with obesity, obesity was an independent risk factor for respiratory failure requiring intubation, intensive care unit admission, and death.[31,34,39–41] Patients with obesity and a BMI of 30 are 1.8 to 6.23 times more likely to be admitted to critical care and 2.6 to 3.45 times more likely to require mechanical ventilation.[35] As BMI increases to greater than 35, the risk associated with these events also increases to greater than 7 times more likely to require mechanical ventilation and almost 8 times more likely to be admitted to a critical care setting.[34] Patients with obesity need respiratory support sooner than patients with normal weight, and the effect of obesity on lung function, lung inflammation, and severity of illness contributed to the need for early mechanical ventilation.[31,33,39,41]

The mechanism between obesity and coronavirus disease 2019 includes a complex process. The effects of obesity on chronic adipose tissue inflammation and altering immune response played a significant role in developing the coronavirus disease 2019 infection and respiratory complications. The most notable changes to immunity involve impairment of lymphocytes, macrophages, and neutrophils, which had a negative impact on immunity from infection and vaccine efficacy.[32,37,39] Furthermore, obesity compromises the immune system by reducing macrophage activation, increasing inflammatory markers, and impairing B- and T-cell activation. This all leads to the inability of the body to fight infection, leading to more severity and complications associated with contracting the coronavirus disease 2019.[32,36,42]

In addition to the physiologic changes to the respiratory system from obesity, the coronavirus disease 2019 leads to decreased perfusion, increased hypoxemia, and limited ventilation through a complex process.[32,36,37] In patients with obesity, there is an increase in adipose tissue and fat deposits, which alters the mechanics of the lungs and chest wall as discussed previously. In addition, these fat deposits increase production of angiotensin-converting enzyme 2, which acts as a host cell for which coronavirus disease 2019 can enter and spread throughout the body to other organs, including the lung.[38,42,43] Also, through this metabolizing process, there is an overproduction of angiotensin II, which causes pulmonary vasoconstriction, inflammation, and lung injury. This leads to further exacerbation of coronavirus disease 2019, resulting in more severe lung injury.[38]

PHARMACOKINETICS

Obesity can affect pharmacokinetics and pharmacodynamics based on the pharmacochemistry of the drug.[1,21] Drugs are either hydrophilic or lipophilic. Hydrophilic drugs are soluble in water found in interstitial fluid and muscle, whereas lipophilic drugs penetrate the lipid bilayer of a cell and are absorbed into adipose tissue.[1,26,30,44] Therefore, as body fat increases with obesity, the absorption of hydrophilic drugs will decrease, and the absorption of lipophilic drugs will increase. In addition, one must consider dose adjustments for medications that are based on body weight.[1,30]

In addition to pharmacokinetics and pharmacodynamics, one must consider the effects of obesity on body systems and how these changes effect dosing. Patients may have cardiovascular compromise, renal dysfunction, liver dysfunction, malabsorption in the gut, and malnutrition.[1,26,44] Gastric emptying and gut permeability have an effect on oral bioavailability of some medications, so intravenous or intramuscular medications may need to be considered.[1,18,26,30] In addition, because medications are processed through the liver and kidneys, dose adjustments should be considered in those who have altered renal and liver perfusion.[1] In patients who have malnutrition, hypoalbuminemia may affect drug clearance because of altered protein binding.[1,44] Multiple factors, including comorbidities, should be considered when adjusting medications to minimize the effects of potential adverse outcomes.

Furthermore, there is evidence that supports patients with obesity may have a decreased response to vaccinations compared with individuals with normal weight. Obesity was associated with a poor antibody response to hepatitis B vaccination and lower antitetanus immunoglobulin G (IgG) antibodies.[18,30] In addition, there is an impaired immune response to influenza vaccination as detected by a greater decline in IgG antibodies in patients with obesity compared with patients with normal weight.[45] Reduced absorption from the injection site owing to increased adipose tissue and impaired immune cell activity are contributing factors for the response to vaccination.[7] In addition, altered metabolism, altered renal excretion, and hepatic metabolism can affect drug clearance and efficacy.[7] Decreased response to vaccination should be considered in the prevention and treatment of subjects with obesity.[30,45] There has been discussion as to whether patients with obesity should receive booster vaccinations, but further studies are warranted at this time.

SUMMARY

Increased consumption of energy-dense foods and a sedentary lifestyle are contributors to obesity. Contrary to belief, excessive caloric intake is not the only factor that causes obesity. The cause of obesity is multifactorial, including pathogenic factors, genetic inheritance, and behavioral and environmental causes, which also contribute to obesity.

Patients with obesity are at an increased risk for morbidity and mortality. Strong evidence shows that obesity impacts immune functions, produces a chronic inflammatory response that disturbs metabolic hormones, which results in sepsis, infections, and changes to respiratory function. Although obesity poses many complications for critically ill patients, these patients have improved mortality compared with patients with normal weight. The chronic low-grade inflammatory process may lead to a lower than expected proinflammatory response during severe infection and respiratory illness, which in turn leads to improved mortality. In addition, the additional adipose tissue in patients with obesity may protect the patient from metabolic syndrome and catabolic states that often occur in patients with normal weight.

In conclusion, although the obesity paradox is not fully understood, underlying comorbidities and how they affect outcomes of the patient with obesity should be considered. Vigilant monitoring, especially in the critical care setting, should be implemented to decrease the risk for the development of sepsis, infections, and respiratory alterations, including the need for mechanical ventilation, increased risk for lung injury, and increased length of intensive care unit stay. Early detection and treatment could lead to a huge financial savings. Upon discharge to home, implementing a nutritional regimen would be important to decrease any lingering metabolic or catabolic states. As always, including a referral to a dietician is warranted, as nutritional needs change when being discharged. Patients with obesity should be referred for treatment of this chronic disease with either their primary care provider or an obesity specialist if the patient has severe disease. Because of the extent of information under the stress of hospitalization, caregivers should be included in the discharge process to assist with lifestyle modifications and implementation of recommendations.

CLINICS CARE POINTS

- When managing an obese patient in the critical care setting, be proactive in monitoring for infection, as obesity increases the risk of sepsis and infection.

- When intubating an obese patient, take into consideration the anatomic changes that can lead to difficulties with intubation and be prepared.

- When adjusting ventilatory settings in critically ill obese patients, use low tidal volumes and moderate to high positive end-expiratory pressure to reduce the occurrence of barotrauma and ventilatory-induced lung injury.

- When starting vasopressor support in critically ill hemodynamically compromised obese patients, avoid using high doses of vasopressor agents and start with lower doses, as obese patients usually require fewer doses to reach hemodynamic goals.

- When vaccinating obese patients, obese patients may have a reduced response to vaccinations, such as hepatitis B and influenza vaccinations, so monitoring immunoglobulin G antibodies may be warranted to detect response to vaccinations.

DISCLOSURE

The authors have nothing to disclose.

REFERENCES

1. Schetz M, De Jong A, Deane AM, et al. Obesity in the critically ill: a narrative review. Intensive Care Med 2019;45(6):757–69.
2. Bochicchio GV, Joshi M, Bochicchio K, et al. Impact of obesity in the critically ill trauma patient: a prospective study. J Am Coll Surg 2006;203(4):533–8.
3. Hainer V, Aldhoon-Hainerová I. Obesity paradox does exist. Diabetes Care 2013; 36(Suppl 2):S276–81.
4. Utzolino S, Ditzel CM, Baier PK, et al. The obesity paradox in surgical intensive care patients with peritonitis. J Crit Care 2014;29(5):887.e1.
5. Dossett LA, Dageforde LA, Swenson BR, et al. Obesity and site-specific nosocomial infection risk in the intensive care unit. Surg Infect 2009;10(2):137–42.
6. Patel JJ, Rosenthal MD, Miller KR, et al. The critical care obesity paradox and implications for nutrition support. Curr Gastroenterol Rep 2016;18(9):1–8.
7. Dhurandhar NV, Bailey D, Thomas D. Interaction of obesity and infections. Obes Rev 2015;16(12):1017–29.
8. Spartalis M, Tzatzaki E, Moris D, et al. Morbidity, mortality, and obesity paradox. Ann Transl Med 2017;5:440.

9. Sakr Y, Madl C, Filipescu D, et al. Obesity is associated with increased morbidity but not mortality in critically ill patients. Intensive Care Med 2008;34(11): 1999–2009.

10. Papadimitriou-Olivgeris M, Aretha D, Zotou A, et al. The role of obesity in sepsis outcome among critically ill patients: a retrospective cohort analysis. Biomed Res Int 2016;2016:5941279.

11. Richard AJ, White U, Elks CM, et al. Adipose tissue: physiology to metabolic dysfunction. Endotext 2020;4(4). Available at: https://www.ncbi.nlm.nih.gov/sites/books/NBK555602/.

12. Green WD, Beck MA. Obesity altered T cell metabolism and the response to infection. Curr Opin Immunol 2017;46:1–7.

13. Desruisseaux MS, Nagajyothi, Trujillo ME, et al. Adipocyte, adipose tissue, and infectious disease. Infect Immun 2007;75(3):1066–78.

14. Robinson J, Swift-Scanlan T, Salyer J. Obesity and 1-year mortality in adults after sepsis: a systematic review. Biol Res Nurs 2020;22(1):103–13.

15. Adams C, Tucker C, Allen B, et al. Disparities in hemodynamic resuscitation of the obese critically ill septic shock patient. J Crit Care 2017;37:219–23.

16. Shashaty M, Stapleton RD. Physiological and management implications of obesity in critical illness. Ann Am Thorac Soc 2014;11(8):1286–97.

17. Kalani C, Venigalla T, Bailey J, et al. Sepsis patients in critical care units with obesity: is obesity protective? Cureus 2020;12(2):e6929.

18. Milner JJ, Beck MA. The impact of obesity on the immune response to infection. Proc Nutr Soc 2012;71(2):298–306.

19. Dobner J, Kaser S. Body mass index and the risk of infection-from underweight to obesity. Clin Microbiol Infect 2018;24(1):24–8.

20. Huttunen R, Syrjänen J. Obesity and the risk and outcome of infection. Int J Obes 2013;37(3):333–40.

21. Huttunen R, Karppelin M, Syrjänen J. Obesity and nosocomial infections. J Hosp Infect 2013;85(1):8–16.

22. Grier WR, Kratimenos P, Singh S, et al. Obesity as a risk factor for urinary tract infection in children. Clin Pediatr 2016;55(10):952–6.

23. Restrepo MI, Sibila O, Anzueto A. Pneumonia in patients with chronic obstructive pulmonary disease. Tuberc Respir Dis (Seoul) 2018;81(3):187–97.

24. Bercault N, Boulain T, Kuteifan K, et al. Obesity-related excess mortality rate in an adult intensive care unit: a risk-adjusted matched cohort study. Crit Care Med 2004;32(4):998–1003.

25. Ashburn DD, DeAntonio A, Reed MJ. Pulmonary system and obesity. Crit Care Clin 2010;26(4):597–602.

26. Parker BK, Manning S, Winters ME. The crashing obese patient. West J Emerg Med 2019;20(2):323.

27. De Jong A, Chanques G, Jaber S. Mechanical ventilation in obese ICU patients: from intubation to extubation. Crit Care 2017;21(1):1–8.

28. Tafelski S, Yi H, Ismaeel F, et al. Obesity in critically ill patients is associated with increased need of mechanical ventilation but not with mortality. J Infect Public Health 2016;9(5):577–85.

29. Mancuso P. Obesity and respiratory infections: does excess adiposity weigh down host defense? Pulm Pharmacol Ther 2013;26(4):412–9.

30. Genoni G, Prodam F, Marolda A, et al. Obesity and infection: two sides of one coin. Eur J Pediatr 2014;173(1):25–32.

31. Kalligeros M, Shehadeh F, Mylona EK, et al. Association of obesity with disease severity among patients with coronavirus disease 2019. Obesity 2020;28(7): 1200–4.
32. Fedele D, De Francesco A, Riso S, et al. Obesity, malnutrition and trace elements deficiency in the COVID19 pandemic: an overview. Nutrition 2020;81:111016.
33. COVID-ICU Group on behalf of the REVA Network and the COVID-ICU Investigators. Clinical characteristics and day-90 outcomes of 4244 critically ill adults with COVID-19: a prospective cohort study. Intensive Care Med 2021;47(1):60–73.
34. Rottoli M, Bernante P, Belvedere A, et al. How important is obesity as a risk factor for respiratory failure, intensive care admission and death in hospitalised COVID-19 patients? Results from a single Italian centre. Eur J Endocrinol 2020;183(4): 389–97.
35. Albashir AAD. The potential impacts of obesity on COVID-19. Clin Med 2020; 20(4):e109.
36. De Lorenzo A, Tarsitano MG, Falcone C, et al. Fat mass affects nutritional status of ICU COVID-19 patients. J Transl Med 2020;18(1):1–8.
37. Richardson S, Hirsch JS, Narasimhan M, et al. Presenting characteristics, comorbidities, and outcomes among 5700 patients hospitalized with COVID-19 in the New York City area. JAMA 2020;323(20):2052–9.
38. Sanchis-Gomar F, Lavie CJ, Mehra MR, et al. Obesity and outcomes in COVID-19: when an epidemic and pandemic collide. In: Mayo clinic proceedings. Elsevier; 2020.
39. Hussain A, Mahawar K, Xia Z, et al. Obesity and mortality of COVID-19. Meta-analysis. Obes Res Clin Pract 2020;14(4):295–300.
40. Frank RC, Mendez SR, Stevenson EK, et al. Obesity and the risk of intubation or death in patients with coronavirus disease 2019. Crit Care Med 2020;48(11): e1097–101.
41. Földi M, Farkas N, Kiss S, et al. Obesity is a risk factor for developing critical condition in COVID-19 patients: a systematic review and meta-analysis. Obes Rev 2020;21(10):e13095.
42. Malik P, Patel U, Patel K, et al. Obesity a predictor of outcomes of COVID-19 hospitalized patients—a systematic review and meta-analysis. J Med Virol 2021; 93(2):1188–93.
43. Soeroto AY, Soetedjo NN, Purwiga A, et al. Effect of increased BMI and obesity on the outcome of COVID19 adult patients: a systematic review and meta-analysis. Diabetes Metab Syndr 2020;14(6):1897–904.
44. Smit C, De Hoogd S, Brüggemann RJ, et al. Obesity and drug pharmacology: a review of the influence of obesity on pharmacokinetic and pharmacodynamic parameters. Expert Opin Drug Metab Toxicol 2018;14(3):275–85.
45. Hainer V, Zamrazilová H, Kunesova M, et al. Obesity and infection: reciprocal causality. Physiol Res 2015;64:S105.

Obesity and Children

Nancy T. Browne, MS, PPCNP-BC

KEYWORDS

- Pediatric • Obesity • Weight stigma • Bullying • Victimization • Pharmacotherapy
- Obesity treatment • Social determinants

KEY POINTS

- Pediatric obesity is a heterogenous, chronic, relapsing disease
- Obesity in childhood is associated with metabolic and psychosocial complications
- Weight-based victimization is common with metabolic and psychosocial implications
- Evidence-based guidelines are available to treat childhood obesity
- Nurses are positioned to positively impact children with obesity by providing affirmation, clinical management, and psychosocial support

INTRODUCTION

The constructs of optimal diet, activity, sleep, and environmental elements are integral to a child's health. The observation that some children with "good health habits" develop obesity, whereas others with "poor health habits" do not, speaks to the complexity of energy dysregulation in children. Ongoing research examines why some children are more susceptible to obesity, why some develop obesity earlier with a steeper trajectory, and why some are more responsive metabolically to therapy than their counterparts. The goal of pediatric obesity disease is prevention; the secondary goal is successful treatment that is the least invasive with minimal consequences.

Optimal treatment strategies are a current research focus. Treatment options and combinations are being explored, studied, and implemented. Personalized, interdisciplinary care is necessary to meet the complexity and wide disease variance found in pediatric obesity. Complications of obesity in children and adolescents encompass a wide range of metabolic and psychosocial conditions, many traditionally only seen in older adults. In particular, weight-based victimization (WBV) threatens the health of children with obesity as much as metabolic obesity–related complications.[1] Nurses play a key role in mitigating this threat to children's physical and psychosocial health. The purpose of this review is to discuss the complexity of pediatric obesity and its unique components and consequences. Evidence-based pediatric guidelines and treatment recommendations are shared that advocate for their implementation in all

25 Andrews Avenue, Falmouth, ME 04105, USA
E-mail address: nancytkacz@sbcglobal.net
Twitter: @nancytbrowne (N.T.B.)

Nurs Clin N Am 56 (2021) 583–597
https://doi.org/10.1016/j.cnur.2021.07.006
0029-6465/21/© 2021 Elsevier Inc. All rights reserved.

levels of pediatric practice. The review shares how nurses in multiple practice areas can make a meaningful impact on the lives of children and adolescents with obesity.

DEFINITION AND PREVALENCE OF PEDIATRIC OBESITY

Obesity in children is measured by body mass index percentiles obtained by plotting weight and height on gender-specific standardized growth charts.[2,3] The Centers for Disease Control and Prevention[4] define adiposity in children as overweight (85th–94th percentiles), obesity (95th–98th percentiles; class 1 obesity), and severe obesity (>99th percentile; class 2 and class 3 obesity). Specific growth charts are available to track severe obesity (percentage of the 95th percentile) classifying greater than or equal to 120% to 140% of the 95th percentile as class II obesity and greater than or equal to 140% of the 95th percentile as class III obesity.[5,6] Growth charts tailored to the needs of children with Down syndrome, achondroplasia, and Turner syndrome are also available.[7–9]

The prevalence of overweight and obesity in children living in the United States currently approaches 33%.[10] The severity of pediatric obesity increases with age: 41.5% of US adolescents 16 to 19 years old are classified with class 1 or 2 obesity and 4.5% meet the criteria for class 3 obesity. Globally, obesity affects more than 337 million children.

HEALTH CONSEQUENCES ASSOCIATED WITH OBESITY IN CHILDREN AND ADOLESCENTS

Obesity-related complications and co-occurring conditions present a challenge to pediatric clinicians. Traditionally, minimal health screening is performed for children and adolescents beyond yearly well child visits, which are heavily scripted for anticipatory guidance and immunizations. With obesity now affecting a third of US children, many will have significant obesity-related disease burden requiring diagnosis and treatment.[11–13] More than 200 obesity-related conditions affecting all organ systems have been identified.[14,15] **Table 1** lists the most common obesity-related complications in children.

Psychosocial and Associated Complications

Psychosocial obesity-related complications are common. Children experiencing weight stigmatizing events are at increased risk for adverse metabolic and psychosocial outcomes.[16,17] In particular, depression and anxiety are increased in children with severe obesity.[18] Chronic stress from ongoing WBV, bullying, and teasing breaks down normal functioning of energy regulatory pathways and weakens normal immune responses.[1,17] Quality of life is significantly affected by these stressors resulting in further threats to mental and cardiometabolic health.[19]

As the understanding of energy regulation physiology and pathophysiology deepens, so does an understanding of other diseases that share the same injured metabolic pathways, particularly in the central nervous system and brain. Diseases sharing these pathways and co-occurring with obesity include attention-deficit/hyperactivity disorder,[20,21] sleep disorders,[22] loss of control eating disorder/binge eating disorder,[23] and anxiety.[24] It is important for nurses to assess for obesity co-occurring conditions regardless of why the child presented for health care.

GENETICS AND EPIGENETICS

Obesity is a complex and heritable disorder, resulting from the interplay between genetic susceptibility, epigenetics, plasticity, and the environment.[25] Genetic involvement

Table 1
Obesity-related complications in children

Medical	Psychosocial
Cancers	Attention-deficit/hyperactivity disorder
Cholelithiasis	Anxiety
Gallbladder disease	Bulimia nervosa
Gastrointestinal reflux	Bullying
Hyperinsulinemia	Depression
Insulin resistance	Low quality of life
Joint disorders (osteoarthritis)	Low self-esteem
Liver disease (nonalcoholic fatty liver disease, nonalcoholic steatohepatitis)	Night eating syndrome
Obstructive sleep apnea	Poor school performance
Thyroid disease	Sleep-related eating disorder
Dyslipidemia	Teasing
Idiopathic intracranial hypertension	Weight bias/discrimination
Metabolic syndrome	
Asthma	
Hypertension	
Sleep disorder syndromes	
Prediabetes	
Polycystic ovary syndrome	
Insulin resistance	
Orthopedic conditions (Blount disease, slipped capital femoral epiphysis)	
Cardiovascular disease	
Type 2 diabetes	

Data from: Skinner AC, Perrin EM, Moss LA, et al. Cardiometabolic risks and severity of obesity in children and young adults. N Engl J Med. 2015;373(14):1307-1317. https://doi.org/10.1056/NEJMoa1502821; Puhl RM, Lessard LM. Weight stigma in youth: Prevalence, consequences, and considerations for clinical practice. Curr Obes Rep. 2020;9(4):402-411. https://doi.org/10.1007/s13679-020-00408-8.

in childhood obesity is defined as monogenic (syndromic and nonsyndromic), polygenic, and epigenetic.[26]

Monogenic obesity disorders consist of a single gene mutation and are less affected by environmental factors. These disorders are rare and typically characterized by severe hyperphagia and steep trajectories in weight gain during early childhood.[27] Monogenic obesity disorders are caused by mutations in leptin–melanocortin hypothalamic pathways, which regulate appetite, hunger, and satiety.

Monogenic obesity is further depicted as syndromic and nonsyndromic. In syndromic obesity, clinical phenotypes, such as intellectual and developmental delays, severe hyperphagia, and dysmorphic features occur in association with obesity.[27] In nonsyndromic obesity, the main symptom is severe obesity. **Figs. 1 and 2** list monogenic nonsyndromic and syndromic conditions associated with pediatric obesity.[27,28]

Polygenic obesity is multifactorial and involves several obesity-related polymorphic genes interacting with environmental factors, such as diet, physical activity, and

Disease	Characteristic Features	Comments
Congenital Leptin Deficiency	Early-onset severe obesity and hyperphagia, altered immune function, delayed puberty	Mutations: *ob* gene Undetectable serum leptin levels Treatment: leptin
Congenital leptin receptor deficiency	Early-onset severe obesity and hyperphagia, altered immune function, delayed puberty	Normal serum leptin levels
Melanocortin 4 receptor (MC4-R) Mutation	Tall stature Rapid growth	Normal mental status
Pro-opiomelanocortin (POMC) Mutation	Red hair, pale skin, low blood pressure or rapid pulse, corticotropin deficiency, adrenal insufficiency	Hypopigmentation Isolated ACTH deficiency

Fig. 1. Monogenic nonsyndromic obesity. ACTH, adrenocorticotropic hormone. (*Data from* Chung WK. An overview of monogenic and syndromic obesities in humans. Pediatr Blood Cancer 2012;58(1):122–8; and Mason K, Page L, Balikcioglu PG. Screening for hormonal, monogenic, and syndromic disorders in obese infants and children. Pediatr Ann 2014;43(9):e218–24.)

endocrine disruptors. Individual responses to these environmental components are influenced by susceptibility genes.[29] In polygenic obesity, a greater number of obesity-related gene mutations increases the risk for obesity phenotypes.[29]

Epigenetics refers to factors that can affect gene function without modifying the gene's DNA sequence. Environmental influences during early life may induce epigenetic variation affecting later metabolism and chronic disease risk including obesity.[30]

CONSIDERATIONS UNIQUE TO CHILDREN IMPACTING OBESITY TREATMENT
Plasticity

Obesity treatment for children is conceptually unique in several ways. The first unique concept is plasticity, which is the ability to reprogram development based on internal

Disease	Key Characteristics	Comments
Prader-Willi Syndrome	Short stature, hypotonia, developmental delay, hyperphagia	Increased ghrelin level
Bardet-Biedl Syndrome (Laurence-Moon)	Retinitis pigmentosa, polydactyly, hypogonadism, hypotonia, developmental delay	Autosomal recessive
Albright Hereditary Osteodystrophy	Developmental delay, short stature, and short fourth and fifth metacarpals, hypocalcemia	Pseudohypoparathyroidism; Precocious puberty
Fragile X	Intellectual disability, large ears, large testes, CCG trinucleotide affecting *FMR-1* gene on X chromosome	FISH Hybridization
Chen Syndrome	Obesity, hypotonia, microcephaly, prominent incisors	Auto Recessive
Beckwith-Wiedemann Syndrome	Macroglossia, macrosomia, hypoglycemia, ear pits, midline abdominal wall defects	Increased cancer incidence (Wilms tumor, hepatoblastoma)
Alström Syndrome	Sensorial hearing loss, blindness, IR and hyperinsulinemia, DM, dilated cardiomyopathy, hepatic and renal failure	Mutation in *ALMS1* gene

Fig. 2. Monogenic syndromic obesity. DM, diabetes mellitus; FISH, fluorescence in situ hybridization; IR, insulin resistance. (*Data from* Chung WK. An overview of monogenic and syndromic obesities in humans. Pediatr Blood Cancer 2012;58(1):122–8; and Mason K, Page L, Balikcioglu PG. Screening for hormonal, monogenic, and syndromic disorders in obese infants and children. Pediatr Ann 2014;43(9):e218–24.)

and external factors affecting the organism.[30,31] There are critical developmental periods for endocrine and metabolic systems where plasticity may exhibit positive and negative effects depending on the child's responses to environmental influences. Questions for ongoing research, particularly for the child with obesity, include can early intervention reset the body's energy set point (preset normal weight range, controlled by genetic DNA) and change accelerated weight trajectory,[32] and is there a point where the plasticity effect is lost and change in trajectory no longer possible?

Adiposity Rebound

In normal growth, adiposity rises rapidly in the first year of life (time of accelerated growth); then growth rate declines, reaching its lowest rate at approximately 6 years of age. Adiposity rebound is the age at which the growth rate rises again.[33] Early adiposity rebound (as early as 2–4 years old) is a marker of later obesity development and an indication for early obesity intervention.

Off-Label: What It is and what It is Not

Off-label is a common concept in pediatric care with implications for pediatric obesity treatment options. Off-label does not mean illegal; rather, it means that there is not enough (or any) evidence from double-blinded, randomized trials to demonstrate the efficacy of a treatment for a particular indication. Therapies for pediatric conditions, including those for obesity treatment, are often guided by clinical practice guidelines and best practice evidence. Pediatric clinicians are guided by the American Academy of Pediatrics (AAP) statement on off-label medication use in children.[34]

PEDIATRIC OBESITY TREATMENT
Goals and Principles of Treatment

The goal of pediatric obesity treatment is to improve the child's health and quality of life. Numerous guidelines, statements, and recommendations from pediatric and obesity specialists are available for the clinician (**Table 2**). In 2007, the AAP outlined a progressive recommendation of four stages of pediatric obesity treatment: primary care with increasing intensity (stages 1 and 2) and interdisciplinary obesity treatment teams (stages 3 and 4).[35] Revised AAP pediatric obesity treatment guidelines are anticipated in 2022.

The Obesity Medicine Association pediatric obesity algorithm reviews pediatric age groups, obesity complications, and pediatric obesity treatment.[36] The Obesity Medicine Association treatment pyramid (**Fig. 3**) depicts the stepwise approach to advanced pediatric obesity care that mirrors AAP stages 2 to 4. All pediatric obesity treatment is built on the standard foundation of evidenced-based dietary, activity, behavioral health, and environmental support (intensive lifestyle therapy [ILT]). All further advanced treatments are additive and administered with ongoing ILT support by an obesity-trained interdisciplinary team.

Clinical Assessment

A focused clinical assessment of the child with suspected obesity is additive to their general clinical examination. The focused areas specific to obesity include particular attention to growth history, accurate weight and height (weight percentile), growth trajectory, and age of onset of increased weight. What has been tried, what has worked, and what has not worked in the management of accelerated weight gain guides the clinician in identifying potential obesity subtypes. A weight graph drawn by the parents or child (if able) is helpful to see the pattern of weight gain (linear in trajectory or

Table 2
Pediatric obesity evidence-based guidance

Citation	Guidance	Organization
Armstrong et al,[49] 2019	Pediatric metabolic and bariatric surgery	American Academy of Pediatrics
Barlow & Expert Committee,[35] 2007	Pediatric staged obesity management and prevention	American Academy of Pediatrics[a]
Cuda et al,[36] 2020	Pediatric obesity treatment algorithm	Obesity Medicine Association
Estrada et al,[40] 2014	Consensus statements on childhood obesity comorbidities	Children's Hospital Association
Frattarelli et al,[34] 2014	Off-label use of drugs in children	American Academy of Pediatrics
Institute for Healthy Childhood Weight,[41,b]	Algorithm for assessment and management of childhood obesity	American Academy of Pediatrics
Jastreboff et al,[15] 2019	Obesity as a disease: Position Statement	The Obesity Society
Pont et al,[56] 2017	Weight stigma experienced by children and adolescents	The Obesity Society
Pratt et al,[50] 2018	Pediatric metabolic and bariatric surgery guidelines	American Society of Metabolic & Bariatric Surgery
Rubino et al,[19] 2020	International consensus statement for ending obesity stigma	International obesity organizations
Rudd Center for Food Policy & Obesity[c]	Weight bias, stigma tool kit for adults and children	Rudd Center for Food Policy & Obesity
Srivastava et al,[51] 2019	Clinical considerations regarding obesity pharmacotherapy in adolescents with obesity	Multicenter expert panel
Styne et al,[42] 2017	Pediatric obesity assessment, treatment, and prevention practice guidelines	The Endocrine Society
US Preventive Services Task Force,[44] 2017	US Preventive Services Task Force Recommendation Best Practice Statement	US Preventive Services Task Force

[a] Revised American Academy of Pediatrics recommendations expected 2022.
[b] https://ihcw.aap.org/resources/Documents/algorithm_brightfutures_032819.pdf/.
[c] www.uconnruddcenter.org/.

intermittent). A complete list of the child's current medications allows for identification of drugs that cause unintentional weight gain. **Table 3** lists focused areas of obesity assessment.

A psychosocial assessment identifies stressors that may exacerbate obesity illness. Bullying, teasing, and weight discrimination are common for children with obesity leading to complications, such as anxiety, depression, decreased self-esteem, and decreased coping skills.[1] Appropriate counseling and referrals for more intense

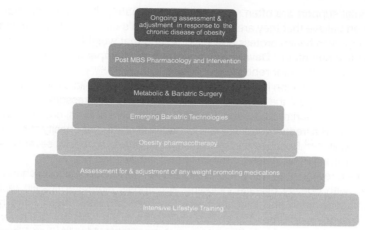

Fig. 3. Building blocks of pediatric obesity treatment. MBS, metabolic and bariatric surgery. (With permission: © Obesity Medicine Association® 2020-2022.)

Table 3
Focused pediatric obesity assessment

Assessment Area	History of
Previous weight management experience	What has worked; what has not When did excessive weight gain begin Discuss weight graph drawn by family
Current medications	Weight promoting, weight neutral, weight decreasing
Diet history	Who shops and cooks Daily and weekly diet routine Fluid intake (water, sugar-sweetened beverages)
Hunger and satiety assessment	"Out of control" related eating "Hungry all the time" "Food hoarding and sneaking" Eating related to emotions?
Food insecurity	Evaluate for food insecurity
Psychological assessment	Past traumas/severe stress Anxiety, depression, psychological diagnosis Bullying/teasing/weight stigma history
Social assessment	Caretakers, guardians With whom does the child live and when Social or racial determinants of health
Obesity-related complications	Metabolic Psychosocial Sleep disturbances
Activity	Daily and weekly pattern Opportunities and limitations Preferences

Data from: Barlow SE, Expert Committee. Expert committee recommendations regarding the prevention, assessment, and treatment of child and adolescent overweight and obesity: summary report. Pediatrics. 2007;120 Suppl 4:S164-S192. https://doi.org/10.1542/peds.2007-2329C; Cuda S, Censani M, O'Hara V, et al. Pediatric Obesity Algorithm, presented by the Obesity Medicine Association. 2020-2022. www.obesitymedicine.org/childhood-obesity (Accessed February 2021).

psychosocial support are often necessary. Unfortunately, it is common that parents and children believe that they are at fault for the child's excess weight with family, educators, and even health professionals suggesting that weight gain is a failure in self-control and/or parenting.[1] Developing a supportive, therapeutic relationship with the child and family allows for rebuilding of trust.

Psychosocial evaluation is conducted in the context of a child's social determinants of health, which impact the child's family and environment. Stressors can include economic instability; discrimination; and threats to health care access, housing, and safety. Food insecurity is a frequent stressor associated with childhood obesity and is screened for at each visit.[37,38] Because chronic stress contributes to obesity severity, efforts to decrease environmental stress for the child and family are a priority.[39]

A complete review of systems and physical examination focuses on characteristics connected with obesity disease including acanthosis nigricans (insulin resistance), joint dysfunction (pain and joint degeneration from physical stress), and hirsutism (polycystic ovary syndrome). For children higher than the 95th percentile for weight, baseline screening includes fasting glucose, hemoglobin A1c, lipid and liver panels, and blood pressure using an age-appropriate cuff size.[40,41] Further testing based on initial screening results may include sleep study, liver scan, and fasting insulin.[36,42] In collaboration with the child and family, a plan of care tailored to the child's specific needs and treatment options is devised.[20]

Clinical Management

Foundational pediatric obesity treatment

The cornerstone of obesity treatment is ILT and management of weight-promoting medications and obesity complications. Childhood and adolescence are dynamic times and principles of growth and development guide all treatment.[43] In collaboration with the family and child, a treatment plan consisting of small, achievable goals is implemented. Coordination with dietitians, activity specialists, and behavioral professionals trained in obesity care is recommended.[35,42] Guided by chronic disease management principles, obesity care is ongoing with expected relapses and times of educational repetition. The US Preventive Services Task Force recommends comprehensive ILT (≥26 hours) over 2 to 12 months for children with obesity disease.[44]

The child's medications are identified as weight promoting, weight neutral, or weight reducing (**Figs. 4 and 5**). The cause of weight gain for many children is often related to

	Significant Weight Gain		Small to Neutral Weight Gain		Weight Loss (neutral to mild)
ADHD			Guanfacine		Atomoxetine Lisdexamfetamine Amphetamine Methylphenidate
Anti-Seizure	Valproate Vigabatrin	Pregabalin Gabapentin	Carbamazepine Oxocarbazepine	Lamotrigine Levetoracetam Phenytoin	Topiramate Zonisamide Felbamate
Migraine	Amitriptyline Divalproex Flunarizine	Gabapentin Metoprolol Propranolol	Timolol Levetiracetam		Zonisamide Topiramate
Diabetic Medications	Insulin and analogs				Liraglutide, Exenatide, Semaglutatide, Dulagulitide Metformin
Other Medications	Glucocorticoids Gleevac Depo Provera		Benzodiazepines Statins Antihistamines (Cyproheptadine) Carvedilol Oral Contraceptive Pills		

Fig. 4. Nonpsychiatric medications that affect weight. ADHD, attention-deficit/hyperactivity disorder. (With permission: © Obesity Medicine Association® 2020-2022.)

	Significant Weight Gain		Small to Neutral Weight Gain	Weight Loss
Antipsychotics	Clozapine Olanzapine Chlorpromazine Quetiapine Risperidone		Aripiprazole Haloperidol Ziprasidone	
Antidepressants	Paroxetine* Amitriptyline Olanzapine Citalopram Nortriptyline Doxepin Mirtazapine	Lithium Desipramine Imipramine Duloxetine Escitalopram	Venlafaxine Fluvoxamine Sertraline Trazodone Fluoxetine	Bupropion*
Mood Stabilizers	Valproate Lithium Gabapentin			Topiramate
Anxiolytics			Lorazepam Diazepam Oxazepam	

Fig. 5. Psychiatric medications that affect weight. (With permission: © Obesity Medicine Association® 2020-2022.)

pharmacotherapy necessary to manage a separate medical condition. Medications as complex as steroids or as commonplace as antihistamines for seasonal allergies may trigger unusual weight gain in susceptible children. Coordination to manage medical conditions with the least weight-promoting side effects is complex but essential to best outcomes.

Advanced pediatric obesity treatment

Advanced treatment of severe obesity and its complications may include antiobesity pharmacotherapy, device therapy, metabolic and bariatric surgery (MBS), or a combination of these modalities.[45] MBS safety and efficacy in adolescents, including psychosocial outcomes, have been demonstrated in single and multi-institutional studies managed by interdisciplinary groups that reinforce ILT throughout preoperative and postoperative care.[46–48] MBS outcomes in adolescents mirror adult weight loss along with improvement of obesity-related conditions and general health.[46] Guidelines for MBS in the pediatric population are available from the AAP and the American Society for Metabolic and Bariatric Surgery.[49,50]

Antiobesity pharmacotherapy also is used as an adjunct to ILT in pediatric obesity care. Antiobesity pharmacotherapy options may be Food and Drug Administration (FDA)-approved for weight loss in certain pediatric age groups or FDA-approved for other indications (type 2 diabetes) and administered using off-label pediatric protocols.[34] Best practice use of antiobesity pharmacotherapy in children and adolescents includes ongoing care by an interdisciplinary team trained in pediatric obesity management.[51,52]

Antiobesity device therapy includes space-occupying devices (intragastric balloons), malabsorptive endoscopic luminal sleeve, vagal nerve stimulation, and aspiration devices. These devices are temporary, removable, and adjustable, which may be an advantage in children and adolescents because of plasticity of pediatric obesity disease.[53] Device therapy is not currently FDA-approved in the pediatric population in the United States.

Chronic disease management principles guide the care of children with obesity.[54] Obesity as a chronic disease tends to improve and relapse, necessitating ongoing assessment of treatment efficacy and adjustment of treatment options. Combination therapy uses ILT and advanced therapies in a multitude of groupings to manage obesity-related complications and maintain optimal health. The interdisciplinary team, particularly obesity-trained counselors, plays an important role in supporting children, adolescents, and their families in the realization and understanding that obesity disease is chronic and requires ongoing care. The principles of patient- and family-centered care are used throughout the spectrum of care.[55]

IMPLEMENTATION INTO PEDIATRIC PRACTICE

Building on concepts discussed throughout this article, this section considers how to maximize the impact of pediatric obesity care at the nursing practice, clinical office, community, and professional nursing levels. Pediatric nurses encounter children and adolescents with obesity in a variety of professional settings. In some encounters, the purpose for the visit is to address concerns regarding weight and obesity-related complications. In other settings, the primary reason for the encounter has a different focus, which challenges the nurse in how to intervene to a health-related concern requiring a timely and sensitive conversation.[19] Effective communication is central to meeting this challenge; perhaps with direct conversation with the child and family or perhaps with the child's primary provider. The key point is that the child with obesity has a chronic disease with obesity-related conditions that threaten overall health.

Pediatric Nursing Specific Strategies

At the individual nursing practice level, in addition to strategies already discussed, education of the family remains a primary goal. The disease of obesity is observable. Frequently, children with obesity and their families receive ongoing, unrelenting variations of weight-related bias, teasing, bullying, unsolicited advice, and outdated theories leading to internalized bias with psychosocial and metabolic consequences.[17] A safe haven clinical space grounded in evidence-based obesity care provides the child and family with optimal clinical and emotional support.[56]

Pediatric Office and Community Considerations

In primary care practice, all members of the office and clinical team play a role in providing optimal care for the child with obesity. Sadly, research demonstrates that health care providers may inadvertently contribute to poor weight-related interactions with patients.[1] Nurses can open conversations with other team members regarding feelings in caring for children with the disease of obesity. Opportunities for education include obesity etiology, psychosocial risks (bullying, teasing), office environment (appropriately sized/weight limit for chairs, examination table, gowns, blood pressure cuffs), and sensitivity around obtaining weights (privacy, permission). Evolving a culture that is sensitive, educated to the disease of obesity, and supportive of person-first language promotes optimal obesity care for the child and family. The nurse plays a key role in educating and modeling these concepts.

Professional Considerations

Professionally, nurses have a multitude of opportunities to advance pediatric obesity care. Education about normal energy regulation, pathophysiology resulting in obesity, phenotypes, obesity treatment options, and risks of weight-promoting medications can be shared within the nursing profession and also in the general community. Evidence-based information about how obesity affects children, along with correction of common obesity myths reduces obesity-related bias and discrimination. Pediatric nurses are respected and positioned to model person first language and actions. Advocacy extends to health care institutions (committees), professional organizations,

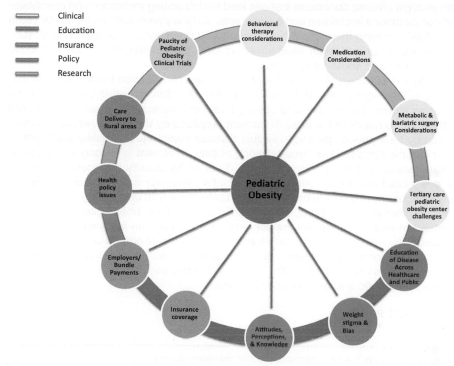

Fig. 6. Twelve barriers to care in pediatric obesity treatment. (With permission: Srivastava G, Kyle T, O'Hara V, et al. Caring for US children: barriers to effective treatment in children with the disease of obesity. Obesity 2021;29(1):46–55.)

and policy makers.[57] The consensus statement for ending obesity stigma includes a call-to-action pledge suitable for office display as a code of conduct.[19]

BARRIERS TO PEDIATRIC OBESITY CARE INCLUDING MYTHS

Barriers to pediatric obesity care include incomplete clinical management, outdated education, poor insurance coverage, insufficient policy advances, and exclusion from research.[58] Central to these barriers is the disparity between current scientific knowledge of energy regulation and impact of dysregulation (obesity) and what is considered "common knowledge" in lay and health care education. WBV is pervasive in every facet of society. From lack of person-first language ("person with obesity" instead of "obese person") to disrespectful portrayals on media channels, negative portrayal of children with obesity results in cultural stereotypes. Insurance coverage for pediatric obesity care is severely hampered by outdated beliefs that obesity treatment is cosmetic and optional. Nurses, through education and behavior modeling, can advocate to dispel these myths allowing for evidence-based care for children and adolescents with the disease of obesity. **Fig. 6** depicts these barriers in the clinical, education, insurance, policy, and research realms.[58]

SUMMARY

Obesity is a heterogenous, chronic, relapsing disease with the strong potential to severely affect a child's physical, mental, and spiritual life. The disease is associated with multiple chronic conditions that can lead to debilitating metabolic and psychosocial complications in children and adolescents. WBV is particularly impactful on youth with obesity putting them at risk for psychosocial conditions, including anxiety, substance abuse, and suicidal ideation along with detrimental effects on academic advancement and social integration.[1]

Evidence-based recommendations offer guidance for stepwise treatment of obesity and associated conditions. Built on a foundation of nutrition, activity, and behavioral therapies supported by advanced obesity treatment, clinical management is tailored to the specific needs of the child. Treatment is guided by the child's response represented by their phenotype and individual disease trajectory. Not unlike treatment of other chronic diseases (eg, hypertension), obesity treatment is lifelong with ongoing therapy adjustment as per clinical needs. Successful obesity treatment is different for every child and family. Although the child's metabolic and psychosocial needs may be equally important to the health care team, WBV with unrelenting microaggressions is often the lens through which children see their obesity-impacted world. Nurses can make a significant impact in the lives of children living with the disease of obesity by listening, offering affirmation that WBV is wrong, providing and facilitating psychosocial support, and offering respite for children to escape the constant barrage of stress-related interactions.[59] By improving psychosocial health, the child receives metabolic and psychosocial benefits.

CLINICS CARE POINTS

- Pediatric obesity is a heterogenous, chronic, relapsing disease
- Obesity in childhood is associated with metabolic and psychosocial complications
- Weight-based victimization is common with metabolic and psychosocial implications
- Evidence-based guidelines are available to treat childhood obesity
- Nurses are positioned to positively impact children with obesity by providing positive affirmation and psychosocial support

DISCLOSURE

The author has nothing to disclose.

REFERENCES

1. Puhl RM, Lessard LM. Weight stigma in youth: prevalence, consequences, and considerations for clinical practice. Curr Obes Rep 2020;9(4):402–11.
2. Kuczmarski RJ, Ogden CL, Grummer-Strawn LM, et al. CDC growth charts: United States. Adv Data 2000;314:1–27.
3. Centers for Disease Control and Prevention, Division of Nutrition, Physical Activity, and Obesity, National Center for Chronic Disease Prevention and Health Promotion (2018). Defining childhood obesity. 2018. Available at: https://www.cdc.gov/obesity/childhood/defining.html. Accessed January 21, 2021.
4. Centers for Disease Control and Prevention, National Centers for Health Statistics (2017). Clinical growth charts. 2017. Available at: https://www.cdc.gov/growthcharts/clinical_charts.htm. Accessed January 21, 2021.
5. Gulati AK, Kaplan DW, Daniels SR. Clinical tracking of severely obese children: a new growth chart. Pediatrics 2012;130(6):1136–40.

6. Kelly AS, Barlow SE, Rao G, et al. Severe obesity in children and adolescents: identification, associated health risks, and treatment approaches: a scientific statement from the American Heart Association. Circulation 2013;128(15): 1689–712.

7. Zemel BS, Pipan M, Stallings VA, et al. Growth charts for children with down syndrome in the United States. Pediatrics 2015;136(5):e1204–11.

8. Hoover-Fong JE, McGready J, Schulze KJ, et al. Weight for age charts for children with achondroplasia. Am J Med Genet 2007;143A:2227–35.

9. Christesen HT, Pedersen BT, Pournara E, et al. Short stature: comparison of WHO and National Growth Standards/References for Height. PLoS One 2016;11(6): e0157277.

10. Skinner AC, Ravanbakht SN, Skelton JA, et al. Prevalence of obesity and severe obesity in US children, 1999-2016. Pediatrics 2018;141(3):e20173459.

11. O'Hara V, Browne N, Fathima S, et al. Obesity cardiometabolic comorbidity prevalence in children in a rural weight-management program. Glob Pediatr Health 2017;4:1–10.

12. Skinner AC, Perrin EM, Moss LA, et al. Cardiometabolic risks and severity of obesity in children and young adults. N Engl J Med 2015;373(14):1307–17.

13. Sharma V, Coleman S, Nixon J, et al. A systematic review and meta-analysis estimating the population prevalence of comorbidities in children and adolescents aged 5 to 18 years. Obes Rev 2019;20(10):1341–9.

14. Güngör NK. Overweight and obesity in children and adolescents. J Clin Res Pediatr Endocrinol 2014;6(3):129–43.

15. Jastreboff AM, Kotz CM, Kahan S, et al. Obesity as a disease: the Obesity Society 2018 position statement. Obesity 2019;27(1):7–9.

16. Palad CJ, Yarlagadda S, Stanford FC. Weight stigma and its impact on paediatric care. Curr Opin Endocrinol Diabetes Obes 2019;26(1):19–24.

17. Puhl RM, Himmelstein MS, Pearl RL. Weight stigma as a psychosocial contributor to obesity. Am Psychol 2020;75(2):274–89.

18. Fox CK, Gross AC, Rudser KD, et al. Depression, anxiety, and severity of obesity in adolescents: is emotional eating the link? Clin Ped 2016;55(12):1120–5.

19. Rubino F, Puhl RM, Cummings DE, et al. Joint international consensus statement for ending stigma of obesity. Nat Med 2020;26(4):485–97.

20. O'Hara VM, Curran JL, Browne NT. The co-occurrence of pediatric obesity and ADHD: an understanding of shared pathophysiology and implications for collaborative management. Curr Obes Rep 2020;9(4):451–61.

21. Cortese S. The association between ADHD and obesity: intriguing, progressively more investigated, but still puzzling. Brain Sci 2019;9(10):256.

22. Geiker NRW, Astrup A, Hjorth MF, et al. Does stress influence sleep patterns, food intake, weight gain, abdominal obesity and weight loss interventions and vice versa? Obes Rev 2018;19(1):81–97.

23. Fang CT, Chen VC, Ma HT, et al. Attentional bias, "cool" and "hot" executive functions in obese patients: roles of body mass index, binge eating, and eating style. J Clin Psychopharmacol 2019;39(2):145–52.

24. Lindberg L, Hagman E, Danielsson P, et al. Anxiety and depression in children and adolescents with obesity: a nationwide study in Sweden. BMC Med 2020; 18(1):30.

25. Pigeyre M, Yazdi FT, Kaur Y, et al. Recent progress in genetics, epigenetics and metagenomics unveils the pathophysiology of human obesity. Clin Sci 2016; 130(12):943–86.

26. Golden A, Kessler C. Obesity and genetics. J Am Assoc Nurse Pract 2020;32(7): 493–6.

27. Mason K, Page L, Balikcioglu PG. Screening for hormonal, monogenic, and syndromic disorders in obese infants and children. Pediatr Ann 2014;43(9):e218–24.

28. Chung WK. An overview of monogenic and syndromic obesities in humans. Pediatr Blood Cancer 2012;58(1):122–8.

29. Stagi S, Bianconi M, Amina Sammarco M, et al. New thoughts on pediatric genetic obesity: pathogenesis, clinical characteristics and treatment approach. In: Gordeladze J, editor. Adiposity: omics and molecular understanding. London: InTechOpen; 2017. p. 1320–678.

30. Hanson MA, Gluckman PD. Early developmental conditioning of later health and disease: physiology or pathophysiology? Physiol Rev 2014;94(4):1027–76.

31. Campbell M. Biological, environmental, and social influences on childhood obesity. Pediatr Res 2016;79:205–11.

32. Farias MM, Cuevas AM, Rodriguez F. Set-point theory and obesity. Metab Syndr Relat Disord 2011;9(2):85–9.

33. Rolland-Cachera MF, Cole TJ. Does the age at adiposity rebound reflect a critical period? Pediatr Obes 2019;14(1).

34. Frattarelli DA, Galinkin JL, Green TP, et al. Off-label use of drugs in children. Pediatrics 2014;133(3):563–7.

35. Barlow SE, Expert Committee. Expert committee recommendations regarding the prevention, assessment, and treatment of child and adolescent overweight and obesity: summary report. Pediatrics 2007;120(Suppl 4):S164–92.

36. Cuda S, Censani M, O'Hara V, et al. Pediatric obesity algorithm, presented by the Obesity Medicine Association. 2020–2022. Available at: www.obesitymedicine. org/childhood-obesity. Accessed August, 2021.

37. Hager ER, Quigg AM, Black MM, et al. Development and validity of a 2-item screen to identify families at risk for food insecurity. Pediatrics 2010;126(1): e26–32.

38. Council on Community Pediatrics; Committee on Nutrition. Promoting food security for all children. Pediatrics 2015;136(5):e1431–8.

39. Tester JM, Rosas LG, Leung CW. Food insecurity and pediatric obesity: a double whammy in the era of COVID-19. Curr Obes Rep 2020;9(4):442–50.

40. Estrada E, Eneli I, Hampl S, et al. Children's Hospital Association consensus statements for comorbidities of childhood obesity. Child Obes 2014;10(4): 304–17.

41. Institute for Healthy Childhood Weight. Algorithm for the assessment and management of childhood obesity in patients 2 years and older. 2015. Available at: https://www.paaap.org/uploads/1/2/4/3/124369935/551b74_5a52cf9033cb48b0 9aba3c0280a15402.pdf. Accessed August, 2021.

42. Styne DM, Arslanian SA, Connor EL, et al. Pediatric obesity-assessment, treatment, and prevention: an Endocrine Society Clinical Practice Guideline. J Clin Endocrinol Metab 2017;102(3):709–57.

43. Davies D, Troy MF. Child development: a practitioners guide. 4th edition. NY: Guilford Press; 2020.

44. US Preventive Services Task Force, Grossman DC, Bibbins-Domingo K, Curry SJ, et al. Screening for obesity in children and adolescents: US Preventive Services Task Force Recommendation Statement. JAMA 2017;317(23):2417–26.

45. Cardel MI, Atkinson MA, Taveras EM, et al. Obesity treatment among adolescents: a review of current evidence and future directions. JAMA Pediatr 2020; 174(6):609–17.

46. Inge TH, Courcoulas AP, Jenkins TM, et al. Five-year outcomes of gastric bypass in adolescents as compared with adults. N Engl J Med 2019;380(22):2136–45.

47. Olbers T, Beamish AJ, Gronowitz E, et al. Laparoscopic Roux-en-Y gastric bypass in adolescents with severe obesity (AMOS): a prospective, 5-year, Swedish nationwide study. Lancet Diabetes Endocrinol 2017;5(3):174–83.

48. Paulus GF, de Vaan LE, Verdam FJ, et al. Bariatric surgery in morbidly obese adolescents: a systematic review and meta-analysis. Obes Surg 2015;25(5): 860–78.

49. Armstrong SC, Bolling CF, Michalsky MP, et al. Pediatric metabolic and bariatric surgery: evidence, barriers, and best practices. Pediatrics 2019;144(6): e20193223.

50. Pratt JSA, Browne A, Browne NT, et al. ASMBS pediatric metabolic and bariatric surgery guidelines, 2018. Surg Obes Relat Dis 2018;14(7):882–901.

51. Srivastava G, Fox CK, Kelly AS, et al. Clinical considerations regarding the use of obesity pharmacotherapy in adolescents with obesity. Obesity 2019;27(2): 190–204.

52. Singhal V, Sella AC, Malhotra S. Pharmacotherapy in pediatric obesity: current evidence and landscape. Curr Opin Endocrinol Diabetes Obes 2021;28(1): 55–63.

53. Reece LJ, Sachdev P, Copeland RJ, et al. Intra-gastric balloon as an adjunct to lifestyle support in severely obese adolescents; impact on weight, physical activity, cardiorespiratory fitness and psychosocial well-being. Int J Obes 2017;41(4): 591–7.

54. Lozano P, Houtrow A. Supporting self-management in children and adolescents with complex chronic conditions. Pediatrics 2018;141(Suppl 3):S233–41.

55. Committee on Hospital Care and Institute for Patient and Family Centered Care. Patient- and family-centered care and the pediatrician's role. Pediatrics 2012; 129(2):394–404.

56. Pont SJ, Puhl R, Cook SR, et al. Stigma experienced by children and adolescents with obesity. Pediatrics 2017;140(6):e20173034.

57. Weight Bias and Stigma: Healthcare. Rudd Center for Food Health and Policy. Available at: http://www.uconnruddcenter.org/weight-bias-stigma-health-care. Accessed January 21, 2021.

58. Srivastava G, Kyle T, O'Hara V, et al. Caring for US children: barriers to effective treatment in children with the disease of obesity. Obesity 2021;29(1):46–55.

59. Sue DW, Alsaidi S, Awad MN, et al. Disarming racial microaggressions: microintervention strategies for targets, white allies, and bystanders. Am Psychol 2019; 74(1):128–42.

Obesity and Men's Health

Ryan Holley-Mallo, PhD, DNP, NP-C, FAANP[a],*,
Angela Golden, DNP, FNP-C, FAANP[b]

KEYWORDS

- Men's health • Health care • Obesity • Masculinity

KEY POINTS

- Obesity is nationwide pandemic that leads to a lower quality of life for men and subsequently leads to health disparity in the lives of women and children.
- Obesity increases the risk of many disease processes noted to be leading causes of death for men throughout the United States.
- Recognizing the difference in obesity impact for men can allow for better treatment.

INTRODUCTION

The National Center for Health Statistics show that men lead in 9 of the top 10 causes of death and women are 100% more likely than men receive health care prevention.[1] There are more than 86 million males within the United States and a plethora of data that supports a lower life expectancy as well as higher costs of managing comorbid conditions for males when compared with females.[2] Obesity plays a key role in many of the leading causes of death in both men and women. Studies support that females are more likely than males to seek primary care services, and 1 study found that 33% of men surveyed responded that they do not have a primary care provider.[3] Moreover, research confirms that only 25% of men have been evaluated by a primary care provider in at least a year, suggesting that underuse of preventive health care and adherence to hegemonic masculine norms are key factors in the higher morbidity and mortality of men.[4]

Economics are key factors that must be considered when evaluating health disparities faced by men. Currently available data reveal that, in 2011, premature morbidity and mortality of men cost the United States a staggering $479 billion with the cost for African and Hispanic men constituting the highest portion of this health care price tag.[5] Men's underuse of primary care services often leads to the use of hospital services and higher costs of secondary or tertiary care, which further drive up the cost of health care.[4]

[a] School of Nursing, Averett University, 420 W. Main Street, Danville, VA 24541, USA; [b] NP from Home, LLC and NP Obesity Treatment Clinic, Flagstaff, AZ, USA
* Corresponding author.
E-mail address: RyanMalloDNP@gmail.com

Nurs Clin N Am 56 (2021) 599–607
https://doi.org/10.1016/j.cnur.2021.07.004
0029-6465/21/© 2021 Elsevier Inc. All rights reserved.

nursing.theclinics.com

PREVALENCE, INCIDENCE, AND UNSUSTAINABILITY

Obesity is increasing in the United States, with the most recent statistics from the National Health and Nutrition Examination Survey show a percentage of 39.6%.[6] The prevalence in men is 37.9% versus 41.1% for women. Among men between the ages of 40 to 59, 40.8% are considered obese, and among men between the ages of 20 and 39, 34.8% are considered obese. Finally, another one-third of adults are listed in the preobesity category.

The poor health of men has ramifications that reach far beyond ones' self; it has a direct impact on the individual's spouse, children, employer, and even the economy through direct and indirect costs.[4] Although it may not seem to be readily evident, indirect costs are a burden on employers when they are forced to train another individual in the work that any given man completes while the employee takes time off secondary to illness.

INSTITUTIONAL INFLUENCES AFFECTING CARE

In addition to interpersonal barriers, men also face institutional barriers when attempting to navigate the health care system. Such barriers often include poor communication regarding testing and treatment options, lengthy wait times to see a provider, judgmental and/or disrespectful treatment from providers, and the expectation that men will discuss their problem with multiple health care providers during the same visit.[7] Certainly, these issues are not unique to men, but the extant literature on men being less likely to access health care in the first place magnifies these issues and becomes quite apparent in terms of morbidity and mortality. Clinicians wishing to care for men have the daunting task of overcoming both interpersonal and institutional barriers.

Physiologic Variations

Adipose tissue and men

Men have a more visceral distribution of adipose tissue.[8] During puberty, men develop this central distribution, whereas women have some protection with estrogen that preferentially deposits adipose tissue in the subcutaneous areas. As discussed in pathophysiology, visceral adiposity is correlated with higher rates of metabolic complications owing to the endocrine dysfunction that results from adipospathy. The rate of lipolysis is higher in visceral adipose tissue, leading to greater amounts of fatty acid deposits in the liver as well as the increase in the inflammatory nature of the disease of obesity, which further increases metabolic disease. Men with obesity also have a lower level of adiponectin compared with women with obesity, promoting greater intra-abdominal adiposity and insulin resistance.[8]

Sex hormones and obesity

A specific complication for men is that of hypogonadism. Obesity is thought to cause hypogonadism through multiple mechanisms.[9] Insulin resistance with the resulting hyperinsulinemia causes a decrease in sex hormone-binding globulin by directly reducing the hepatic production of sex hormone-binding globulin. Normally, testosterone is bound to sex hormone-binding globulin with approximately 2% bound to albumin. The low binding protein decreases the bioavailable hormone. Additionally, adipose tissue increases the conversion of free testosterone to estrogen adding to testosterone deficiency. Leptin also suppresses gonadal steroidogenesis.[10] Although the Endocrine Society does not recommend routine screening; patients with a history and/or physical that identify symptoms or signs of androgen insufficiency should be screened. The American Association of Clinical Endocrinologists and the Endocrine Society recommend screening with serum total testosterone (by mass spectrometry whenever possible) and calculated free testosterone from total testosterone as well as sex hormone-binding globulin measurement.[11,12] Testosterone replacement is only recommended for consideration with biochemical and clinical evidence of hypogonadism.

As men age, there is a decreasing level of testosterone and an increase in adipose mass even without obesity. Research demonstrates with hypotestosteronism treated with testosterone there is an increase in lean mass, insulin sensitivity, and a decrease in visceral fat mass.[13]

Fat as an energy source

Genetically, men may have a predisposition to visceral adiposity because it is more readily available for energy needs. Ross and colleagues[14] demonstrated that, when men exercised, they lost visceral fat first. This nature allows for a rapid transport from the liver to the peripheral tissues.

There is also evidence that men's brains respond differently to a high-fat diet. The evidence has been shown in mice studies and now in a small human study.[15] Increases in markers of inflammation and angiogenesis occurred after a high-fat meal was consumed more so in older inactive men.[16]

Obesity-related complications

Obesity has many complications and comorbidities for men and women. A study by Censin and colleagues[17] demonstrated that men with obesity have a higher risk of chronic kidney disease. An increased waist height ratio was associated with a greater risk of chronic obstructive pulmonary disease for men than women. Women had a higher risk for type 2 diabetes. There was no difference identified with nonalcoholic fatty liver disease, colorectal cancer, dementia, stroke, or infertility between men and women with obesity.

Approach Variations

Bias and stigma affecting care

To provide optimal care for men, clinicians need to better understand barriers that may preclude participation in health care. Bias and stress of bias are very similar between men and women. Forty percent of men have reported experiencing stigma related to their weight. Men described verbal mistreatment being experienced throughout their lives, with physical mistreatment more likely to occur during their child and adolescent years.[18] Weight bias internalization for men has been associated with a higher body mass index and more binge episodes.[19]

The primary reasons men reported seeking weight loss or obesity treatment were for a decreased sex drive and orthopedic issues.[20] Men are less likely to take part in a weight loss program, perceiving them to be for women.[21] Few programs are designed specifically for men.[22]

Treatment Variations

Eating plans

In approaches to eating plans, the evidence does not provide one eating plan that works better than another for men. What is known is that men will have a higher caloric and protein need than their female counterparts owing to their higher muscle and bone proportion. There is also a need for higher magnesium. Calorie needs for men tend to be 2000 to 2500 per day. The protein needs are 1 to 1.2 g/kg per day. The magnesium needs are 400 to 420 mg/d, thought to assist with heart health in men and support testosterone levels.[23]

The ROMEO systematic review recommends that the program delivery may be more important than any specific eating plan.[21] Men prefer more fact-based language. They also prefer individual program delivery versus group programming.

Activity

Physical activity is the second component of treatment for obesity in all patients. In men, studies have demonstrated that aerobic resistance exercise may increase the fat-free mass of the arms and trunk while decreasing the fat mass in the trunk.[24] Additionally, the longer duration of physical activity has been shown to increase fat loss in men.[25] This process may be occurring because visceral adipose tissue has a higher response to physical activity, as well as weight loss increases testosterone levels in men, which has been shown to increase lipolysis.[26]

Behavior intervention

Delivering care in places men naturally congregate, such as work (eg, worksite health promotion) or barber shops, has been shown to increase men's likelihood to enter into care.[27] In a factory, for example, if there is a provider on site, people can come in off the factory floor and receive chronic care for obesity and access health resources without having to take time off or make peers and supervisors aware of their health challenges. Holding a health fair or taking clinics to remote places where men are known to congregate, such as college campuses, youth programs, barbershops, sporting events, job training sites, local mosques, homeless shelters, soccer clubs, bars, dance clubs, and through mobile units, also likely will encourage participation.[28] Fear of receiving bad news, being judged by a health care provider, perceived or actual negative reactions from family and/or friends, and fear of what their partner may think also are interpersonal barriers that clinicians caring for men need to be ready to navigate.[29] This point calls into question how we socialize males in the health care system and emphasize education via coping strategies, cultivating support systems, and discussion and training on how to explain what is going on to support systems. Deficits in being properly educated in health are a substantial interpersonal barrier that men face when seeking primordial and primary preventive care.

A lack of knowledge about when and where to seek health care, especially when no signs and symptoms are present, often delays or precludes seeking help.[30] Maximizing time and topics must be viewed as imperative during the visit. When talking with male patients about obesity, health care providers need to make health care choices easy and appealing. Additionally, telehealth provides an avenue for ease of interacting with the health care providers, as well as providing time-sensitive treatment. However, providers should be aware that some apps and online virtual appointments could hinder patients from engaging in holistic, primary, preventive health care if technology is a barrier.

TARGETED INTERVENTIONS TO REACH MEN IN THE HEALTH CARE SETTING

Ensuring that the most current testing modalities and treatment options are understood is essential. This goal will require each professional to stay up to date with the current literature to provide evidence-based care. Ideally, this education should be tracked, monitored, and assessed periodically.

Modern facilities, nearby locations, short or no waiting times, same-day appointments, not having to give a reason for the appointment, and availability to receive multiple health care services at the same location are all factors that have been noted to be appealing to men entering into care.[31] Removing cumbersome processes before entering into care, such as multipage registration forms, also are favored by men. Scheduling patients immediately for appointments is essential and, if such scheduling is not possible, then the health care provider or facility should refer them to someone with immediate availability and do a follow-up to confirm that their needs were addressed sufficiently.

Individualizing the health care provider–patient approach and using a style that men are responsive to and being flexible in the delivery of health care in a nonclinical environment are requisite in the successful implementation of health care delivery to men.[32] Research has illustrated that males respond best to direct communication and a frank approach. They appreciate the thoughtful use of humor as well as the use of empathy and have a high regard for clinical competence.[33] Clinicians also can help to reframe the experience positively by encouraging men on their decision to seek help and pursue healthy lifestyles (ie, shared decision-making).[34] Providers also need to create positive first impressions and male-friendly spaces in which health care is offered. Waiting rooms that have male interest magazines, health education materials that target men's issues, and TV programming of interest to men are immediate and simple steps offices can take in welcoming men into the primary care arena.

Out-of-clinic interventions are built on the premise that men are not as likely as women to enter a health care setting both nationally and internationally. Men who are unengaged or underengaged in the health care system are not generally disinterested in their health, but rather the forum in which health care is delivered.[28] An example is worksite health promotion programs that have been found to decrease medical costs by more than 25%, and advocates for companies to offer such programs argue that they elicit a higher return on investment from the employee. Such programs have been shown to decrease health system charges by as much as $300,000 in an 18-month period.[35]

Offering a holistic and respectful approach to health care in conjunction with targeted messaging that empowers men such as "sexual health care is a way to be stronger" or "taking care of your health is cool" has been noted to increase office visits by young men.[36] Provider compassion and empathy toward men helps them with the acceptance of health-promoting behavior.[37]

Realizing that men often are drawn to technology (eg, mHealth, online discussion forums, online doctors, telehealth, telemental health), leveraging curiosity in the use of the latest technology and testing devices can help to spur interest in primary preventive care.[37] Online virtual visits, patient portals, or phone apps would be examples. One example of a successful, targeted message is that of cell phone applications that will send weekly tips and education on preventive practices and sexual health, in addition to notifications regarding health care directly to the patient via their mobile device.[37] For men who are less technologically inclined, tailoring health care messages to patient populations in formats they interface with regularly, such as sporting events, barbershops, or other social venues, these platforms can be successful in engaging patients in health-promoting behaviors.[38]

Finally, tailoring health care messages to men's spouses or partners may prove beneficial; data from national health surveys have found that partnered men were more likely than unpartnered men to undergo a primary health care visit and screenings the last 12 months.[27] Other research suggests that it is critical to be cognizant of interpersonal partner communication techniques and how best to foster effective discourse. Perhaps some attention should be paid to how we can more effectively communicate to a spouse or partner about their role in their partners' health maintenance and give them some helpful tools to promote optimal well-being among their husbands/partners. Although not an "only" strategy to reach men, further research on partners and other relationship dynamics also could provide rich data to integrate in health care practice when engaging males.[27]

Even the positioning of the provider can influence how a man may receive health information. Side-by-side communication and engagement seem to be more efficacious in promoting health-based conversations with men than face-to-face or the health care provider standing while the man is seated or lying down.[39] Educational reform in the training of all health care providers (particularly pediatric physicians in working with parents of boys), the use of men's health services in the workplace, and campaigns to target marginalized men and vulnerable male populations are key to improving men's health on a global scale.[40]

SUMMARY

Obesity is a chronic, progressive, relapsing and treatable disease for everyone. There are some unique points to consider for men with obesity. They have different experiences of bias and stigma. Physiologically, men deposit adipose tissue viscerally at an earlier age than women. There are differences in macro and micronutrient requirements beyond just size differences to consider. Men approach health care differently than women do and to impact their treatment of obesity health care providers must be aware of these differences and approach the care with these issues in mind to allow for the best possible outcomes.

CLINICS CARE POINTS

- The identification of men as an at-risk population for obesity is important.
- Provide care where men congregate if possible.
- Recognize the differences in physiology and treatment for men to address obesity with the best outcomes.

DISCLOSURE

The authors have nothing to disclose

REFERENCES

1. National Center for Health Statistics. Men's health. 2021. Available at: CDC.gov. Accessed May 26, 2021.

2. Bruce MA, Griffith DM, Thorpe RJ Jr. Stress and the kidney. Adv Chronic Kidney Dis 2015;22(1):46–53.
3. Garfield CF, Isacco A, Rogers TE. A review of men's health and masculinity. Am J Lifestyle Med 2008;2(6):474–87.
4. Baker P, Shand T. Men's health: time for a new approach to policy and practice? J Glob Health 2017;7(1):010306.
5. Heidelbaugh JJ. Objectivity and compassion. Prim Care 2016;43(2):xiii–xiv.
6. Hales CM, Carroll MD, Fryar CD, et al. Prevalence of obesity among adults and youth: United States, 2015-2016. NCHS Data Brief 2017;(288):1–8.
7. Powell W, Adams LB, Cole-Lewis Y, et al. Masculinity and race-related factors as barriers to health help-seeking among African American men. Behav Med 2016; 42(3):150–63.
8. Chang E, Varghese M, Singer K. Gender and sex differences in adipose tissue. Curr Diab Rep 2018;18(9):69.
9. Fernandez CJ, Chacko EC, Pappachan JM. Male obesity-related secondary hypogonadism - pathophysiology, clinical implications and management. Eur Endocrinol 2019;15(2):83–90.
10. Odle AK, Akhter N, Syed MM, et al. Leptin regulation of gonadotrope gonadotropin-releasing hormone receptors as a metabolic checkpoint and gateway to reproductive competence. Front Endocrinol (Lausanne) 2018;8:367.
11. Bhasin S, Brito JP, Cunningham GR, et al. Testosterone therapy in men with hypogonadism: an endocrine society clinical practice guideline. J Clin Endocrinol Metab 2018;103(5):1715–44.
12. Garvey WT, Mechanick JI, Brett EM, et al. American Association of Clinical Endocrinologists and American College of Endocrinology comprehensive clinical practice guidelines for medical care of patients with obesity. Endocr Pract 2016;22(Suppl 3):1–203.
13. Jones TH, Arver S, Behre HM, et al. Testosterone replacement in hypogonadal men with type 2 diabetes and/or metabolic syndrome (the TIMES2 study). Diabetes Care 2011;34(4):828–37.
14. Ross R, Dagnone D, Jones PJ, et al. Reduction in obesity and related comorbid conditions after diet-induced weight loss or exercise-induced weight loss in men. A randomized, controlled trial. Ann Intern Med 2000;133(2):92–103.
15. Morselli E, Fuente-Martin E, Finan B, et al. Hypothalamic PGC-1α protects against high-fat diet exposure by regulating ERα. Cell Rep 2014;9(2):633–45.
16. Emerson SR, Sciarrillo CM, Kurti SP, et al. High-fat meal–induced changes in markers of inflammation and angiogenesis in healthy adults who differ by age and physical activity level. Curr Dev Nutr 2019;3(1):nzy098.
17. Censin JC, Peters SAE, Bovijn J, et al. Causal relationships between obesity and the leading causes of death in women and men. PLoS Genet 2019;15(10): e1008405.
18. Himmelstein M, Puhl R, Quinn D. Weight stigma in men: what, when, and by whom? Weight stigma in men. Obesity 2018;26:968–76.
19. Boswell RG, White MA. Gender differences in weight bias internalisation and eating pathology in overweight individuals. Adv Eat Disord 2015;3(3):259–68.
20. Elliott M, Gillison F, Barnett J. Exploring the influences on men's engagement with weight loss services: a qualitative study. BMC Public Health 2020;20(1):1–11.

21. Robertson C, Archibald D, Avenell A, et al. Systematic reviews of and integrated report on the quantitative, qualitative and economic evidence base for the management of obesity in men. Health Technol Assess 2014;18(35):v–424.
22. Young MD, Morgan PJ, Plotnikoff RC, et al. Effectiveness of male-only weight loss and weight loss maintenance interventions: a systematic review with meta-analysis. Obes Rev 2012;13(5):393–408.
23. Magnesium fact sheet for health professionals. ods.od.nih.gov. 2021. Available at: https://ods.od.nih.gov/factsheets/Magnesium-HealthProfessional/. Accessed May 26, 2021.
24. Sanal E, Ardic F, Kirac S. Effects of aerobic or combined aerobic resistance exercise on body composition in overweight and obese adults: gender differences. A randomized intervention study. Eur J Phys Rehabil Med 2013;49(1):1–11.
25. Aadland E, Jepsen R, Andersen JR, et al. Differences in fat loss in response to physical activity among severely obese men and women. J Rehabil Med 2014;46(4):363–9.
26. Grossmann M. Low testosterone in men with type 2 diabetes: significance and treatment. J Clin Endocrinol Metab 2011;96(8):2341–53.
27. Leone JE, Rovito MJ, Gray KA, et al. Practical strategies for improving men's health: Maximizing the patient-provider encounter. J Mens Soc Community Health 2021;4(1):e1–16.
28. Cordier R, Wilson NJ. Community-based men's sheds: promoting male health, well-being and social inclusion in an international context. Health Promo Int 2013;29(3):483–93.
29. Evans J, Frank B, Oliffe JL, et al. Health, illness, men and masculinities (HIMM): a theoretical framework for understanding men and their health. J Mens Health 2011;8(1):7–15.
30. Cohn L, Murray SB, Walen A, et al. Including the excluded: males and gender minorities in eating disorder prevention. Eat Disord 2016;24(1):114–20.
31. National Academies of Sciences, Engineering, and Medicine; Health and Medicine Division; Board on Health Care Services; Committee on Health Care Utilization and Adults with Disabilities. Health-care utilization as a proxy in disability determination. Washington (DC): National Academies Press (US); 2018. Factors That Affect Health-Care Utilization. Available at: https://www.ncbi.nlm.nih.gov/books/NBK500097/.
32. National Academy of Engineering (US) and Institute of Medicine (US) Committee on Engineering and the Health Care System. Building a better delivery system: a new engineering/health care partnership. In: Reid PP, Compton WD, Grossman JH, et al, editors. Washington (DC): National Academies Press (US); 2005. A Framework for a Systems Approach to Health Care Delivery. Available at: https://www.ncbi.nlm.nih.gov/books/NBK22878/.
33. Witty K, White A. Tackling men's health: implementation of a male health service in a rugby stadium setting. Comm Pract 2011;84(4):29–32.
34. Sagar-Ouriaghli I, Godfrey E, Bridge L, et al. Improving mental health service utilization among men: a systematic review and synthesis of behavior change techniques within interventions targeting help-seeking. Am J Mens Health 2019;13(3). 1557988319857009.
35. Control Health Care Costs. Workplace health programs can impact health care costs. CDC.gov. 2015. Available at: https://www.cdc.gov/

workplacehealthpromotion/model/control-costs/index.html. Accessed May 26, 2021.

36. Committee on the Learning Health Care System in America; Institute of Medicine. Best care at lower cost: the path to continuously learning health care in America. In: Smith M, Saunders R, Stuckhardt L, et al, editors. Washington (DC): National Academies Press (US); 2013. Engaging Patients, Families, and Communities. Available at: https://www.ncbi.nlm.nih.gov/books/NBK207234/.

37. Springer KW, Mouzon DM. "Macho men" and preventive healthcare: implications for older men in different social classes. J Health Soc Behav 2011;52(2):212–27.

38. Cohen CE, Coyne KM, Mandalia S, et al. Time to use text reminders in genitourinary medicine clinics. Int J STD AIDS 2008;19(1):12–3.

39. Manchester A. Men are dying from self-induced illnesses. Nurs N Z 2015; 21(6):13–4.

40. Yousaf O, Grunfeld EA, Hunter MS. A systematic review of the factors associated with delays in medical and psychological help-seeking among men. Heal Psychol Rev 2015;9(2):264–76.

Obesity in Women
Paying a High Price

Denise G. Link, PhD, WHNP-BC

KEYWORDS

- Obesity • Women • Polycystic ovary syndrome • Infertility • Stigma
- Patient counseling

KEY POINTS

- Obesity affects women in ways that are different from the experience of men.
- The physiologic processes of pregnancy in obese women may result in an increased risk of obesity for the future child.
- Polycystic ovary syndrome is a condition that can be exacerbated by obesity.
- Insulin excess in obesity interferes with processes necessary for ovulation and conception.
- Patient-centered care and collaboration with the patient are key to success in improving health in women with obesity.

In the Shakespearean play *The Merchant of Venice*, the antagonist, Shylock, is a shrewd money lender. He makes a loan to a man, Antonio, with a condition that, if the loan is not repaid on time, Shylock would be entitled to take a pound of Antonio's flesh from anywhere on Antonio's body. This penalty, if allowed to take place, would likely inflict a mortal wound; a high price for a loan. In modern times, the phrase "getting (one's) pound of flesh" has come to mean 1 person gaining some recompense regardless of the consequences on another person. If we think of obesity as an antagonist in the realm of human health to which humans become indebted (by no fault of their own or by behavior), it has certainly collected its pound of flesh from those affected by obesity, especially women. Obesity and associated chronic and acute health conditions are responsible for a significant amount of human suffering. There is a robust body of evidence to support that having overweight or obesity puts both men and women at greater risk for the development of cardiovascular disease, several types of cancer, type 2 diabetes, and other conditions. Based on data from 2017 and 2018, the Centers for Disease Control and Prevention estimates that more than 42% of US adults have obesity.[1] When comparing the prevalence of obesity between men

Arizona State University Edson College of Nursing and Health Innovation, 4015 North 12th Avenue, Phoenix, AZ 85013, USA
E-mail address: Denise.Link@asu.edu

Nurs Clin N Am 56 (2021) 609–617
https://doi.org/10.1016/j.cnur.2021.07.005
0029-6465/21/© 2021 Elsevier Inc. All rights reserved.

and women, the difference is small. However, the prevalence of class 3 obesity (body mass index [BMI] of ≥40) in women has been reported at 9.9%, compared with 5.5% in men.[2] Obesity-related disorders that include some of the leading causes of chronic disease and preventable death also disproportionately affect women.[2] Between 1988 and 2012, the metabolic syndrome—a cluster of conditions including hypertension, elevated serum glucose levels, excess body fat around the waist, and abnormal serum lipids—has increased in non-Latina White and Black women by 44% and 41%, respectively.[3] At age 70 and older, the prevalence of the metabolic syndrome in women increases to almost 70%.[3] Consumer cost share, inpatient and community care expenditures, prescription drug charges, and emergency department fees combined result in health care expenses related to obesity and associated conditions that are 31% higher in women than in men.[2]

CONSEQUENCES OF OBESITY LABELS AND MEASURES

In 2013, there was an intense debate at the annual meeting of the American Medical Association over whether to classify obesity as a disease; some argued that obesity is a condition that can be identified and treated independent of other health problems. Those opposed to affixing the disease label cited the inability to identify a clear pathogenesis and universally effective treatments. Eventually, the delegates were able to come to consensus and obesity was assigned a unique diagnosis code. This development may sound like a trivial achievement, but in our society and the health care system that assigns insurance coverage and financial value to human conditions, it is a rite of passage. Recognizing and defining human physical and mental states, whether physiologic or pathologic, raises their status to problems and leads to the assignment of a code in the *International Classification of Diagnoses*, currently in its tenth edition. This process in turn facilitates standardization in clinical research to identify the physiologic pathways of the condition, investigate effective pharmacologic and behavioral interventions, compare outcomes data, and justify health insurance coverage for the care processes involved in their diagnosis and management. Bestowing the label of disease on a condition that affects a large segment of the population stimulates a response in the form of a demand for services and products to identify, prevent, cure, or manage the disease. All of this attention has, in fact, led to investigations for more effective strategies to decrease the incidence of obesity and its associated human and financial costs. However, researchers have shown that women pay a higher price for bearing the label obese. Based on their literature review for evidence about the stigmatization of women related to weight, Fikkan and Rothblum[4] opined that fat should be the term used to describe women who have excess adipose tissue. Their rationale is that obese is a medical term that emphasizes pathology. The authors believe that overweight is likewise unfavorable because it implies deviance from some arbitrary acceptable standard of normal. When persons with obesity themselves were asked to rate terms used to refer to their weight, the participants identified "excess weight," "weight problem," and "BMI" as being the preferred descriptors.[5] The words obese and obesity were chosen for this article because they are more universally used in the professional literature and because of the association of obesity with an increased risk for morbidity and mortality. This author acknowledges, however, that, when interacting with patients, it is desirable for the clinician to ask patients about their preferences and use the terms with which the person is most comfortable regardless of the topic under discussion.

The knowledge about obesity generated by research is limited by the use of the BMI as a means to quantify excess adipose tissue and judge the efficacy of the outcomes of the tested interventions. This point may be especially true when analyzing results in studies involving women. BMI, which has been standard for determining obesity, has been deemed an unreliable measure of adipose tissue volume.[6,7] The BMI was introduced in the early nineteenth century by a Belgian mathematician Lambert A.J. Quetelet.[6] The calculation of BMI assumes a low muscle mass and high relative fat content, and makes no allowance for the relative proportions of bone, muscle, and fat in the body. What Quetelet did not know (and is now known) is that type of fat and where it is located are additional important variables for determining what constitutes a healthy level of body fat. Although these variations occur in both men and women, young adult women start with less visceral fat, bone, and muscle mass than men. As women age, they will lose an average of 13 pounds of bone and muscle mass and their visceral fat will increase 4-fold. Visceral fat in men also increases, but only by a factor of 2.[8] It has been suggested that using abdominal waist circumference or hip/waist ratio may be better surrogates for assessing the proportion of adipose tissue that contributes to weight in women. However, it is important to keep in mind that using only one of any of these measures to diagnose obesity fails to consider the multiple other factors that must be considered when assessing women for obesity and risk for health problems. The current practice of using BMI as the sole diagnostic criteria for obesity is inconsistent with the evidence that obesity is a complex condition that involves biology, heredity, and environmental influences, many of which are only partially under the control of the person living with the disease.

OBESITY IN CHILDBEARING

Linkages between maternal obesity and the development of obesity in offspring beyond the influence of heredity have been described. The insulin resistance and inflammation that lead to the increased storage of fat (adipogenesis) and breakdown of fat tissue (lipolysis) are characteristics of both obesity and pregnancy. An abnormal increase in circulating lipids in the mother during pregnancy can lead to an increased risk of the metabolic syndrome in their offspring.[9] There is a body of evidence to support that infant feeding practices also impact a child's risk for having obesity later in life. Arenz and colleagues[10] completed a metanalysis to look for an association between breastfeeding and the risk of the children having overweight. In the analysis of combined data from 9 studies involving more than 69,000 participants the researchers were able to show that breastfeeding significantly decreased the risk of obesity in childhood.[10] Other researchers have had similar findings, including benefits from longer duration of breastfeeding.[11,12]

IMPACT OF OBESITY ON THE FEMALE REPRODUCTIVE SYSTEM

Overweight and obesity have been associated with disruption of the menstrual cycle through several interacting mechanisms. An excess in central adipose tissue (fat centered around the waist) is associated with an increase in resistance to the action of insulin for transporting glucose into cells for the energy needed to perform various cellular and metabolic functions. As a result of this resistance to the action of insulin, the system sends out signals to initiate corrective action to overcome insulin resistance by producing more insulin. The increased insulin, still unable to move glucose into working cells, resorts to lowering circulating glucose through storage as triglycerides in fat tissue. These activities can result in interference with the communication among the hypothalamus, pituitary, and ovary (hypothalamic–pituitary–ovarian axis) that regulates the processes of effective ovulation. The result is unpredictable menstrual cycles (abnormal uterine bleeding), longer cycles with short duration of menses (oligomenorrhea), and the prolonged absence of menstruation (amenorrhea). The relationship between obesity and interference with menstrual cycles and reproduction is thought to be related to the effect of high levels of insulin in women with obesity on the production of luteinizing hormone. The overproduction of luteinizing hormone owing to hyperinsulinemia overstimulates the theca cells of the ovary that produce androgens, creating an excess of circulating androgens. Hyperandrogenism (HA) disrupts the effective function of the feedback loop between the pituitary gland and the ovary that is necessary for regulation of the menstrual cycle and ovulation. All of these conditions contribute to infertility or subfertility in women with obesity and decrease the likelihood that natural conception or conception involving assisted reproductive technology will result in a pregnancy.

Women with obesity or overweight may also have one or more signs or symptoms of an endocrine disorder called polycystic ovary syndrome (PCOS). PCOS is the most common endocrinopathy in women of childbearing age. The prevalence of PCOS has been estimated to be between 5% and 20%[13] in the total population of women depending on the criteria used for diagnosis. The exact cause of PCOS is unknown, but there is evidence of a genetic component owing to the tendency of the condition to run in families through both maternal and paternal lineages. Because genetic variants similar to those observed in women with PCOS have been detected in populations of people of ancient Chinese and European decent, it is suggested that the disorder may have developed at least 60,000 years ago. Therefore, PCOS is not a result of the increasing global occurrence of obesity. Although it has been reported that 30% to 60% of women with PCOS have obesity, the prevalence of obesity in women with PCOS is about the same as in women without PCOS within the same population.[13] In other words, although these 2 conditions have similar pathophysiologic characteristics that involve heredity, hyperinsulinemia, and inflammatory processes, they are distinct conditions that require different approaches to diagnosis and management. Obesity does not cause PCOS; rather, it can amplify the clinical and biochemical changes, the symptoms of menstrual cycle disruption, and interference with fertility that characterizes PCOS.[13] A BMI of greater than 30 is not one of the criteria for the diagnosis of PCOS and women with a BMI of 26 or less have been confirmed to have PCOS. Women with PCOS who also have obesity have a higher rate of spontaneous abortion (miscarriage), pregnancy-related hypertension, gestational diabetes, premature births, type 2 diabetes, and metabolic syndrome.[14] Multiple developing follicles that are part of the pathophysiology of PCOS are visualized as cysts on imaging studies and are antral follicles. When overstimulated, the antral follicles produce abnormally high amounts of hormones (androgens) that disrupt the normal physiologic process of follicular development that should result in ovulation. The antral follicles are different from functional ovarian cysts. Functional ovarian cysts occur as larger single cysts, usually resolve on their own, and do not produce hormones that disrupt reproductive function.

The diagnostic criteria for PCOS include the presence of at least 2 of the 3 following conditions: clinical or biochemical HA, or both, infrequent or no ovulation (oligoanovulation [OA]), and polycystic ovarian morphology (PCOM). PCOM is further defined as (1) the enlargement of 1 or both ovaries measuring 10 cm^3 or more or (2) having 12 or more antral follicles that are 2 to 9 mm in diameter. Some references include menstrual irregularity as a defining feature of PCOS. At 1 time, unpredictable or prolonged absence of menses (amenorrhea) was included as a criterion. However, because the disturbance of the menstrual cycle is actually a manifestation of infrequent or anovulation, OA is the more precise criterion. In an attempt to more accurately document the features of PCOS experienced by women, 4 different combinations of the consensus diagnostic criteria are used. These variations in how the criteria are applied account for the wide variance in estimates of the prevalence of PCOS that are reported in research. The criteria grouping that is used most often for clinical diagnosis and in research is one that was developed by experts in reproductive endocrinology and other women's health specialists at a joint meeting of the European Society for Human Reproduction and Embryology and the American Society of Reproductive Medicine. The standard is referred to as the Rotterdam criteria, after the location where the joint meeting took place in 2003. In the intervening time since the dissemination of the Rotterdam criteria, further refinement was recommended based on recognition that there are as many as 4 distinct groupings of the main clinical and biochemical characteristics observed in women with PCOS. The clinical and biochemical manifestations of PCOS are arranged in different pairings and labeled as phenotypes as A, B, C, or D, respectively. Based on these additional refinements for guiding diagnosis and management, authors of the National Institutes of Health Consensus Statement from 2012 recommended that clinicians use the Rotterdam criteria along with documentation of which phenotype most closely matches the patient presentation when confirming a diagnosis of PCOS. PCOS phenotype A includes HA, OA, and PCOM. Phenotype B is HA and OA alone. Phenotype C is HA and PCOM alone, and phenotype D is OA and PCOM alone.[13]

SOCIAL STIGMA FOR WOMEN

Simply being identified as having a disease can instigate stigma, particularly if the condition is chronic. The stigma associated with obesity has been demonstrated to adversely affect women with obesity disproportionately both in comparison with thin women and men who also have obesity.[4] Until the early twentieth century, stoutness was associated with health, wealth, and higher social status. At the turn of the last century, excess weight began to be linked to sinful behavior as in a moral weakness and gluttony. In times of war and the accompanying imposition of food rationing and shortages, gaining weight was considered unpatriotic. These changes in societal attitudes transformed being overweight from a desirable characteristic to one of shame. An industry was spawned for the development of products and interventions to fight obesity. Because the rates of obesity are increasing, researchers have found that the level of stigmatization of people who have overweight and obesity has also increased in the last 20 years. The level of negative stereotypes present in advertising, entertainment, and the literature has been positively correlated with low self-esteem and the social devaluation of people who have overweight or obesity.[15,16] In 1 study, women reported that the highest number of "nasty comments" related to in some way to their weight that occurred in their daily human interactions were made by spouses, family, and friends (74%).[15] Both males and females experience weight-related shaming, discrimination in the workplace, and physical barriers like the size of chairs in health care facilities and transportation. However, public shaming related to their body, humiliation in academic settings, stereotyping when seeking physical or mental health care, fewer romantic relationships, and being passed over for a job or promotion are experienced significantly more often by women.[4,15] Along with the social consequences of weight stigma, researchers have documented psychological, behavioral, and physical effects in women. In addition to lowered self-esteem, the consequences of stigmatization include depression, binge eating, and physical activity avoidance.[16–18] The stigma for women of having obesity is so powerful that it can affect how male partners are treated or judged. In 1 study, researchers reported that simply being seen with a woman with obesity before an interview resulted in the male being perceived more negatively.[19] Living in a community where there are few or no places to engage in safe or socially comfortable physical activity can compound the reluctance on the part of women to exercise.

APPROACHES TO THE DIAGNOSIS AND MANAGEMENT OF OBESITY IN WOMEN

The US Preventive Services Task Force recommends that all adults should be screened for obesity.[20] As mentioned elsewhere in this article, although the BMI measurement is a relatively simple way to initially screen men and women for obesity in a clinical setting, it should not be the sole means to assess for excess adipose tissue. The American Academy of Family Physicians published a comprehensive monograph detailing the diagnosis and management of obesity, including pharmacologic, surgical, and nonpharmacologic approaches to working with patients to meet their health goals related to their weight and reducing health risks.[21] Although the publication does not focus specifically on women, it is a good primer on the topic. In combination with other more current resources, it is a reliable resource for nurses and other clinicians who want to learn more about the approach to patients and apply the principles to their routine practice. It is beyond the scope of this article to discuss the content of the monograph in detail. Remarks are limited to interventions that may help to decrease risk and improve quality and quantity of life for women living with obesity and associated conditions. The frequent contact with the health care system during pregnancy and postpartum offers opportunities for initiating discussions with women about healthy lifestyle behaviors and goal setting. For the majority of women, pregnancy is a time when the motivation for optimal personal and fetal health encourages them to make positive changes. It is important to communicate the benefits of healthy eating and physical activity for both the woman and for her baby during fetal development that will have lifelong impact. Healthy habits that begin in pregnancy may be sustained after birth and also applied for other family members. Well woman visits for the full range of health promotion and disease prevention services that are particular to women, such as family planning and cervical and breast cancer screenings, should include screening for obesity and counseling. Finally, women who have obesity may develop other chronic health conditions that require frequent follow-up for physical and biochemical monitoring. In all of these encounters, clinicians caring for women with obesity should be clear that, although the decisions are hers, the professional is ready and willing to help her. In the same way that we offer the full range of options to women to manage hypertension or other chronic health conditions and support while encouraging self-care between visits, we do not (or should not) place the full responsibility on the woman alone for managing her obesity. Even small successes can have measurable positive effects. In women whose BMI is 26 or higher and waist circumference is greater than 35 inches, other assessments such as blood pressure, and lipid and fasting glucose levels should be measured. Women who have obesity are at greater risk for 13 different types of cancer, most notably in the breast, uterus, and ovaries. Although there is no screening test for ovarian cancer, mammography for the early detection of breast cancer and sampling of the lining of the uterus (endometrium) through endometrial biopsy are available and should be completed as recommended by expert panels and consultation with a clinician. Treating modifiable risk factors for cardiovascular diseases like hypertension, high lipid levels, and diabetes through lifestyle changes and medication management can positively impact health outcomes for women.

In women with obesity suspected of having PCOS, the diagnosis of the endocrine dysfunction is best accomplished by systematically ruling out other causes for the woman's clinical signs and symptoms and confirming findings consistent with PCOS criteria. Specifically, tests for thyroid-stimulating hormone and prolactin levels must be done to rule out thyroid disorder and hyperprolactinemia. A 17-hydroxyprogesterone level should be obtained to detect adrenal hyperplasia. For women who exhibit hirsutism, an elevated dehydroepiandrosterone sulfate can establish HA. An oral glucose tolerance test and fasting insulin levels will identify problems with glucose metabolism. Last, a transvaginal ultrasound examination of the ovaries to quantify the number of antral follicles and to measure the total volume of the ovary should be completed. If the findings are consistent with the Rotterdam criteria for PCOS, a treatment plan can be selected by the clinician and woman, based on phenotype, health goals, and preferences. The initial intervention is attempting weight loss through nutritional changes and physical activity. For many women with PCOS, as little as a 5% decrease in weight will improve their menstrual symptoms. For women who have had prolonged amenorrhea, an endometrial biopsy may be completed to rule out endometrial hyperplasia (a risk for endometrial cancer) or cancer. Women who do not want to conceive and have irregular or no periods may use a combined low-dose oral contraceptive, if there are no contraindications, to prevent pregnancy and induce regular withdrawal bleeding. Metformin is prescribed to assist with menstrual dysfunction and has been associated with some weight loss. Spironolactone is often prescribed along with the oral contraceptives in women who are also hirsute; it can take as long as 6 months of treatment to noticeably decrease male pattern hair growth on the trunk and thighs. For women who want to conceive, ovulation stimulation can be accomplished by clomiphene citrate or letrozole. Some clinicians will also add metformin to the regimen, but its effect on ovulation is believed to be modest at best.[13]

It is understandable that women may find it difficult to discuss their weight given the relationship of obesity and significant health risks and the negative social messages that are now present in nearly every aspect of western culture. Yet, the evidence of the association between obesity and preventable disease is too strong for clinicians to avoid the discussion of weight with patients. The National Institute of Diabetes and Digestive and Kidney Diseases provides some guidance for talking with patients about their weight and constructively assisting them to set a goal for healthy lifestyle behavior changes that focus on nutrition and fitness, and not on weight.[22] The Joint International Statement on Obesity and Stigma[23] provides some foundational information for forming or reforming one's attitudes about obesity and those living with it that can help clinicians to approach the conversation in a more patient-first manner. Start the visit by addressing the patient's primary reason for the appointment before approaching a discussion about weight. This practice will help to avoid sending a message that the clinician assumes that the patient's problem is due to weight. Find out if your patient is willing to talk about the issue – "Ms. Smith, your BMI is above the healthy range. I would like to help you to reduce your risk for some health problems. Do you mind if we talk about it?" Identify and use the patient's preferences for terms to use when discussing weight. Explore with patients how ready they are to make changes in food choices and becoming more physically active. When they express readiness to change, let them take the lead in choosing specific actions and measurable goals. A 5% to 7% weight loss over a 6-month time period at a rate of ½ to 2 pounds per week is reasonable and safe. Document the discussion so that, when they return, you can check on progress on their goals and help them to develop strategies to overcome any barriers they may have encountered. Use data other than weight to provide evidence of progress, such as changes in blood pressure, blood sugar, and cholesterol levels to provide encouragement to stick with their plan.

The character, Shylock, in *The Merchant of Venice* did not collect his pound of flesh from Antonio owing to clever intervention on the part of the judge in the case. Using evidence-based, patient-centered strategies to help women, we may be able to prevent obesity from exacting its high price from women by decreasing their risk for preventable disease and increasing quality and quantity of life.

CLINICS CARE POINTS

- BMI should be paired with waist circumference and waist/hip ratio measurements when assessing and monitoring obesity in women.
- Many of the factors contributing to obesity are not under the control of women.
- Obesity during pregnancy can increase the risk of obesity in the child.
- A weight loss of as little as 5% can improve some of the symptoms experienced by women owing to obesity.
- Obesity can intensify the signs and symptoms associated with PCOS.
- Obese women who have infrequent or no menses should be screened for endometrial cancer.
- Lifestyle behavior counseling and interventions related to nutrition and physical activity are the cornerstones of obesity management.

DISCLOSURE

The author has no commercial or financial conflicts of interest related to this article. The author received no funding for the preparation of this article.

REFERENCES

1. Centers for Disease Control and Prevention [CDC]. Prevalence of obesity and severe obesity among adults: United States, 2017 - 2018. 2020. Available at: https://www.cdc.gov/nchs/products/databriefs/db360.htm#:~:text=Among%20women%2C%20the%20prevalence%20of,overall%20or%20by%20age%20group. Accessed March 30, 2021.
2. Tauqeer Z, Gomez G, Cody Stanford F. Obesity in women: insights for the clinician. J Womens Health 2018;27:444–57.
3. Moore JX, Chaudhary N, Akinyemiju T. Metabolic syndrome prevalence by race/ethnicity and sex in the United States, National Health and Nutrition Examination Survey, 1988–2012. Prev Chronic Dis 2017;14:160287.
4. Fikkan JL, Rothblum ED. Is fat a feminist issue? Exploring the gendered nature of weight bias. Sex Roles 2012;66:575–92.
5. Volger S, Vetter M, Dougherty M, et al. Patients' preferred terms for describing their excess weight: discussing obesity in clinical practice. Obesity 2012;20:147–50.
6. Karasu S. Adolphe Quetelet and the evolution of body mass index. 2016. Available at: https://www.psychologytoday.com/us/blog/the-gravity-weight/201603/adolphe-quetelet-and-the-evolution-body-mass-index-bmi. Accessed March 30, 2021.
7. Romero-Corral A, Somers V, Sierra-Johnson J, et al. Accuracy of body mass index to diagnose obesity in the US population. Int J Obes 2008;32:958–66.

8. Rubin R. Postmenopausal women with a "normal" BMI might be overweight or even obese. JAMA 2018;319:1185–7.

9. Heerwagen MJ, Miller MR, Barbour LA, et al. Maternal obesity and fetal metabolic programming: a fertile epigenetic soil. Am J Phys Reg Integ Comp Phys 2010; 299:R711–22.

10. Arenz S, Ruckerl R, Koletzko B, et al. Breastfeeding and childhood obesity: a systematic review. Int J Obes Relat Metab Disord 2004;28:1247–56.

11. Horta BL, Loret de Mola C, Victora CG. Long-term consequences of breastfeeding on cholesterol, obesity, systolic blood pressure and type 2 diabetes: a systematic review and meta-analysis. Acta Paediatr 2015;104:30–7.

12. Yan J, Liu L, Zhu Y, et al. The association between breastfeeding and childhood obesity: a metanalysis. BMC Pub Health 2014. Available at. https://bmcpublichealth.biomedcentral.com/track/pdf/10.1186/1471-2458-14-1267.pdf. Accessed March 30, 2021.

13. Azziz R. Polycystic ovary syndrome. Obstet Gynecol 2018;132:321–36.

14. Glueck C, Goldenberg N. Characteristics of obesity in polycystic ovarian syndrome: Etiology, treatment, and genetics. Metabolism 2018;92(Supplement 7). https://doi.org/10.1016/j.metabol.2018.11.002.

15. Seacat J, Dougal S, Roy D. A daily diary assessment of female weight stigmatization. J Health Psych 2014;21:228–40.

16. Friedman K, Reichman S, Costanzo P, et al. Weight stigmatization and ideological beliefs: relation to psychological functioning in obese adults. Obes Res 2005;13:907–16.

17. Vartanian L, Novak S. Internalized societal attitudes moderate the impact of weight stigma on avoidance of exercise. Obesity 2011;19:757–62.

18. Seacat J, Mickelson K. Stereotype threat and the exercise/dietary health intentions of overweight women. J Health Psychol 2009;14:556–67.

19. Hebl M, Mannix L. The weight of obesity in evaluating others. Pers Soc Psychol Bull 2003;29:28–38.

20. U.S. Preventive Services Task Force. Screening for obesity in adults: recommendations and rationale. Ann Int Med 2012;139:930–2.

21. American Academy of Family Physicians. Diagnosis and management of obesity in adults. 2013. Available at: https://www.aafp.org/dam/AAFP/documents/patient_care/fitness/obesity-diagnosis-mono.pdf. Accessed March 30, 2021.

22. National Institutes of Health. Talking with patients about weight loss: tips for primary care professionals. 2017. Available at: https://www.niddk.nih.gov/health-information/professionals/clinical-tools-patient-management/weight-management/talking-adult-patients-tips-primary-care-clinicians. Accessed March 30, 2021.

23. Joint International Consensus Statement. The clinician's guide on talking with patients about obesity. 2020. Available at: https://www.endocrineweb.com/professional/resource-centers/clinicians-guide-talking-patients-about-obesity. Accessed March 30, 2021.

Systemic and Environmental Contributors to Obesity Inequities in Marginalized Racial and Ethnic Groups

Faith A. Newsome, BA[a],*, Clarence C. Gravlee, PhD[b],
Michelle I. Cardel, PhD, MS, RD[a,c]

KEYWORDS

- Social determinants of health • Health inequities • Health equity

KEY POINTS

- Racism and discrimination, socioeconomic status, and increased levels of stress are systemic, and these environmental factors can influence obesity development, maintenance, and treatment among marginalized racial and ethnic groups.
- Within the health care delivery system, access to care and clinician bias can further contribute to health inequities.
- Current prevention and treatment options for obesity are not equally effective across racial and ethnic groups. More work related to implementation science and pragmatic trials among diverse populations is necessary to identify and implement effective interventions tailored to specific groups.
- There are several actionable steps health care providers can take to understand and address systemic contributors and offer personalized recommendations.

INTRODUCTION

Health inequities are preventable, unjust differences in disease burden that adversely impact oppressed, stigmatized, or medically underserved groups, such as people with lower socioeconomic status, people with disabilities, members of the LGBTQ community, individuals in rural areas, and marginalized racial and ethnic groups.[1] Racial and ethnic health inequities in the United States are pervasive, because of the harms of structural racism.[2] These harms include higher rates of heart disease, cancer, diabetes, HIV/AIDS, and other leading causes of death among marginalized racial and

[a] Department of Health Outcomes and Biomedical Informatics, University of Florida College of Medicine, 2197 Mowry Road, Gainesville, FL 32610, USA; [b] Department of Anthropology, University of Florida College of Liberal Arts and Sciences, 1112 Turlington Hall, PO Box 117305, Gainesville, FL 32611, USA; [c] WW International, Inc, New York, NY, USA
* Corresponding author.
E-mail address: fnewsome@ufl.edu

Nurs Clin N Am 56 (2021) 619–634
https://doi.org/10.1016/j.cnur.2021.07.003
0029-6465/21/© 2021 Elsevier Inc. All rights reserved.

ethnic groups, as compared with White patients.[3] In the United States, these inequities are attributed largely to long-standing, systemic inequalities in health care, interpersonal discrimination, and structural racism in housing, education, banking, law
enforcement, and other policy domains.[2,4] We recognize race and ethnicity as social
classifications rooted in a political system of racialized oppression, not as proxies for
genetic differences among people or populations.

This review focuses on racial and ethnic inequities in obesity. Hispanic, Black,
Native American, and Alaskan Native patients experience obesity at disproportionately higher rates than non-Hispanic Whites.[5] Obesity is a complex, multifactorial disease influenced by genetic, behavioral, metabolic, physiologic, and hormonal factors.[6]
Although behavioral factors are perceived to be within an individual's control, they
may be complicated by forces outside their control.[7,8] In many ways, the health
care delivery system and broader society contribute to these inequities, and this article
discusses factors that contribute to the disproportionate incidence of obesity among
marginalized groups, including existing treatment options, socioeconomic status,
racism and discrimination, access to care, and stigma within the health care system.

INEQUITIES IN RESEARCH

The basis of clinical care is evidence-based treatments supported by research. There
are several treatment options available for obesity, but they are not equally effective or
equally accessible across patient populations. The main treatment options for obesity
include lifestyle or behavioral interventions, pharmacotherapy, and bariatric surgery,
or a combination of these options.

Lifestyle interventions are often the first step in treating obesity, because they are
the least invasive, focusing on diet, physical activity, and behavioral change strategies.[9] Samples in studies of lifestyle interventions generally include mostly White females; therefore, there is less evidence on the efficacy of lifestyle interventions in
samples diverse in race, ethnicity, gender identity, and sex.[10] Because of limitations
in the design of these interventions to meet the needs of diverse groups of people,
there are differences in outcomes, specifically weight loss. In general, non-Hispanic
Black, Hispanic, and American Indian/Alaskan Natives patients lose less weight
than do Whites exposed to the same behavioral interventions.[11,12] Even among interventions tailored for lower-income individuals with a high percentage of Black adults
(67.2%), Black participants lost less weight than White patients. Specifically, Black patients had a 6% body weight loss at 6 months postintervention, compared with an 8%
body weight loss for those in other racialized groups.[13] When assessing the currently
available literature, it seems behavioral interventions for obesity are not as effective
among non-Hispanic Black, Hispanic, Native American and Alaskan Native patients
relative to Whites, suggesting the lack of provision of a level of care that is tailored
to address racial/ethnic inequities in outcomes and/or able to address the larger systemic issues contributing to observed differences. More research to better understand
differential outcomes and how these gaps in care can be addressed is critical.

For those who do not respond optimally to lifestyle intervention alone, pharmacologic intervention is appropriate. Currently, Food and Drug Administration–approved
antiobesity medications include phentermine, orlistat, phentermine/topiramate
extended release, naltrexone sustained release/bupropion SR, and liraglutide.[14] Prescriptions for antiobesity medications are more common among Black, Native Hawaiian or Pacific Islander, and American Indian or Alaskan Native patients.[15] Although
there are scarce data evaluating the extent to which pharmacotherapy outcomes differ
by race and ethnicity, limited evidence suggests differential responses to

pharmacotherapy options because of differences in social contexts that impact clinical presentation, adherence, and physiology.[16] For example, metformin usage among Black patients resulted in better glycemic control compared with White patients.[17] Yet, several medications including sibutramine and orlistat, result in higher weight loss, ranging from 0.5 kg to 1.7 kg, for White patients compared with Black and Hispanic patients.[16,18,19] Thus, findings are mixed based on which pharmacotherapy option is provided, in addition to other yet unidentified predictors. This suggests that although Black, Native Hawaiian or Pacific Islander, and American Indian or Alaskan Native patients are more likely to be prescribed antiobesity medication, it is unclear whether pharmacologic interventions have comparable effects across diverse populations or what accounts for potential differences.[15]

Bariatric surgery is the most invasive but also the most effective form of treatment of obesity. Bariatric surgery includes malabsorptive or restrictive procedures, such as Roux-en-Y gastric bypass and gastric sleeve.[20] Racial and ethnic inequities persist at this level of care, including inequities in access and referral to this effective intervention, increased risk of procedural complications, and poorer postoperative outcomes. Significantly more White than non-White patients receive bariatric surgery, with 60% of bariatric surgery patients identifying as White, 11% as Black, 5% as Hispanic, 0.2% as Native American, and 0.1% as Asian (race/ethnicity not reported for 25% of the sample).[21] Racial inequities in access to and receiving bariatric surgery may be caused, in part, by recommendations from physicians, which were lower for Black patients and men.[21–24] In terms of procedural complications, readmission, reintervention, and mortality rates following bariatric surgery are more likely in Black patients, and surgical complications are more common in Hispanic patients compared with Whites.[22,25,26] Postoperatively, Hispanic and Black patients lose less weight compared with Whites, and Hispanic, Black, and Asian patients do not experience the same level of cardiometabolic improvements compared with Whites.[27,28]

ENVIRONMENTAL FACTORS CONTRIBUTING TO OBESITY-RELATED INEQUITIES

It is not possible to understand how race relates to health without considering environmental factors through the lens of structural racism. Structural racism, including institutions, ideologies, and additional macrolevel forces, is a fundamental cause that contributes to racial inequities in obesity risk and treatment outcomes through several pathways.[4] These pathways include environmental factors, such as socioeconomic status, food insecurity, racism and interpersonal discrimination, and unequal access to health care.

Socioeconomic Status

Socioeconomic status attainment is limited for communities of color because of racist policies related to residential segregation, education, and employment opportunities.[3,29–31] Consequently, low neighborhood-level socioeconomic status can result in a clustering of a variety of risk factors including food insecurity, lack of access to safe housing, obesogenic living environments, and lack of community resources.

Food insecurity is associated with increased odds of having overweight or obesity in the United States and this relationship is stronger among racial and ethnic groups, such as Black and Hispanic patients, and women.[32–34] The insurance hypothesis/resource scarcity hypothesis, which assumes that perceived food insecurity and access to calorie-dense foods can result in excess calorie consumption and increased fat storage for individuals with lower social status, has been posited as an underlying contributor for the relationship between obesity and food insecurity.[35–37] Additionally, research involving experimentally manipulated social status revealed food insecure individuals consumed a greater percentage of their daily energy needs during a mealtime compared with food secure individuals. Moreover, individuals randomized to a low social status condition produce higher levels of ghrelin, priming individuals to consume more calories, than when placed in a high social status condition.[38,39] This suggests that marginalized racial and ethnic groups are at increased risk of developing obesity as a result of physiologic changes that can occur with food insecurity and subjugated social status.

Aspects of the built environment related to physical activity and diet also vary according to neighborhood-level socioeconomic status and race-based residential segregation. There is increased density of fast-food restaurants, with concordant decreased access to fresh foods in lower-income neighborhoods that predominately consisted of marginalized racial and ethnic groups, but not among low-income neighborhoods comprised primarily of non-Hispanic Whites.[40–42] Similarly, parks and recreational centers are also more likely to be absent or of poor quality in low-income or predominately Black and Hispanic neighborhoods.[43] Other aspects of the built environment that have been linked to the risk of obesity include connectivity of transportation networks, walkability, land-use mix, access to outdoor recreational spaces, and concentrated marketing of unhealthful foods.[44] The combination of reduced access to community resources and increased access to calorically dense foods can play a role in making racially segregated neighborhoods vulnerable to living in positive energy balance, which contributes to developing and maintaining obesity.

Thus, socioeconomic inequalities rooted in structural racism partially explain unequal risk of obesity among racial and ethnic groups because of inequities in food security, the food environment, and available community resources.[3,13,29,32,34,39,40,44] Clinicians need to consider and address these obstacles and opportunities when developing and discussing obesity treatment plans with patients.

Racism, Discrimination, and Stress

Beyond the independent effects of structural racism on health outcomes, the stress of interpersonal discrimination has effects on obesity development and maintenance. Interpersonal discrimination includes exposure to chronic and acute stressors in everyday social interactions, which can result in psychological and physiologic risk factors for the development of obesity.[45] Physiologic stress responses to interpersonal discrimination can have multiple impacts on cardiometabolic outcomes, because the experience of racism can lead to higher stress reactivity, resulting in increased risk of developing stress-induced diseases, such as hypertension and obesity.[29,46,47] According to the weathering hypothesis, racial disparities in health outcomes are a result of continued exposure to social disadvantage, through racism and discrimination, which contribute to declines in physical health.[46] Given that racial and ethnic groups, such as Black, Hispanic, Native American, American Indian, and Alaskan Natives, experience significantly more racism and discrimination over their lifetime relative to Whites, these populations are at increased risk for the development of cardiometabolic disease. For these reasons, understanding and addressing how stress resulting from interpersonal discrimination can impact obesity development, maintenance, and treatment is necessary.

Stress has additional effects on metabolic outcomes and obesity. Moderate levels of stress in Black men and high levels of stress in Black women increases the severity of metabolic syndrome.[47,48] Additionally, there is also a relationship between stress and obesity among Hispanic, Latino, Native American, and Alaskan Native patients such that those with chronic and high levels of perceived stress have increased energy intake and lower diet quality.[49,50] Thus, because the aforementioned racial and ethnic groups experience higher levels of stress as a result of discrimination, and this stress has effects on metabolic outcomes and obesity, these patient groups are at higher risk of stress-induced adverse cardiometabolic and weight-related outcomes.

Additionally, weight-based discrimination is well-documented, and the prevalence of weight-based discrimination is similar to rates of race-based discrimination, particularly for women.[51] Similar to racism, perceived weight-based discrimination results in adverse physiologic outcomes, such as increased cortisol and increased levels of C-reactive protein levels and psychological outcomes, such as depression, anxiety, and self-esteem.[52,53] Weight discrimination also results in increased stress, thus the intersection between race and weight-based discrimination may have compounding effects for marginalized racial/ethnic groups at higher weight status.

Western Thin Ideal

A thin ideal can result in disordered eating behaviors, therefore impacting obesity development and treatment. The thin ideal is not universal, because it is based on a Western, White supremacist ideal.[54] Awareness and internalization of the thin ideal is a predictor of weight gain and disordered eating, and should be considered in the context of weight management because disordered eating behavior is common in patients with obesity.[55] The relationship between internalization of a thin ideal and disordered eating varies by race and ethnicity. For example, internalization of a thin ideal served as a mediator between awareness of the ideal and a drive for thinness, thus increasing disordered eating risk among Black patients.[56] However, among some Hispanic subgroups, cultural norms for body size and shape serve as a protective factor against internalizing a thin ideal.[57] Thus, although there is variance in response to internalization of the ideal, there is a potential for the thin ideal to result in adverse outcomes in some racial groups.

Access to Care

Equitable access to care is critical for receiving quality, evidence-based treatment of obesity and achieving desired outcomes across populations. Rural communities are often believed to be predominately White[58]; therefore, diverse racial and ethnic groups in rural areas are often overlooked, including Native American reservations that are located in rural areas.[58] However, resources for weight management are usually located in academic, tertiary-care centers, often leaving rural communities with reduced access. Identification of scalable and easily disseminated ways to reach rural populations for obesity-related care is essential.

In addition to the location of comprehensive weight-management clinics, insurance coverage can also prevent access to care. Rates of insurance coverage are lower among Black, Hispanic, Asian, and Latino populations.[59] Although the Affordable Care Act has slightly reduced these inequities in public and private insurance coverage, there is still limited coverage for obesity treatment, because evidence-based treatments are not consistently covered across all states.[60,61] Thus, the combination of lower insurance rates and lack of consistent coverage can contribute to racial inequities, such that there is an increased risk of being unable to access and receive insurance coverage for evidence-based obesity treatments.

Because geography and insurance coverage limit access to obesity care, patients may seek information on the Internet. Internet searches for diet information are cyclical in nature and typically consist of current fads, undermining the sustained interest over time necessary for improving weight loss outcomes.[62] Patients seeking health information from the Internet trust its accuracy, regardless of the source.[63] However, disparities exist between the validity and accuracy of resources accessed by White patients versus other racial and ethnic groups. Specifically, the quality of content of weight loss information is lower for Spanish Web sites, relative to those cited in English.[64] This pattern suggests that Spanish-speakers seeking weight loss information on the Internet are likely to come across unreliable information, potentially leading to further inequities.

BIAS IN HEALTH CARE

Health care professionals have been shown to exhibit race, ethnicity, and weight-based biases.[65–68] This bias impacts the quality of care patient groups receive, thus peripherally impacting health-related outcomes and negatively affecting the relationship between the provider and patient.[68–70] Similar to the compounding impacts of multiple layers of stress, the intersection of race-based and weight-based stigma in health care has the potential to contribute disproportionately to racial inequities among diverse patients living with obesity. Specifically, poor relationships with or mistrust of health care professionals can result in avoiding or delaying seeking health care, particularly among diverse racial and ethnic groups who have experienced previous discrimination based on the intersection of race, ethnicity, and weight-based biases.[71,72] Therefore, addressing bias in health care delivery is an essential first step to addressing inequities in health care settings. It is difficult to tailor recommendations or effectively engage with diverse patient groups to address obesity unless they feel comfortable visiting health care professionals.

CONTROLLABLE VERSUS UNCONTROLLABLE FACTORS

As clinicians, when discussing obesity with patients who are racially and ethnically marginalized, it is crucial to differentiate between factors that are within a person's control, and factors that are outside that person's control. Overestimating a patient's autonomy to act on certain behavioral prescriptions (eg, eat more fruits and vegetables, increase sleep duration) can harm patients by placing the blame on them, rather than acknowledging how behavioral choices are constrained by the environmental pathways of structural racism. Some contributing factors to the development of obesity, such as family history or genetics, are more obviously outside the person's control. However, some behavioral factors that may initially seem to be within an individual's control are actually socially patterned behaviors impacted by environmental factors. We must take environmental constraints into consideration when making recommendations.

One example of a behavior that initially seems to be within an individual's control is sleep. Shorter sleep duration is generally associated with obesity, and Black, Hispanic, Latino, and Asian patients report shorter sleep duration than do Whites, increasing their risk.[73] Additionally, individuals with lower socioeconomic status disproportionately exhibit sleep patterns that contribute to adverse health outcomes and mortality.[73–75] Yet these patterns reflect social context, not just individual choice. Sleep is impacted by cultural norms, job type, and stress reactivity resulting from chronic exposure to racism.[47,76–78] For example, a patient with high blood pressure and obesity who works the night shift and experiences racial discrimination at work may experience shorter sleep duration and lower sleep quality. Therefore, opening a discussion with patients regarding their barriers to sleep quality and duration can assist in making personalized recommendations pertaining to sleep attuned to social context.

Food-related choices also initially seem to be within an individual's control but are often complicated by many factors including geographic location, access, social interactions, and the built environment.[79] The decisions people make are based on the choices they have. Thus, when environmental factors affecting marginalized racial and ethnic groups (eg, food insecurity, decreased access to fresh foods, and increased density of fast-food restaurants) impact the dietary choices that are available, it impacts people's ability to adhere to nutritional recommendations.[35,40,42,79] As an example, a provider may wish to place a patient with type 2 diabetes and obesity on a ketogenic diet. However, the patient's ability to follow that recommendation depends on many contextual factors, including access to transportation to grocery stores with high-quality, affordable fresh fruits and vegetables and lean sources of protein, a refrigerator to store those items, a stove or oven to cook these foods, and time to acquire and prepare recommended meals. Thus, it is essential to assess (not assume) whether patients have access to healthful foods and resources to purchase, store, and cook those foods.

These are just a few examples of factors that may initially seem within an individual's control but are constrained by societal and economic inequalities and material deprivation. It is critical to consider the complicated nature of autonomy in factors related to obesity development, maintenance, and treatment when working with patients to improve personalized recommendations. Additional questions to consider in patient interactions that can aid in understanding social determinants of health that impact the individual are found in **Table 1**.

ACTIONABLE STEPS

Treatments and assessments that consider the aforementioned barriers are necessary to reduce racial inequities in obesity development and treatment. Suggestions for improving clinical care through consideration of these factors are categorized by domain (research, clinical care, and policy) and are outlined next.

Investigating racial inequities in obesity treatment accessibility and outcomes among diverse racial and ethnic groups through research is imperative to achieving equitable outcomes among all patient populations. Specifically, culturally tailoring existing interventions to address the needs of diverse populations can improve outcomes through increased effect sizes; however, this work among Native American, Alaskan Native, Hispanic, and Latino patients remains limited or in formative stages.[80-82] Using implementation science strategies, such as community-based participatory research, to culturally tailor interventions encourages participation of marginalized racial and ethnic groups in the research process by offering shared decision-making in the development of research questions, data collection methods, and dissemination of findings thus resulting in increased levels of acceptability, feasibility, and effectiveness.[83] Equity must be a guiding principle of implementation science approaches.[84] There are increased effect sizes shown in lifestyle interventions that include tailored components, such as the inclusion of culturally appropriate recipes, community feedback regarding specific barriers of adherence, peer leaders or community health workers as instructors and facilitators of educational materials, translation of material into participant's native language, and modification of text for lower literacy levels.[85] Therefore, using implementation science and encouraging the participation of diverse racial and ethnic groups in research through community-based techniques can reduce inequities by appropriately culturally tailoring interventions, thus increasing effect sizes.

In the domain of clinical care actionable steps include attention to barriers, such as food insecurity, racism and discrimination, and stress. Generally, quantitative assessment of environmental factors can improve outcomes through personalized

Table 1
Questions to ask during clinical encounters with diverse racial/ethnic patients with obesity to personalize recommendations and assess social determinants of health

Social Determinant of Health	Suggested Questions
Food insecurity	Have you ever you worried that food would run out before you and your family were able to get money to buy more?[86,99]
	Did the food that you bought not last and did you not have money to get more?[86,99]
	In the last month, has it been difficult to afford balanced meals?[99]
	Where do you purchase groceries?
	How do you prepare foods?
Socioeconomic status	Is it difficult to pay for basics, such as food, medications, health care, and housing?[99]
Support system	In a typical week, how often do you spend time with friends and family?[99]
	How often do you spend time using technology, such as email or social media, to connect with friends and family?[99]
	Do you ever feel isolated or lonely?[99]
	Do you feel supported in your weight management journey?
Stress	In the past month have you felt a lot of stress, a moderate amount of stress, little stress, or almost no stress at all?[99]
	What are the biggest sources of stress in your life?
Sleep	Does your stress impact your sleep?
	Are there any barriers you experience that prevent you from sleeping 7–9 hours a night?
	Do you find it difficult to fall asleep or stay asleep?
Community resources	Are there sidewalks or places to exercise in your neighborhood or in the surrounding area?
	Is there anything about your community, or neighborhood, that prevents you from participating in physical activity outside?
	(If patient experiences food insecurity) Are you aware of local resources, such as food banks?
	Is there anything about your community or neighborhood that makes it difficult to follow the physical activity recommendations discussed today?
Goals	What health-related goals would you like to discuss today?
	Do you feel like you have access to resources that will help you achieve your goals? How can we help?
	What do you think is a realistic goal? What are the steps we can take to achieve it?

recommendations for diverse patient groups seeking obesity treatment. Conventional recommendations for diet and physical activity may not consider pertinent social determinants of health. Suggestions for clinical measures to quantitatively assess environmental factors include the assessment of food insecurity, a social determinants questionnaire, and the inclusion of social determinants of health in electronic health records.[86–88]

Qualitative assessments also have value. One way to guide discussion of environmental factors is to use the equity-oriented obesity prevention framework.[89] This framework focuses on four components: (1) increasing healthy options, (2) improving social and economic resources, (3) reducing deterrents, and (4) building community capacity. Additionally, the framework offers guidance on addressing factors that drive racial inequities, such as food insecurity and community resources, to cater to people with lower socioeconomic status and in marginalized racial and ethnic groups. This framework is used to guide conversation about available resources and needs in the community (**Fig. 1**).

Including information on social determinants of health in clinical assessments allows providers to offer personalized recommendations based on the specific needs of the patient. These personalized recommendations differ based on the most pervasive environmental factors affecting the patient at that time. Thus, the priority for a patient experiencing food insecurity may include offering information and discussing community or federal resources. The priority for a patient experiencing increased levels of stress and sleep disturbances as a result of racism or discrimination may include discussing stress management techniques or referral to a psychologist, which is a beneficial component of obesity treatment among medically underserved groups experiencing high levels of stress.[90,91] Additionally, for patient groups at risk for internalizing the Western thin ideal, screening for disordered eating and discussion of realistic goals of 5% to 10% body weight loss to improve cardiometabolic risk factors also contribute to patient-centered care.[91] Cumulatively, these quantitative and qualitative assessments can result in personalized treatment plans and shared goals that consider the needs of the patient, their social determinants of health, and realistic recommendations (**Table 1**).

Changes in the clinical environment itself are also necessary. It is imperative to recognize the systemic nature of racial bias in health care, listen extensively to patients in marginalized groups, and implement system-wide interventions to combat inequities in care.[92] Thus, a comprehensive approach to improving workforce diversity and provider training is necessary. Racial/ethnic and language concordance among

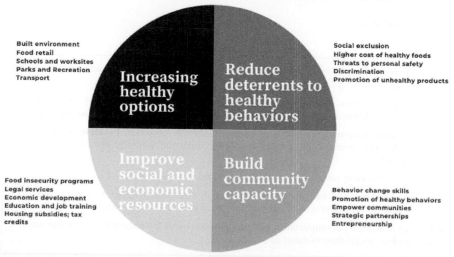

Fig. 1. Equity-oriented obesity prevention for guiding discussion with patients on community resources. (Kumanyika, S. 2017. Getting to Equity in Obesity Prevention: A New Framework. NAM Perspectives. Discussion Paper, National Academy of Medicine, Washington, DC. https://doi.org/10.31478/201701c. Adapted and reproduced with permission from the National Academy of Sciences, Courtesy of the National Academies Press, Washington, D.C.)

patient and provider is demonstrated to improve the relationship between provider and patient and improve health outcomes.[93,94] For providers who do not identify as a part of marginalized racial or ethnic groups, limited evidence suggests that cultural education for health care professionals can result in low to moderate improvements in patient outcomes.[95,96] In addition to cultural and linguistic competency, it is also important to increase structural competency among health care providers to combat stigma and improve health equity.[97]

Finally, the larger environmental factors discussed in this review continually serve as barriers that require attention through the domain of policy. Although these factors are beyond the scope of direct patient contact, health care providers have a role to play in advocating for policy change. For example, potential solutions for addressing food insecurity include community-level interventions, such as supplementary food and food banks, in combination with federal-level interventions, such as food subsidies and cash transfers. More work is necessary to identify and implement effective and accessible interventions for food insecurity.[32,98] Generally speaking, policy changes tied to institutional racism (ranging from racist and discriminatory policies in housing, education, and employment that affect socioeconomic status attainment, wealth accumulation, and resource allocation among communities) are crucial to reducing racial inequities in health and increasing access to care. Clinicians and researchers can advocate for patients by sharing their expertise and participating in science communication with policymakers to explain how policy influences health outcomes and contributes to inequities. Ultimately, the collaboration of health care and policy is necessary to address systematic health racial inequities in the United States.

Addressing pervasive racial inequities in obesity prevalence and treatment demands integration of research, clinical care, and policy. The actionable steps described in this article are only a few of many ways that individuals working in health care, including researchers, clinicians, and policymakers, can contribute to reducing inequities. Much work remains to be done across all three domains to achieve equity in obesity risk, treatment, and care.

CLINICS CARE POINTS

Based on this review, we recommend incorporating the following steps to address diverse and marginalized patient groups.

- Recognize multiple environmental pathways through which structural racism shapes inequities in obesity risk, access to care, and adherence to provider recommendations.
- Assess social determinants of health using questions provided in **Table 1** to provide personalized recommendations that consider the individual patients' need and their environment.
- Focus on increasing racial and ethnic representation in health care.
- Provide cross-cultural education and training in structural competency, particularly for providers who do not identify with marginalized racial or ethnic groups.
- Engage in science communication with policymakers and legislators to encourage policies that address social determinants of health.

CONCLUSION

Obesity is more prevalent among patients in marginalized racial and ethnic groups in the United States. Currently, available treatment options are not as accessible, feasible, and effective in diverse patient groups, resulting in racial inequities in treating obesity and cardiometabolic improvements. Structural racism contributes to these inequities through multiple pathways including food insecurity, obesogenic living environments, socioeconomic inequalities, inequitable access to care, and psychological and physiologic consequences of stress related to weight- and race-based discrimination. These complex, intersecting factors place patients in marginalized racial and ethnic groups at increased risk for developing and maintaining obesity. Thus, it is imperative for the health care delivery system, from researchers to clinicians, to acknowledge the structural basis of racial inequities and take concrete steps toward eliminating them.

DISCLOSURE

FAN reports personal fees from Novo Nordisk, outside the submitted work. MIC reports grants from NIH NHLBI, grants from WellCare Health Plans, Inc, during the conduct of the study; personal fees and income from WW International, Inc, consulting with NovoNordisk where personal fees were not accepted, outside the submitted work. CCG has no conflicts to disclose.

REFERENCES

1. Braveman P. Health disparities and health equity: concepts and measurement. Annu Rev Public Health 2006;27(1):167–94.
2. Bailey ZD, Krieger N, Agénor M, et al. Structural racism and health inequities in the USA: evidence and interventions. Lancet 2017;389(10077):1453–63.
3. Williams DR. Race, socioeconomic status, and health the added effects of racism and discrimination. Ann N Y Acad Sci 1999;896(1):173–88.
4. Gee GC, Ford CL. Structural racism and health inequities. Du Bois Rev 2011;8(1): 115–32.
5. Petersen R, Pan L, Blanck HM. Racial and ethnic disparities in adult obesity in the United States: CDC's tracking to inform state and local action. Prev Chronic Dis 2019;16:E46.
6. Cardel MI, Atkinson MA, Taveras EM, et al. Obesity treatment among adolescents: a review of current evidence and future directions. JAMA Pediatr 2020; 174(6):609–17.
7. St-Onge MP. Sleep–obesity relation: underlying mechanisms and consequences for treatment. Obes Rev 2017;18(Suppl 1):34–9.
8. Wang Y, Beydoun MA. The obesity epidemic in the united states gender, age, socioeconomic, racial/ethnic, and geographic characteristics: a systematic review and meta-regression analysis. Epidemiol Rev 2007;29(1):6–28.
9. Looney SM, Raynor HA. Behavioral lifestyle intervention in the treatment of obesity. Health Serv Insights 2013;6:15–31.
10. Haughton CF, Silfee VJ, Wang ML, et al. Racial/ethnic representation in lifestyle weight loss intervention studies in the United States: a systematic review. Prev Med Rep Mar 2018;9:131–7.
11. Wingo BC, Carson TL, Ard J. Differences in weight loss and health outcomes among African Americans and whites in multicentre trials. Obes Rev 2014;15: 46–61.
12. Eight-year weight losses with an intensive lifestyle intervention: the look AHEAD study. Obesity 2014;22(1):5–13.
13. Katzmarzyk PT, Martin CK, Newton R, et al. Weight loss in underserved patients: a cluster-randomized trial. N Engl J Med 2020;383(10):909–18.

14. Srivastava G, Apovian CM. Current pharmacotherapy for obesity. Nat Rev Endocrinol 2018;14(1):12–24.
15. Saxon DR, Iwamoto SJ, Mettenbrink CJ, et al. Antiobesity medication use in 2.2 million adults across eight large health care organizations: 2009-2015. Obesity 2019;27(12):1975–81.
16. Egan BM, White K. Weight loss pharmacotherapy: brief summary of the clinical literature. Ethn Dis 2015;25(4):511.
17. Williams LK, Padhukasahasram B, Ahmedani BK, et al. Differing effects of metformin on glycemic control by race-ethnicity. J Clin Endocrinol Metab 2014;99(9): 3160–8.
18. Yanovski SZ, Yanovski JA. Long-term drug treatment for obesity. JAMA 2014; 311(1):74.
19. Osei-Assibey G, Adi YKI, Kumar S, et al. Pharmacotherapy for overweight/obesity in ethnic minorities and White Caucasians: a systematic review and meta-analysis. Diabetes Obes Metab 2011;13(5):385–93.
20. Piché M, Auclair A, Harvey J, et al. How to choose and use bariatric surgery in 2015. Can J Cardiol 2015;31(2):153–66.
21. Pratt GM, Learn CA, Hughes GD, et al. Demographics and outcomes at American Society for Metabolic and Bariatric Surgery centers of excellence. Surg Endosc 2009;23(4):795–9.
22. Sheka A, Kizy S, Wirth K, et al. Racial disparities in perioperative outcomes after bariatric surgery. Surg Obes Relat Dis 2019;15(5):786–93.
23. Wee CC, Huskey KW, Bolcic-Jankovic D, et al. Sex, race, and consideration of bariatric surgery among primary care patients with moderate to severe obesity. J Gen Intern Med 2014;29(1):68–75.
24. Worni M, Guller U, Maciejewski ML, et al. Racial differences among patients undergoing laparoscopic gastric bypass surgery: a population-based trend analysis from 2002 to 2008. Obes Surg 2013;23(2):226–33.
25. Welsh LK, Luhrs AR, Davalos G, et al. Racial disparities in bariatric surgery complications and mortality using the MBSAQIP data registry. Obes Surg 2020;30(8): 3099–110.
26. Kizy S, Jahansouz C, Downey MC, et al. National trends in bariatric surgery 2012–2015: demographics, procedure selection, readmissions, and cost. Obes Surg 2017;27(11):2933–9.
27. Coleman K, Huang Y, Hendee F, et al. Three-year weight outcomes from a bariatric surgery registry in a large integrated healthcare system. Surg Obes Relat Dis 2014;10(3):396–403.
28. Valencia A, Garcia L, Morton J. The impact of ethnicity on metabolic outcomes after bariatric surgery. J Surg Res 2019;236:345–51.
29. Loury G. The anatomy of racial inequality. Cambridge (MA): Harvard University Press; 2002.
30. Din- Dzietham R, Nembhard W, Collins R, et al. Perceived stress following race-based discrimination at work is associated with hypertension in African-Americans. The metro Atlanta Heart Disease Study, 1999-2001. Soc Sci Med 2004;58(3):449–61.
31. Williams DR. Racial residential segregation: a fundamental cause of racial disparities in health. Public Health Rep 2001;116(5):404–16.
32. Visser J, Mclachlan MH, Maayan N, et al. Community-based supplementary feeding for food insecure, vulnerable and malnourished populations: an overview of systematic reviews. Cochrane Database Syst Rev 2018;11(11):CD010578.

33. Martin K, Ferris A. Food insecurity and gender are risk factors for obesity. J Nutr Educ Behav 2007;39(1):31–6.
34. Papas MA, Trabulsi JC, Dahl A, et al. Food insecurity increases the odds of obesity among young Hispanic children. J Immigrant Minor Health 2016;18(5): 1046–52.
35. Myers A, Painter M. Food insecurity in the United States of America: an examination of race/ethnicity and nativity. Food Security 2017;9(6):1419–32.
36. Dhurandhar EJ. The food-insecurity obesity paradox: a resource scarcity hypothesis. Physiol Behav 2016;162:88–92.
37. Nettle D, Andrews C, Bateson M. Food insecurity as a driver of obesity in humans: the insurance hypothesis. Behav Brain Sci 2017;40:1–34.
38. Cardel M, Pavela G, Janicke D, et al. Experimentally manipulated low social status and food insecurity alter eating behavior among adolescents: a randomized controlled trial. Obesity 2020;28(11):2010–9.
39. Sim A, Lim E, Leow M, et al. Low subjective socioeconomic status stimulates orexigenic hormone ghrelin: a randomised trial. Psychoneuroendocrinology 2018;89:103–12.
40. Larson NI, Story MT, Nelson MC. Neighborhood environments. Am J Prev Med 2009;36(1):74–81.e10.
41. Zenk SN, Schulz AJ, Israel BA, et al. Neighborhood racial composition, neighborhood poverty, and the spatial accessibility of supermarkets in metropolitan Detroit. Am J Public Health 2005;95(4):660–7.
42. Block JP, Scribner RA, Desalvo KB. Fast food, race/ethnicity, and income. Am J Prev Med 2004;27(3):211–7.
43. Moore LV, Diez Roux AV, Evenson KR, et al. Availability of recreational resources in minority and low socioeconomic status areas. Am J Prev Med Jan 2008;34(1): 16–22.
44. Booth KM, Pinkston MM, Poston WSC. Obesity and the built environment. J Am Diet Assoc 2005;105(5):110–7.
45. Tull S, Wickramasuriya T, Taylor J, et al. Relationships of internalized racism to abdominal obesity and blood pressure in Afro-Caribbean women. J Natl Med Assoc 1999;91:447–52.
46. Forde AT, Crookes DM, Suglia SF, et al. The weathering hypothesis as an explanation for racial disparities in health: a systematic review. Ann Epidemiol 2019;33: 1–18.e13.
47. Tomiyama AJ. Stress and obesity. Annu Rev Psychol 2019;70:703–18.
48. Cardel MI, Min Y-I, Sims M, et al. Association of psychosocial stressors with metabolic syndrome severity among African Americans in the Jackson Heart Study. Psychoneuroendocrinology 2018;90:141–7.
49. Barrington WE, Beresford SAA, Mcgregor BA, et al. Perceived stress and eating behaviors by sex, obesity status, and stress vulnerability: findings from the vitamins and lifestyle (VITAL) study. J Acad Nutr Diet 2014;114(11):1791–9.
50. Isasi CR, Parrinello CM, Jung MM, et al. Psychosocial stress is associated with obesity and diet quality in Hispanic/Latino adults. Ann Epidemiol 2015; 25(2):84–9.
51. Puhl RM, Andreyeva T, Brownell KD. Perceptions of weight discrimination: prevalence and comparison to race and gender discrimination in America. Int J Obes 2008;32(6):992–1000.
52. Jackson SE, Steptoe A. Obesity, perceived weight discrimination, and hair cortisol: a population-based study. Psychoneuroendocrinology 2018;98:67–73.

53. Wu Y, Berry D. Impact of weight stigma on physiological and psychological health outcomes for overweight and obese adults: a systematic review. J Adv Nurs 2018;74(5):1030–42.

54. Witcomb G, Arcelus J, Chen J. Can cognitive dissonance methods developed in the west for combatting the 'thin ideal' help slow the rapidly increasing prevalence of eating disorders in non-Western cultures? Shanghai Arch Psychiatry 2013;25(6):332–40.

55. Juarascio A, Forman E, Timko C, et al. Implicit internalization of the thin ideal as a predictor of increases in weight, body dissatisfaction, and disordered eating. Eat Behav 2011;12(3):207–13.

56. Gilbert S, Crump S, Madhere S, et al. Internalization of the thin ideal as a predictor of body dissatisfaction and disordered eating in African, African-American, and Afro-Caribbean female college students. J Coll Student Psychotherapy 2009;23(3):196–211.

57. Warren C, Gleaves D, Cepeda-Benito A, et al. Ethnicity as a protective factor against internalization of a thin ideal and body dissatisfaction. Int J Eat Disord 2005;37(3):241–9.

58. Lichter DT. Immigration and the new racial diversity in rural America. Rural Soc 2012;77(1):3–35.

59. National Research Council (US) Panel on Race E, and Health in Later Life. Understanding racial and ethnic differences in health in late life: a research agenda. Washington (DC): National Academies Press (US); 2004.

60. Buchmueller T, Levinson Z, Levy H, et al. Effect of the affordable care act on racial and ethnic disparities in health insurance coverage. Am J Public Health 2016; 106(8):1416–21.

61. Jannah N, Hild J, Gallagher C, et al. Coverage for obesity prevention and treatment services: analysis of Medicaid and state employee health insurance programs. Obes (Silver Spring) 2018;26(12):1834–40.

62. Passos JA, Vasconcellos-Silva PR, Santos LADS. Ciclos de atenção a dietas da moda e tendências de busca na internet pelo Google trends. Ciên Saúde Colet 2020;25(7):2615–31.

63. Bennett GG, Glasgow RE. The delivery of public health interventions via the Internet: actualizing their potential. Annu Rev Public Health 2009;30(1):273–92.

64. Cardel MI, Chavez S, Bian J, et al. Accuracy of weight loss information in Spanish search engine results on the Internet. Obesity 2016;24(11):2422–34.

65. Van Ryn M, Burgess DJ, Dovidio JF, et al. The impact of racism on clinician cognition, behavior, and clinical decision making. Du Bois Rev 2011;8(1):199–218.

66. Tajeu G, Halanych J, Juarez L, et al. Exploring the association of healthcare worker race and occupation with implicit and explicit racial bias. J Natl Med Assoc 2018;110(5):464–72.

67. Fitzgerald C, Hurst S. Implicit bias in healthcare professionals: a systematic review. BMC Med Ethics 2017;18(1):19.

68. Phelan SM, Burgess DJ, Yeazel MW, et al. Impact of weight bias and stigma on quality of care and outcomes for patients with obesity. Obes Rev 2015;16(4): 319–26.

69. Fiscella K, Franks P, Gold M, et al. Inequality in quality: addressing socioeconomic, racial, and ethnic disparities in health care. JAMA 2000;283(19):2579–84.

70. Benkert R, Peters R, Clark R, et al. Effects of perceived racism, cultural mistrust and trust in providers on satisfaction with care. J Natl Med Assoc 2006;98(9): 1532–40.

71. Alberga AS, Edache IY, Forhan M, et al. Weight bias and health care utilization: a scoping review. Prim Health Care Res Dev 2019;20:e116.
72. Spleen AM, Lengerich EJ, Camacho FT, et al. Health care avoidance among rural populations: results from a nationally representative survey. J Rural Health 2014; 30(1):79–88.
73. Whinnery J, Jackson N, Rattanaumpawan P, et al. Short and long sleep duration associated with race/ethnicity, sociodemographics, and socioeconomic position. Sleep 2014;37(3):601–11.
74. Hale L, Do DP. Racial differences in self-reports of sleep duration in a population-based study. Sleep 2007;30(9):1096–103.
75. Van Cauter E, Spiegel K. Sleep as a mediator of the relationship between socio-economic status and health: a hypothesis. Ann N Y Acad Sci 1999;896:254–61.
76. Juda M, Vetter C, Roenneberg T. Chronotype modulates sleep duration, sleep quality, and social jet lag in shift-workers. J Biol Rhythms 2013;28(2):141–51.
77. Williams NJ, Grandner MA, Snipes SA, et al. Racial/ethnic disparities in sleep health and health care: importance of the sociocultural context. Sleep Health 2015;1(1):28–35.
78. Hicken M, Lee H, Ailshire J, et al. "Every shut eye ain't sleep": the role of racism-related vigilance in racial/ethnic disparities in sleep difficulty. Race Soc Probl 2013;5(2):100–12.
79. Drewnowski A, Kawachi I. Diets and health: how food decisions are shaped by biology, economics, geography, and social interactions. Big Data 2015;3(3): 193–7.
80. Lindberg N, Stevens V. Review: weight-loss interventions with Hispanic populations. Ethn Dis 2007;17(2):397–402.
81. Perez LG, Arredondo EM, Elder JP, et al. Evidence-based obesity treatment interventions for Latino adults in the U.S. Am J Prev Med 2013;44(5):550–60.
82. Rosas LG, Vasquez JJ, Naderi R, et al. Development and evaluation of an enhanced diabetes prevention program with psychosocial support for urban American Indians and Alaska natives: a randomized controlled trial. Contemp Clin Trials 2016;50:28–36.
83. Las Nueces D, Hacker K, Digirolamo A, et al. A systematic review of community-based participatory research to enhance clinical trials in racial and ethnic minority groups. Health Serv Res 2012;47(3pt2):1363–86.
84. Brownson RC, Kumanyika SK, Kreuter MW, et al. Implementation science should give higher priority to health equity. Implement Sci 2021;16(1):28.
85. Mccurley JL, Gutierrez AP, Gallo LC. Diabetes prevention in U.S. Hispanic adults: a systematic review of culturally tailored interventions. Am J Prev Med 2017;52(4): 519–29.
86. Lee A, Cardel M, Donahoo W. In: Feingold K, Anawalt B, Boyce A, et al, editors. Social and environmental factors influencing obesity. South Dartmouth (MA): MDText.com, INC; 2019.
87. Pérez-Stable EJ, El-Toukhy S. Communicating with diverse patients: how patient and clinician factors affect disparities. Patient Educ Couns 2018;101(12): 2186–94.
88. Bazemore AW, Cottrell EK, Gold R, et al. "Community vital signs": incorporating geocoded social determinants into electronic records to promote patient and population health. J Am Med Inform Assoc 2016;23(2):407–12.
89. Kumanyika S. Getting to equity in obesity prevention: a new framework. NAM Perspect; 2017. Available at: https://nam.edu/getting-to-equity-in-obesity-prevention-a-new-framework/.

90. Kushner R, Ryan D. Assessment and lifestyle management of patients with obesity: clinical recommendations from systematic reviews. JAMA 2014;312(9): 943–52.

91. Chacko SA, Chiodi SN, Wee CC. Recognizing disordered eating in primary care patients with obesity. Prev Med 2015;72:89–94.

92. Jones RA, Lawlor ER, Birch JM, et al. The impact of adult behavioural weight management interventions on mental health: a systematic review and meta-analysis. Obes Rev 2020;22(4):e13150.

93. Fernandez A, Schillinger D, Warton ME, et al. Language barriers, physician-patient language concordance, and glycemic control among insured Latinos with diabetes: the diabetes study of Northern California (DISTANCE). J Gen Intern Med 2010;26(2):70–6.

94. Saha S, Komaromy M, Koepsell TD, et al. Patient-physician racial concordance and the perceived quality and use of health care. Arch Intern Med 1999; 159(9):997.

95. Betancourt JR. Defining cultural competence: a practical framework for addressing racial/ethnic disparities in health and health care. Public Health Rep 2003; 118(4):293–302.

96. Lie DA, Lee-Rey E, Gomez A, et al. Does cultural competency training of health professionals improve patient outcomes? A systematic review and proposed algorithm for future research. J Gen Intern Med 2011;26(3):317–25.

97. Metzl JM, Hansen H. Structural competency: theorizing a new medical engagement with stigma and inequality. Soc Sci Med 2014;103:126–33.

98. Walker RJ, Campbell JA, Egede LE. Differential impact of food insecurity, distress, and stress on self-care behaviors and glycemic control using path analysis. J Gen Intern Med 2019;34(12):2779–85.

99. Gold R, Bunce A, Cowburn S, et al. Adoption of social determinants of health EHR tools by community health centers. Ann Fam Med 2018;16(5):399–407.

Moving Toward Health Policy that Respects Both Science and People Living with Obesity

Theodore K. Kyle, RPh, MBA[a],*,
Fatima Cody Stanford, MD, MPH, MPA, MBA[b,c]

KEYWORDS

- Obesity • Health policy • Access to care • Scientific rigor • Objectivity
- Population health • Prevention

KEY POINTS

- Despite considerable efforts to address obesity through health policy, trends of rising prevalence have continued relentlessly.
- The failure to reverse these trends is in part due to pervasive bias about obesity and the people living with this condition.
- Weight bias and stigma increased the harm of obesity for the people living with it.
- More effective policies will come from applying obesity science, new research to fill knowledge gaps, and patient-centered care that respects people living with this disease.

INTRODUCTION

The last four decades of health policy have yielded disappointing results with regard to the effects of obesity on health. This failure is easily measured by relentless growth in the prevalence of obesity. Options for evidence-based care of obesity have improved, but access to those options remains poor. Disparities in the health impact of obesity

Funding: National Institutes of Health and Massachusetts General Hospital Executive Committee on Research (ECOR) (F.C. Stanford), National Institutes of Health NIDDK P30 DK040561 (F.C. Stanford) and L30 DK118710 (F.C. Stanford).
Conflicts of Interest: T.K. Kyle, personal fees from Gelesis, Johnson & Johnson, Nutrisystem, Novo Nordisk; FCS, none.
[a] ConscienHealth, 2270 Country Club Drive, Pittsburgh, PA 15241, USA; [b] Department of Medicine, Division of Endocrinology-Neuroendocrine, Massachusetts General Hospital, MGH Weight Center, 50 Staniford Street, Boston, MA 02114, USA; [c] Department of Pediatrics, Division of Endocrinology, Nutrition Obesity Research Center at Harvard (NORCH), 50 Staniford Street, Boston, MA 02114, USA
* Corresponding author.
E-mail address: ted.kyle@conscienhealth.org

have grown wider. Most recently, the COVID-19 pandemic has made it plain that failures to address the rising prevalence of obesity have been costly for the public health of America and, indeed, for countries throughout the world.

Untreated obesity has emerged as one of the top risk factors for severe illness and death with COVID-19. In countries such as the United States, with high obesity prevalence, the morbidity and mortality toll from the pandemic has been especially high.

In short, efforts to address obesity until now have fallen short because prevention strategies have been ineffective and persons affected by obesity have been denied effective medical care for this chronic disease. Thus, an important opportunity exists to move toward health policy that respects the humanity of people living with obesity, as well as the emerging science of obesity. Scientific curiosity about obesity, objectivity about what works for prevention and treatment of obesity, and better care for the people affected by obesity will be necessary to claim that opportunity.

HISTORICAL PERSPECTIVE

More than four decades ago, editors of the *Lancet* identified obesity as "the most important nutritional disease in the affluent countries of the world."[1] In subsequent decades, policy efforts intended to blunt the rise of obesity prevalence have succeeded in elevating the visibility of obesity as a public health issue. However, the prevalence has continued to rise without relief. Viewing obesity as a purely nutritional disease, policymakers invested considerable effort in promoting low-fat diets through the 1980s and 1990s. This concept had a central role in *Dietary Guidelines for Americans* first issued in 1980.[2] Food manufacturers responded by formulating packaged foods that could be marketed as healthy because they were low in fat. The US Food and Drug Administration defined low-fat content as a criterion for marketing a food product as "healthy" in 1993 and persisted with this guidance until 2016.[3]

In the late 1990s, popular thinking about nutrition began to move away from a focus on total dietary fat and toward a focus on sugar and refined carbohydrates. As that happened, consumption of sugar and caloric sweeteners began to decline. That decline is still evident in the most recent available data from the US Department of Agriculture (USDA) reports on food produced for US consumption (**Fig. 1**).[4] Though the shift in consumer behaviors away from low-fat diets started earlier, it was not until

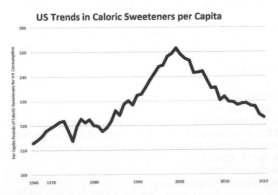

Fig. 1. US Trends in Caloric Sweeteners per Capita. (*Data from* Food Availability (Per Capita) Data System. USDA Economic Research Service. https://www.ers.usda.gov/data-products/food-availability-per-capita-data-system/.)

2015 that USDA removed a recommended upper limit on total dietary fat consumption from *Dietary Guidelines for Americans.*

At the same time as efforts for promoting individual choices about healthy foods continued, health policy also promoted healthy individual choices with regard to physical activity. In 2008, the US Department of Health and Human Services (HHS) issued the first-ever empirical guidelines for physical activity. They provided guidance for healthy physical activity appropriate for individuals from the age of 6 years—and they included people with chronic health conditions and disabilities. An update to those guidelines emerged in 2018. Although the primary audience for these guidelines is health professionals and policymakers, HHS has also developed consumer campaigns to promote them to the public.

In 2010, the ethos of dietary and physical activity guidelines came together in the Obama Administration's *Let's Move!* campaign.

In similar fashion, the clinical guidelines for obesity treatment issued by National Institutes of Health (NIH) in 1998 also emphasized diet and physical activity for the treatment of obesity. Those guidelines cautioned that antiobesity pharmacotherapy should be reserved for "carefully selected patients" and "never be used without concomitant lifestyle modifications." Likewise, the guidelines advised that metabolic and bariatric surgery (MBS) should be an option only for "a limited number of patients" and "reserved for patients in whom medical therapy had failed and who are suffering from the complications of extreme obesity."

But obesity prevalence grew despite a "war on obesity"[5] and pressure for people to make healthy choices. Thus, recognition began to grow that obesity might be a disease caused by social and biological factors more powerful than individual conscious behavioral choices. In 1997, Egger and Swinburne proposed an ecological model for the obesity pandemic.[6] Their model explains the rising prevalence of obesity as the result of a pathologic, obesogenic environment—not as the result of individual behavioral choices.

Finally, the American Medical Association resolved in 2013 that obesity is a complex chronic disease. This resolution explicitly acknowledged the need for both treatment and prevention strategies that account for the pathophysiology of obesity. Since then, more options for antiobesity pharmacotherapy have begun to emerge.[7] MBS has won wider acceptance—both for treating obesity in adults and adolescents[8] and for controlling complications of obesity, such as type 2 diabetes.[9]

Nonetheless, bias about obesity and against the people affected remains prevalent. The dominant public view is that this is a problem of individual choices[10]—more so than biology and an increasingly obesogenic environment. Unfortunately, many policies still reflect such thinking.

SCIENTIFIC RIGOR AND OBJECTIVITY

Scientific rigor in the study of obesity is bringing a deeper understanding of the biological basis for this disease. Decades of research have shown that obesity is a highly heritable condition. The genetic risk for obesity derives from thousands of DNA variants.[11] A few specific and rare variants can cause severe obesity and offer promising targets for treatment. Setmelanotide is an example of a new therapy that works well to rare forms of obesity caused by genetic defects that include pro-opiomelanocortin (POMC), Proprotein Convertase Subtilisin/Kexin Type 1 (PSCK1), and leptin receptor (LEPR) deficiency.[12]

However, obesity prevalence is more fully explained by environmental influences that trigger obesity in genetically susceptible individuals. Obesity prevalence has grown over the last four decades because environmental factors that cause obesity in susceptible individuals have become more common and potent. These factors are numerous, but they fall into 3 broad categories: food, physical activity, and environmental stressors.[13]

Calorie-dense and highly palatable food has grown more ubiquitous in the food supply. Though most scholars agree that these changes are broadly important for triggering a rise in the prevalence of obesity, they disagree about the specifics. For example, the carbohydrate-insulin model of obesity holds that refined carbohydrates are responsible in large measure for rising obesity rates.[14] This model has strong advocates and strong detractors.[15] Other research suggests that ultraprocessed foods have contributed to obesity prevalence as these types of products have become more dominant in the food supply.[16]

Technology, transportation, and work environments have made routine physical activity less common in daily patterns of life. The number of American adults who meet guidelines for physical activity in leisure time has risen only modestly since those guidelines were released in 2008.[16] However, occupation-related physical activity had declined for decades.[17] This decline has the potential for a synergistic effect on obesity prevalence because lower levels of physical activity can lead to dysregulation of energy intake as well as lower levels of energy expenditure.[18]

The environmental stressors that can promote obesity in susceptible persons include sleep disruptions, toxic stress, racism, endocrine-disrupting pollution, medicines, microbes, and other factors.[19,20]

At the same time, scientific inquiry has brought a deeper understanding of obesity, it has also brought a better understanding of effective treatment. Where clinicians once relied heavily upon behavior and lifestyle modification alone, evidence-based guidelines for obesity treatment now emphasize a multidisciplinary approach with the complementary use of pharmacotherapy and surgery to provide better health outcomes. Earlier guidelines emphasized weight reduction as the primary goal. Newer guidelines place a primary emphasis on health outcomes, including health-related quality of life.[21]

Translation of new scientific knowledge and clinical guidelines for obesity into routine practice and policy is, however, a slow process. In part, this is because of pervasive biases about the nature of obesity itself. Myths, presumptions, and facts about obesity are often confused.[22] Most people presume that self-directed diet and exercise are far more effective than they are. Childhood obesity interventions often rely upon presumptions that positive changes in diet and exercise will be sufficient to reduce obesity, rather than empirical evidence from rigorous studies.[23]

However, many obesity prevention programs have failed to yield objective results that indicate a reduction in obesity prevalence. Recently, the *Lancet* Commission on Obesity expressed this plainly: "The current approach to obesity prevention is failing."[24]

Not long ago, policy advocates hailed policies to reduce and prevent obesity in Chile as a prototype for other countries to follow:

> *Nearly 30 years into the ongoing global epidemic of obesity and chronic diseases, Chile has taken the lead in identifying and implementing obesity-control strategies that could prove to be the beginning of the end of the epidemic.*[25]

However, 4 years later, the outcomes from these model strategies are not clearly positive. A recent analysis by Jensen and colleagues concluded that they had reduced the exposure of adolescents to television advertising for unhealthy foods, but no changes in dietary behaviors were evident.[26] Other policies have elicited positive changes in dietary behaviors, but even so, we have yet to see those changes bring meaningful reductions in obesity prevalence.

Thus, the *Lancet* Commission is correct. A new approach is needed. Richardson and colleagues suggest that developing evidence to support more effective policies for obesity "will benefit from a greater emphasis on probative research."[27] Scientific rigor and objectivity would help to overcome the common error of confusing nutrition policy with obesity policy.[28]

BIAS AND STIGMA

Pervasive bias and stigma interfere with effective responses to obesity in 2 ways. First, intellectual biases about obesity itself interfere with making policy decisions regarding obesity that are grounded in sound evidence. Prevalent myths and presumptions about obesity, its causes, prevention, and treatment make it difficult to agree on a common set of facts from which sound policy decisions can be made. The second factor is weight bias and stigma directed at people living with obesity.

Intellectual bias about obesity explains why, as described earlier, the history of policies to address obesity is filled with initiatives that have not had their intended effects. In some cases, they have been counterproductive.

Such is the case with body mass index (BMI) screening in public education.[29] Those screening programs relied on the fundamental bias that obesity could be overcome through personal effort and discipline. The popular misunderstanding of obesity dismissed the more potent influence of genetic susceptibility to obesity and environmental triggers in susceptible individuals. Thus, advocates for BMI screening presumed that measuring BMI in schools and notifying parents of a child's obesity status would serve to motivate parent and child to change behavior and overcome obesity.

This presumption, though it is consistent with prevailing biases about obesity, proved to be incorrect. A recent randomized controlled trial of BMI screening in California schools demonstrated no clinical benefit and the potential for harm to the mental health of students who were singled out for increased weight stigma.[30] For families who live with obesity, this outcome is unsurprising. For policymakers who do not have that lived experience, biased mental models of obesity made it possible to overlook the possibility for unintended negative consequences.

In a critical analysis of obesity prevention policies and strategies, Ximena Ramos Salas and colleagues found the following 5 prevailing narratives:[31]

1. Childhood obesity threatens the health of future generations.
2. Healthy eating and physical activity are sufficient to prevent it.
3. Obesity is a problem of individual behavior.
4. Healthy weight should be a population-wide health goal.
5. Obesity is a risk factor for other diseases, but not a disease itself.

Taken together, Salas and colleagues found that these themes often contribute to weight bias and obesity stigma.

Weight bias can be defined as negative attitudes, beliefs, judgments, stereotypes, or acts of discrimination based solely on a person's weight. It can be subtle or overt, implicit or explicit. Harvard's Project Implicit tracks bias about sexuality, race, skin tone, age, disability, and weight. Over the last decade, this tracking shows that weight bias is the only form of implicit bias becoming more common (**Fig. 2**).[32]

A body of research, summarized by Tomiyama,[33] suggests that the experience of weight stigma adds to the biological stress of people living with obesity, which in

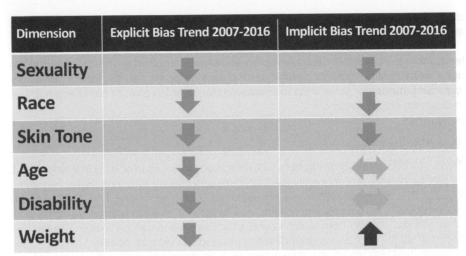

Dimension	Explicit Bias Trend 2007-2016	Implicit Bias Trend 2007-2016
Sexuality	⬇	⬇
Race	⬇	⬇
Skin Tone	⬇	⬇
Age	⬇	⬌
Disability	⬇	⬌
Weight	⬇	⬆

Fig. 2. Trends in implicit and explicit bias, 2007 to 2016. (*Data from* Charlesworth and Banaji, 2018, Patterns of implicit and explicit attitudes: Long-term change and stability from 2007 to 2016.)

turn contributes to progression of obesity to more severe forms. Physiology, biochemistry, cognition, and behavior are linked in this vicious cycle. In this way, weight stigma serves to amplify the health harms of obesity. So, to the extent that health policy has added to the stigma attached to obesity, poorly chosen public health policies can have the unintended consequence of adding to the health burden of obesity.[5]

ACCESS TO CARE

Medical care for obesity requires a multidisciplinary approach that uses a range of clinical tools, including lifestyle therapy, pharmacotherapy, bariatric surgery, and postsurgical care.[34,35] Brief advice to lose weight is ineffective in comparison to intensive lifestyle therapy (ILT).[36] ILT can be modestly effective, producing an additional 5 to 7% total body weight loss. MBS is generally the most effective single option, but even with MBS, some regain is common and postsurgical care is essential to ensure long-term control of this chronic disease.[37] Recent research suggests that pharmacotherapy can be useful after bariatric surgery to maintain ongoing control of obesity and prevent weight regain.[38,39]

However, access to care with these evidence-based treatments is often not available to people living with obesity. Physicians report that they do not provide ILT for obesity because most health plans provide limited compensation for this time-intensive treatment.[40] Among people who have health insurance plans through employment, only 13% report that their insurance will cover medical obesity treatment.[41] Medicare will cover ILT and MBS, but not antiobesity medicines. Antiobesity medication is often not covered under the Affordable Care Act (ACA) despite the notion that the ACA covers care for pre-existing conditions.[42] Utilization of ILT under Medicare remains exceedingly low because reimbursement is poor.[43] Individual states administer Medicaid programs and coverage of obesity care is limited.[44]

Though private insurers often do cover MBS, policies for preauthorization can be quite restrictive and serve to limit utilization. Most insurers restrict coverage of adolescent bariatric surgery through policies that current evidence does not support.[44] Only about 1% of the eligible population undergoes surgical treatment for obesity and insurance coverage policies are a contributing factor for low utilization.[45,46]

In short, health plans provide limited coverage for effective obesity care, which leads most people with obesity to rely upon ineffective methods for treatment based upon self-directed diets and ineffective dietary supplements.[47] The result is an increasing burden of other chronic diseases that result from untreated obesity.[48]

DISPARITIES

Obesity exerts a disparate impact on the health of racial and ethnic minority populations. However, we must also acknowledge that current BMI standards did not consider racial and ethnic minority populations.[49] Despite the lack of inclusion of racial and ethnic minorities in these standards, we note that Black women, along with Mexican American men and women live with the highest prevalence of obesity in the United States. In recent years, the growth in obesity prevalence among adolescents has been almost entirely among Black and Mexican American youth.[50]

A recent analysis of the life course of BMI trajectories from adolescence to old age provides an objective description of these disparities. Disparities for Black persons have become greater in recent birth cohorts. Disparities linked to race and education are greater for women than for men.[51]

Disparities in access to care, both health care generally and obesity care specifically, also contribute a disproportionate impact of obesity on the health of racial and ethnic minority populations. Further exacerbating these disparities are differences in treatment outcomes that favor White persons with obesity.[52] Historically, people of color have been underrepresented in clinical trials of obesity treatment.[53]

Finally, it is noteworthy that policymakers have done little to reduce the disproportionate harm racial and ethnic minority populations suffer from obesity. Aaron and Stanford outline actions needed to reduce the synergistic effects of systemic racism and obesity.[20]

OBESITY IN THE COVID-19 PANDEMIC

The pandemic of COVID-19 revealed special vulnerabilities for the public health of populations with high prevalence of obesity. Obesity is one of the most important and prevalent risk factors for poor outcomes and death after infection with severe acute respiratory syndrome coronavirus 2 (SARS-CoV-2). Only age was more important.[54] Disparities in obesity overlapped with economic and social disparities to further amplify this risk.

Data on variations in COVID-19 death rates among countries suggest that obesity prevalence was an important factor. In a multivariate model published by Gardiner, Oben, and Sutcliffe, obesity prevalence was the one factor most strongly associated with COVID-19 death rates in 30 industrialized countries.[55]

SUMMARY

Through four decades of rising obesity prevalence, health policy to address this pandemic has been mostly ineffective. Prevention policies repeatedly fail to reverse trends of rising obesity prevalence, in part because they are often based on biased mental models[56] about what should work to prevent obesity, rather than empiric evidence for what does work.

Bias toward people living with obesity compounds the harm to their health, while contributing to poor access to effective care that might serve to improve it.

Better public policy will come from an increased application of objective obesity science, curiosity and research to fill knowledge gaps, and greater respect for the human dignity of people who live with this chronic disease.

CLINICS CARE POINTS

- Respect patients
- Counsel patients on the nature of the disease and the full range of options for dealing with it.
- Advocate for policy that respects both science and people living with obesity

REFERENCES

1. Editorial: infant and adult obesity. Lancet 1974;1(7845):17–8.
2. Nutrition and your health: dietary guidelines for Americans [Internet]. 1st edition. USDA/HHS; 1980. Available at: https://www.dietaryguidelines.gov/about-dietary-guidelines/previous-editions/1980-dietary-guidelines-americans. Accessed June 5, 2021.
3. Guidance for industry: use of the term "healthy" in the labeling of human food products [Internet]. U.S. Food and Drug Administration Center for Food Safety and Applied Nutrition; 2020. Available at: https://www.fda.gov/regulatory-information/search-fda-guidance-documents/guidance-industry-use-term-healthy-labeling-human-food-products. Accessed June 5, 2021.
4. Food availability (per capita) data system. USDA Economic Research Service; 2021. Available at: https://www.ers.usda.gov/data-products/food-availability-per-capita-data-system/. Accessed June 15, 2021.
5. Ramos Salas X. The ineffectiveness and unintended consequences of the public health war on obesity. Can J Public Health 2015;106(2):e79–81.
6. Egger G, Swinburn B. An "ecological" approach to the obesity pandemic. Bmj 1997;315(7106):477–80.
7. Gargallo-Vaamonde J, Frühbeck G, Salvador J. New advances and novel approaches in obesity pharmacotherapy. Curr Opin Endocr Metab Res 2019;4: 75–82.
8. Armstrong SC, Bolling CF, Michalsky MP, et al. Pediatric metabolic and bariatric surgery: evidence, barriers, and best practices. Pediatrics 2019;144(6): e20193223.
9. Rubino F, Nathan DM, Eckel RH, et al, Delegates of the 2nd Diabetes Surgery Summit. Metabolic surgery in the treatment algorithm for type 2 diabetes: a joint statement by international diabetes organizations. Diabetes Care 2016;39(6): 861–77.
10. Grannell A, Fallon F, Al-Najim W, et al. Obesity and responsibility: is it time to rethink agency? Obes Rev 2021;22(8):e13270.
11. Bouchard C. Genetics of obesity: what we have learned over decades of research. Obesity 2021;29(5):802–20.
12. Farooqi S, Miller JL, Ohayon O, et al. Effects of setmelanotide in patients with POMC, PCSK1, or LEPR heterozygous deficiency obesity in a phase 2 study. J Endocr Soc 2021;5(Supplement_1):A669–70.
13. Ravussin E, Ryan DH. Three new perspectives on the perfect storm: what's behind the obesity epidemic? Obesity 2018;26(1):9–10.

14. Ludwig DS, Ebbeling CB. The carbohydrate-insulin model of obesity: beyond "calories in, calories out". JAMA Intern Med 2018;178(8):1098–103.

15. Speakman JR, Hall KD. Carbohydrates, insulin, and obesity. Science 2021; 372(6542):577–8.

16. Whitfield GP, Carlson SA, Ussery EN, et al. Trends in meeting physical activity guidelines among urban and rural dwelling adults—United States, 2008–2017. MMWR Morb Mortal Wkly Rep 2019;68(23):513.

17. Church TS, Thomas DM, Tudor-Locke C, et al. Trends over 5 decades in US occupation-related physical activity and their associations with obesity. PloS one 2011;6(5):e19657.

18. Church T, Martin CK. The obesity epidemic: a consequence of reduced energy expenditure and the uncoupling of energy intake? Obesity 2018;26(1):14–6.

19. Davis RA, Plaisance EP, Allison DB. Complementary hypotheses on contributors to the obesity epidemic. Obesity 2018;26(1):17–21.

20. Aaron DG, Stanford FC. Is obesity a manifestation of systemic racism? A ten-point strategy for study and intervention. J Intern Med 2021;290(2):416–20.

21. Wharton S, Lau DC, Vallis M, et al. Obesity in adults: a clinical practice guideline. CMAJ 2020;192(31):E875–91.

22. Casazza K, Fontaine KR, Astrup A, et al. Myths, presumptions, and facts about obesity. New Engl J Med 2013;368(5):446–54.

23. Brown AW, Altman DG, Baranowski T, et al. Childhood obesity intervention studies: a narrative review and guide for investigators, authors, editors, reviewers, journalists, and readers to guard against exaggerated effectiveness claims. Obes Rev 2019;20(11):1523–41.

24. Swinburn BA, Kraak VI, Allender S, et al. The global syndemic of obesity, undernutrition, and climate change: the lancet commission report. Lancet 2019; 393(10173):791–846.

25. Cohen D. Combat obesity like chile. U.S. News & World Report. 2017. Available at: https://www.usnews.com/opinion/policy-dose/articles/2017-12-26/what-the-us-can-learn-from-chiles-strategies-to-control-obesity. Accessed June 5, 2021.

26. Jensen ML, Carpentier FR, Adair L, et al. TV advertising and dietary intake in adolescents: a pre-and post-study of Chile's food marketing policy. Int J Behav Nutr Phys Act 2021;18(1):1.

27. Richardson MB, Williams MS, Fontaine KR, et al. The development of scientific evidence for health policies for obesity: why and how? Int J Obes 2017;41(6): 840–8.

28. Stanford FC, Kyle TK. Why food policy and obesity policy are not synonymous: the need to establish clear obesity policy in the United States. Int J Obes 2015;39(12):1667–8.

29. Kyle TK, Armstrong S. Is it time to remove bmi screening from school settings? Child Obes 2021;17(2):77–8.

30. Madsen KA, Thompson HR, Linchey J, et al. Effect of school-based body mass index reporting in California public schools: a randomized clinical trial. JAMA Pediatr 2021;175(3):251–9.

31. Salas XR, Forhan M, Caulfield T, et al. A critical analysis of obesity prevention policies and strategies. Can J Public Health 2017;108(5):e598–608.

32. Charlesworth TE, Banaji MR. Patterns of implicit and explicit attitudes: I. Longterm change and stability from 2007 to 2016. Psychol Sci 2019;30(2):174–92.

33. Tomiyama AJ. Stress and obesity. Annu Rev Psychol 2019;70:703–18.

34. Bray GA, Ryan DH. Evidence-based weight loss interventions: Individualized treatment options to maximize patient outcomes. Diabetes Obes Metab 2021; 23(Suppl 1):50–62. https://doi.org/10.1111/dom.14200.

35. Parretti HM, Hughes CA, Jones LL. 'The rollercoaster of follow-up care' after bariatric surgery: a rapid review and qualitative synthesis. Obes Rev 2019;20(1): 88–107.

36. Knowler WC, Barrett-Connor E, Fowler SE, et al. Reduction in the incidence of type 2 diabetes with lifestyle intervention or metformin. N Engl J Med 2002; 346(6):393–403.

37. Velapati SR, Shah M, Kuchkuntla AR, et al. Weight regain after bariatric surgery: prevalence, etiology, and treatment. Curr Nutr Rep 2018;7(4):329–34.

38. Stanford FC, Alfaris N, Gomez G, et al. The utility of weight loss medications after bariatric surgery for weight regain or inadequate weight loss: a multi-center study. Surg Obes Relat Dis 2017;13(3):491–500.

39. Hanipah ZN, Nasr EC, Bucak E, et al. Efficacy of adjuvant weight loss medication after bariatric surgery. Surg Obes Relat Dis 2018;14(1):93–8.

40. Nederveld A, Phimphasone-Brady P, Connelly L, et al. The Joys and Challenges of Delivering Obesity Care: a Qualitative Study of US Primary Care Practices. J Gen Intern Med 2021;36(9):2709–16. https://doi.org/10.1007/s11606-020-06548-w.

41. Kaplan LM, Golden A, Jinnett K, et al. Perceptions of barriers to effective obesity care: results from the national ACTION study. Obesity 2018;26(1):61–9.

42. Gomez G, Stanford FC. US health policy and prescription drug coverage of FDA-approved medications for the treatment of obesity. Int J Obes 2018;42(3): 495–500.

43. Luo Z, Gritz M, Connelly L, et al. A survey of primary care practices on their use of the intensive behavioral therapy for obese medicare patients. J Gen Intern Med 2021;36(9):2700–8. https://doi.org/10.1007/s11606-021-06596-w.

44. Jannah N, Hild J, Gallagher C, et al. Coverage for obesity prevention and treatment services: analysis of medicaid and state employee health insurance programs. Obesity 2018;26(12):1834–40.

45. Gebran SG, Knighton B, Ngaage LM, et al. Insurance coverage criteria for bariatric surgery: a survey of policies. Obes Surg 2020;30(2):707–13.

46. Gasoyan H, Soans R, Ibrahim JK, et al. Do insurance-mandated precertification criteria and insurance plan type determine the utilization of bariatric surgery among individuals with private insurance? Med Care 2020;58(11):952–7.

47. Bessell E, Maunder A, Lauche R, et al. Efficacy of dietary supplements containing isolated organic compounds for weight loss: a systematic review and meta-analysis of randomised placebo-controlled trials. Int J Obes (Lond) 2021;45(8): 1631–43. https://doi.org/10.1038/s41366-021-00839-w.

48. GBD 2015 Obesity Collaborators. Health effects of overweight and obesity in 195 countries over 25 years. N Engl J Med 2017;377(1):13–27.

49. Stanford FC, Lee M, Hur C. Race, ethnicity, sex, and obesity: is it time to personalize the scale? Mayo Clin Proc 2019;94(2):362–3.

50. Ogden CL, Fryar CD, Martin CB, et al. Trends in obesity prevalence by race and hispanic origin—1999-2000 to 2017-2018. JAMA 2020;324(12):1208–10.

51. Yang YC, Walsh CE, Johnson MP, et al. Life-course trajectories of body mass index from adolescence to old age: racial and educational disparities. Proc Natl Acad Sci U S A 2021;118(17). e2020167118.

52. Byrd AS, Toth AT, Stanford FC. Racial disparities in obesity treatment. Curr Obes Rep 2018;7(2):130–8.

53. Haughton CF, Silfee VJ, Wang ML, et al. Racial/ethnic representation in lifestyle weight loss intervention studies in the United States: a systematic review. Prev Med Rep 2018;9:131–7.
54. Gao M, Piernas C, Astbury NM, et al. Associations between body-mass index and COVID-19 severity in 6· 9 million people in England: a prospective, community-based, cohort study. Lancet Diabetes Endocrinol 2021;9(6):350–9.
55. Gardiner J, Oben J, Sutcliffe A. Obesity as a driver of international differences in COVID-19 death rates. Diabetes Obes Metab 2021;23(7):1463–70. https://doi.org/10.1111/dom.14357.
56. Hovmand PS, Pronk NP, Kyle TK, et al. Obesity, biased mental models, and stigma in the context of the obesity COVID-19 syndemic. NAM Perspect 2021. https://doi.org/10.31478/202104a.

UNITED STATES POSTAL SERVICE® Statement of Ownership, Management, and Circulation
(All Periodicals Publications Except Requester Publications)

1. Publication Title	2. Publication Number	3. Filing Date
NURSING CLINICS OF NORTH AMERICA	598 – 960	9/18/2021

4. Issue Frequency	5. Number of Issues Published Annually	6. Annual Subscription Price
MAR, JUN, SEP, DEC	4	$163

7. Complete Mailing Address of Known Office of Publication (Not printer) (Street, city, county, state, and ZIP+4®)

ELSEVIER INC.
230 Park Avenue, Suite 800
New York, NY 10169

Contact Person: Malathi Samayan
Telephone (Include area code): 91-44-4299-4507

8. Complete Mailing Address of Headquarters or General Business Office of Publisher (Not printer)

ELSEVIER INC.
230 Park Avenue, Suite 800
New York, NY 10169

9. Full Names and Complete Mailing Addresses of Publisher, Editor, and Managing Editor (Do not leave blank)

Publisher (Name and complete mailing address)
DOLORES MELONI, ELSEVIER INC.
1600 JOHN F KENNEDY BLVD. SUITE 1800
PHILADELPHIA, PA 19103-2899

Editor (Name and complete mailing address)
KERRY HOLLAND, ELSEVIER INC.
1600 JOHN F KENNEDY BLVD. SUITE 1800
PHILADELPHIA, PA 19103-2899

Managing Editor (Name and complete mailing address)
PATRICK MANLEY, ELSEVIER INC.
1600 JOHN F KENNEDY BLVD. SUITE 1800
PHILADELPHIA, PA 19103-2899

10. Owner (Do not leave blank. If the publication is owned by a corporation, give the name and address of the corporation immediately followed by the names and addresses of all stockholders owning or holding 1 percent or more of the total amount of stock. If not owned by a corporation, give the names and addresses of the individual owners. If owned by a partnership or other unincorporated firm, give its name and address as well as those of each individual owner. If the publication is published by a nonprofit organization, give its name and address.)

Full Name	Complete Mailing Address
WHOLLY OWNED SUBSIDIARY OF REED/ELSEVIER US HOLDINGS	1600 JOHN F KENNEDY BLVD. SUITE 1800 PHILADELPHIA, PA 19103-2899

11. Known Bondholders, Mortgagees, and Other Security Holders Owning or Holding 1 Percent or More of Total Amount of Bonds, Mortgages, or Other Securities. If none, check box ▶ ☐ None

Full Name	Complete Mailing Address
N/A	

12. Tax Status (For completion by nonprofit organizations authorized to mail at nonprofit rates) (Check one)
The purpose, function, and nonprofit status of this organization and the exempt status for federal income tax purposes:
☒ Has Not Changed During Preceding 12 Months
☐ Has Changed During Preceding 12 Months (Publisher must submit explanation of change with this statement)

PS Form 3526, July 2014 [Page 1 of 4 (see instructions page 4)] PSN: 7530-01-000-9931 PRIVACY NOTICE: See our privacy policy on www.usps.com

---

13. Publication Title	14. Issue Date for Circulation Data Below
NURSING CLINICS OF NORTH AMERICA	JUNE 2021

15. Extent and Nature of Circulation		Average No. Copies Each Issue During Preceding 12 Months	No. Copies of Single Issue Published Nearest to Filing Date
a. Total Number of Copies (Net press run)		401	335
b. Paid Circulation (By Mail and Outside the Mail)	(1) Mailed Outside-County Paid Subscriptions Stated on PS Form 3541 (Include paid distribution above nominal rate, advertiser's proof copies, and exchange copies)	261	230
	(2) Mailed In-County Paid Subscriptions Stated on PS Form 3541 (Include paid distribution above nominal rate, advertiser's proof copies, and exchange copies)	0	0
	(3) Paid Distribution Outside the Mails Including Sales Through Dealers and Carriers, Street Vendors, Counter Sales, and Other Paid Distribution Outside USPS®	83	75
	(4) Paid Distribution by Other Classes of Mail Through the USPS (e.g., First-Class Mail®)	0	0
c. Total Paid Distribution (Sum of 15b (1), (2), (3), and (4)) ▶		354	305
d. Free or Nominal Rate Distribution (By Mail and Outside the Mail)	(1) Free or Nominal Rate Outside-County Copies Included on PS Form 3541	37	30
	(2) Free or Nominal Rate In-County Copies Included on PS Form 3541	0	0
	(3) Free or Nominal Rate Copies Mailed at Other Classes Through the USPS (e.g., First-Class Mail)	0	0
	(4) Free or Nominal Rate Distribution Outside the Mail (Carriers or other means)	0	0
e. Total Free or Nominal Rate Distribution (Sum of 15d (1), (2), (3) and (4)) ▶		37	30
f. Total Distribution (Sum of 15c and 15e) ▶		401	335
g. Copies not Distributed (See Instructions to Publishers #4 (page #3)) ▶		0	0
h. Total (Sum of 15f and g) ▶		401	335
i. Percent Paid (15c divided by 15f times 100) ▶		90.77%	91.04%

* If you are claiming electronic copies, go to line 16 on page 3. If you are not claiming electronic copies, skip to line 17 on page 3.

16. Electronic Copy Circulation	Average No. Copies Each Issue During Preceding 12 Months	No. Copies of Single Issue Published Nearest to Filing Date
a. Paid Electronic Copies ▶		
b. Total Paid Print Copies (Line 15c) + Paid Electronic Copies (Line 16a) ▶		
c. Total Print Distribution (Line 15f) + Paid Electronic Copies (Line 16a) ▶		
d. Percent Paid (Both Print & Electronic Copies) (16b divided by 16c × 100) ▶		

☒ I certify that 50% of all my distributed copies (electronic and print) are paid above a nominal price.

17. Publication of Statement of Ownership
☒ If the publication is a general publication, publication of this statement is required. Will be printed in the DECEMBER 2021 issue of this publication.
☐ Publication not required.

18. Signature and Title of Editor, Publisher, Business Manager, or Owner	Date
Malathi Samayan - Distribution Controller *Malathi Samayan*	9/18/2021

I certify that all information furnished on this form is true and complete. I understand that anyone who furnishes false or misleading information on this form or who omits material or information requested on the form may be subject to criminal sanctions (including fines and imprisonment) and/or civil sanctions (including civil penalties).

PS Form 3526, July 2014 (Page 2 of 4) PRIVACY NOTICE: See our privacy policy on www.usps.com

Moving?

Make sure your subscription moves with you!

To notify us of your new address, find your **Clinics Account Number** (located on your mailing label above your name), and contact customer service at:

Email: **journalscustomerservice-usa@elsevier.com**

800-654-2452 (subscribers in the U.S. & Canada)
314-447-8871 (subscribers outside of the U.S. & Canada)

Fax number: **314-447-8029**

Elsevier Health Sciences Division
Subscription Customer Service
3251 Riverport Lane
Maryland Heights, MO 63043

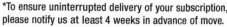

*To ensure uninterrupted delivery of your subscription, please notify us at least 4 weeks in advance of move.

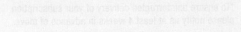

Printed and bound by CPI Group (UK) Ltd, Croydon, CR0 4YY

24/10/2024

01778553-0001